made INCREDIBLY

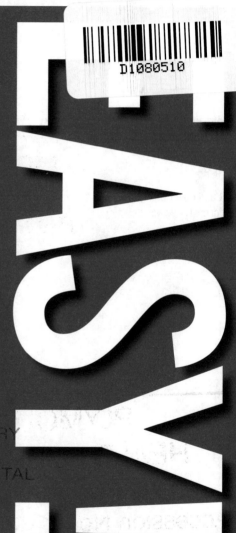

Maternal–Neonatal Care Made Incredibly Easy!

Adapted for the UK by

Sharon Nurse, RN, RM, RCNT, BSc (Hons)

Senior Teaching Fellow Midwifery,
School of Nursing & Midwifery,
The Queen's University,
Belfast

First UK Edition

 Wolters Kluwer | Lippincott Williams & Wilkins
Health

Philadelphia • Baltimore • New York • London
Buenos Aires • Hong Kong • Sydney • Tokyo

Staff

Director, Global Publishing
Cathy Peck

Production Director
Chris Curtis

Acquisitions Editor
Rachel Hendrick

Academic Marketing Executive
Alison Major

Proofreader
Ann Stevens

Illustrator
Bot Roda

Text and Cover Design
Designers Collective

Printed and bound by Euradius in The Netherlands. Typeset by Macmillan Publishing Solutions, New Delhi, India

For information, write to Lippincott Williams & Wilkins, 250 Waterloo Road, London SE1 8RD.

British Library Cataloguing in Publication Data. A catalogue record for this book is available from the British Library.

ISBN-13: 978-1-901831-08-5
ISBN-10: 1-901831 08-6

Contents

Acknowledgements

Reviewers of the UK edition

Maureen Brown, RN, RM, ADM, BSc (Hons), MA, SoM
Lead Midwife for Education, Coventry University, UK

Mabel Simms, MSc, BSc (Hons) RM, SRN
Senior Lecturer (Midwifery & Women's Health) at Birmingham City University, UK

Bernadette Gregory RGN, RM, ADM, PGCEA, BA, MMid
Senior Lecturer in Midwifery, De Montfort University, UK

Ashley Cupples
Direct Entry Midwifery Student, Queen's University Belfast, UK

Sharon Nurse provided some of the illustrations in the Neonatal chapter.

Foreword

Midwifery and nursing educators have long been challenged with making midwifery and neonatal knowledge factual and evidence-based as well as stimulating for the student. For this reason, we often find ourselves asking what it takes for midwifery and nursing concepts, facts and research findings to embed themselves in the brain, resulting in well-reasoned utilisation of caring processes and knowledgeable, critical thinking. A couple of answers come to mind.

First, learning more readily occurs if there's a catalyst to assist it. Educators now realise that by encouraging students' active involvement in the learning process and using various adult-learning methodologies, they can facilitate knowledge acquisition and application. Some of these methods include various forms of testing, case scenarios and simulations.

Second, any way in which the educator can combine a fun experience with the learning process is a positive one. These experiences can come in the form of cartoons, funny poems, puzzles, humorous or clever analogies. There are no limits to the methods.

As a midwifery and neonatal lecturer, I'm drawn to resources that blend the elements of active learning and fun. This combination is what enticed me to adapt the latest American edition of Maternal–Neonatal Nursing Made Incredibly Easy into the British version – Maternal–Neonatal Care Made Incredibly Easy.

Those familiar with the second edition will be pleased to encounter the same well-loved features that helped make it an excellent resource. Comprehensive information is still conveyed succinctly in multiple forms that actively engage the reader. Original content has been updated and enhanced with tables, charts, diagrams, illustrations, quizzes and delightful cartoons that help the reader focus on key facts. Included are content areas on postnatal depression, alternative therapies and substance abuse. I have also included sections on areas which are more relevant to British midwives such as antenatal screening, neonatal screening and midwifery examination of the newborn and neonatal sepsis.

In addition, icons draw your attention to important issues:

Advice from the experts – tips and tricks from the people who know best – midwives and neonatal nurses

Education edge – client-teaching tips and checklists that help the midwife pass along information that can be vital to promoting a healthy pregnancy and preventing complications

Bridging the gap – details on cultural differences that may affect care

Weighing the evidence – evidence-based practice pointers

Websites – there are some really useful website links for you to access

Enjoy this comprehensive resource that doesn't separate learning from fun. With the third British edition of Maternal–Neonatal Care Made Incredibly Easy, it's a packaged deal!

Sharon Nurse, RN, RM, RCNT, BSc (Hons)
Senior Teaching Fellow
School of Nursing & Midwifery
The Queen's University
Belfast BT9 6AZ
Northern Ireland

Contributors and consultants to the US edition

Christine C. Askham, RN, BSN
VN Faculty
Unitek College
Fremont, CA

Kimberly Attwood, RN, PhD(c)
Instructor
DeSales University
Center Valley, PA

Beatrice Beth Benda, RNC, MSN
Staff Nurse
Allina Hospitals & Clinics
University of Minnesota Fairview Riverside
Maternal Fetal Medicine Clinic
Minneapolis, MN

Anita Carroll, EdD, MSN
Nursing Instructor
West Texas A&M University
Canyon, TX

Marsha L. Conroy, RN, MSN, APN
Nursing Instructor
Cuyahoga Community College
Cleveland, OH

Kim Cooper, RN, MSN
Nursing Department Program Chair
Ivy Tech Community College of Indiana
Terre Haute, IN

Patti F. Gardner, MSN, CNM, IBCLC
Clinical Nurse Specialist: Women's Health
& Lactation
United Medical Center
Cheyenne, WY

Valera A. Hascup, RNC, MSN, PhD (c), CCES, CTN
Assistant Professor of Nursing and Director
of the Transcultural Nursing Institute
Kean University
Union, NJ

Vivian Haughton, RN, MSN, CCE, IBCLC
Clinical Nurse Specialist–Maternal/Child
Health
Good Samaritan Health System
Lebanon, PA

Dana M. L. Hinds, RN, MSN, FNP
Nursing Instructor, Family Nurse
Practitioner
Central Maine Medical Center School of
Nursing
Lewiston, ME

Beverly Kass, RNC, MS
Faculty
William Paterson University
Wayne, NJ

Randy S. Miller, RNC, BS, MSN
Student Coordinator
Regional Healthcare, Orlando, FL

James F. Murphy, RNC, MS
Educator/Instructor
ViaHealth/Rochester General Hospital
Isabella Graham Hart School of Nursing
Rochester, NY

Noel C. Piano, RN, MS
Instructor/Coordinator
Lafayette School of Practical Nursing
Adjunct Faculty
Thomas Nelson Community College
Williamsburg, VA

Janet Somlyay, RN, MSN, CNS, CPNP
Clinical Nurse Specialist – Pediatrics and
Nursery
United Medical Center
Cheyenne, WY

Robin R. Wilkerson, RN, PhD
Associate Professor of Nursing
University of Mississippi
Jackson, MS

Just the facts

In this chapter, you'll learn:

♦ roles of midwives and other health professionals

♦ dynamics of family-centred midwifery care

♦ structures and functions of families

♦ factors that influence a family's response to pregnancy

♦ legal and ethical issues associated with maternity care

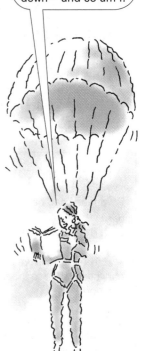

Infant and maternal mortality rates are going down – and so am I!

A look at midwifery care

In the UK, midwives are caring for over 680,000 pregnant women each year. Providing this care can be challenging and rewarding. After all, you must develop your clinical skills, use technology efficiently and effectively, offer thorough client teaching and remain sensitive to and supportive of women's emotional needs.

Going down!

In recent decades, infant and maternal mortality rates have progressively declined. Factors responsible for this decline include better screening and management of disorders such as pre-eclampsia and diabetes, and prevention of related complications. Better control of complications associated with gestational hypertension and decreased use of anaesthesia with childbirth may also contribute to this decline.

Room for improvement

Despite these advances, there's still room for improvement in maternal and neonatal health care. Infant and maternal mortality rates remain high for poor clients, ethnic minorities and teenage mothers – largely because of a lack of good antenatal care or not identifying high-risk cases.

In 2005 in the UK, there were 3,676 stillbirths and 5,496 perinatal deaths. The main risks for infants were prematurity, congenital abnormality, intrapartum factors and infection.

Between 2000 and 2005 in the UK, 238 mothers died. Maternal risk factors were mainly age and social deprivation amongst others. Teenage pregnancy rates in the UK are some of the highest in Europe – you can access these on some of the government websites or access local figures from your own Department of Health statistics website.

These statistics will change every year and so it is useful to access the most recent figures by going online to the following websites:
- Government statistics: www.statistics.gov.uk
- Confidential Enquiry into Maternal and Child Health: www.cemach.org.uk
- Royal College of Midwives: www.rcm.org

The role of the Midwife in providing midwifery care

The primary role of the midwife is to provide comprehensive family-centred care to the pregnant woman and her unborn baby throughout pregnancy, childbirth and in the weeks following (the postnatal period).

Setting the standards

In 1902, the Midwives Registration Act established the state regulation of midwives. The Briggs Committee, established in 1970, reported a number of changes to professional education. Six years later, the Nurses, Midwives and Health Visitors Act 1979 was passed. In 1983, the United Kingdom Central

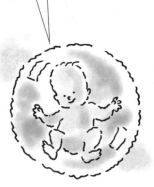

Your job is to take care of me and my mum and the rest of my family. I'll thank you when I arrive!

Three pregnancy periods

Pregnancy can be broken down into three periods:

The *antepartum period* refers to the period from conception to the onset of labour.

The *intrapartum period* extends from the onset of contractions that cause cervical dilation to the first 1–4 hours after the birth of the neonate and delivery of the placenta.

The *postpartum* period refers to the 6 weeks after delivery of the baby and the placenta. Also known as the *puerperium*, this stage ends when the reproductive organs return to the nonpregnant state.

Council (UKCC) was set up. Its core functions were to maintain a register of nurses, midwives and health visitors, provide guidance to registrants and handle professional misconduct complaints. In 2002, the UKCC ceased to exist and was replaced by the Nursing & Midwifery Council (NMC). The functions and powers of the NMC can be viewed in full on the website: www.nmc-uk.org

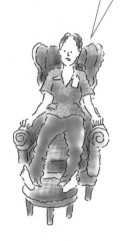

For some families, there's no place like home (or a home-like hospital setting) for having a baby

Practice settings

Midwives practise in various settings. These include community-based health centres, maternity units and birthing centres and as independent midwives they practise mainly in the community.

There's no place like home . . .

For many years most births occurred in hospitals. Today, an increasing number of families are choosing to have their babies in alternative birth settings, such as birthing centres or their homes. These alternative settings may give families more control over their birth experiences by allowing them to become more involved in the process.

. . . or a home away from home

In response to consumer demands for more relaxed, family-friendly birthing environments, hospitals have revamped their labour and delivery units to create more natural childbirth environments. Labour, delivery and postpartum suites are now found in most hospitals. In these home-like settings, partners, family members and other support people may remain in the room throughout the birth experience. The mother then spends the postpartum-recovery period in the same room where she gave birth. These home-like environments allow for a more holistic and family-centred approach to maternal and neonatal health care.

Professionals in Maternity Care

The Midwife

A midwife is a person who, having been regularly admitted to a midwifery educational programme, duly recognised in the country in which it is located, has successfully completed the prescribed course of studies in midwifery and has acquired the requisite qualifications to be registered and/or legally licensed to practise midwifery.

The midwife is recognised as a responsible and accountable professional who works in partnership with women to give the necessary support, care and advice during pregnancy, labour and the postpartum period, to conduct births on her own responsibility and to provide care for the newborn and the infant. This care includes preventative measures, the promotion of normal birth, the detection of complications in mother and child, the accessing of medical care or other appropriate assistance and the carrying out of emergency measures.

The midwife has an important task in health counselling and education, not only for the women, but also within the family and the community. This work should involve antenatal education and preparation for parenthood and may extend to women's health, sexual or reproductive health and childcare. The promotion of breastfeeding has become an even greater aspect of the midwife's role in recent times, particularly with the rise in childhood obesity and the need to encourage healthier lifestyles for the woman and her newborn infant.

A midwife may practise in any setting including the home, community, hospitals, clinics or health units. (Adopted by the International Confederation of Midwives Council meeting, 19 July 2005, Brisbane, Australia.)

The European Midwives Association serves as a valuable link for midwives working within the European Community (EC). It also provides information about legislation relevant to midwives practising in the UK who may wish to work within the EC. Midwifery education and practice are regulated through one single European Directive 2005/36/EC. The information specifically relevant to midwives is available on the NMC website (Council Directives 80/154/EEC and 80/155/EEC): www.nmc-uk.org

Some of the specialised roles within midwifery:

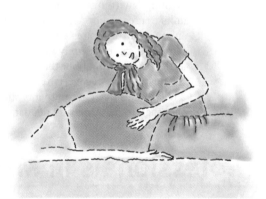

- Breastfeeding coordinator
- Health promotion midwife
- Antenatal and newborn screening
- Reproductive and sexual health
- Diabetes
- Parentcraft education
- Bereavement support
- Assessment units – ultrasound scanning/ fetal development/amniocentesis
- Research development
- Quality assurance
- Education – both in University and in the clinical setting

Registered nurse

Once qualified, many nurses take extra courses to specialise in areas such as cancer care, women's health, accident and emergency, critical care, practice nursing, health visiting or school nursing. Some registered nurses may work in gynae wards, neonatal units or obstetric theatres but have very specific roles – they are not qualified to care for mothers and babies in the same capacity as a registered midwife.

Nursing & Midwifery Council (NMC)

To work in the UK, all nurses, midwives and specialist community public health nurses must register with the NMC. Practitioners have to renew their registration every 3 years. The NMC website (www.nmc-uk.org) contains advice and information on all aspects of registration and professional development issues.

Meeting PREP, continuing professional development (CPD) and practice standard

When nurses, midwives and specialist community public health nurses re-register, they must have undertaken at least 5 days (35 hours) of learning in the previous 3 years. This is called the PREP (CPD) standard. Practitioners can complete this 35 hours of learning in a wide variety of ways; it does not have to cost you any money. Basically, any activity that maintains and develops your professional competence is suitable.

Practitioners must also have completed a minimum 450 hours of practice, in each area of practice, during the 3 years prior to renewal of registration. This is the PREP (practice) standard. This method of registration is only valid for up to 3 months from your expiry date.

If you do not renew your registration prior to your expiry date your registration will lapse and you should not be practising in a position which requires you to be a registered practitioner in the UK.

For more information about this please read *The PREP Handbook* – available from www.nmc-uk.org

Health visitor

A health visitor is a qualified and registered <u>nurse</u> or <u>midwife</u> who has undertaken further (post registration) training in order to be able to work as a member of the primary health care team. The role of the health visitor is about the promotion of health and the prevention of illness in all age groups. Health visitors work with mothers of young babies – advising on such areas as feeding, safety, physical and emotional development and other aspects of health and childcare. They also work with people of any age who suffer from a chronic illness or live with a disability. The health visitor works quite closely with community midwives in providing continuity of care in the community for families of young babies and children, making contact with general practitioners and social workers when appropriate.

Advanced neonatal nurse practitioner

An advanced neonatal nurse practitioner (ANNP) is highly skilled in the care of neonates and can work in practice settings with various care levels, from special care baby units to neonatal intensive care units (NICUs) or neonatal follow-up clinics. The ANNP will have completed a degree/higher degree and a year's study of theory and practice, enabling her to work on the senior house officer's rota in the neonatal unit. Her responsibilities include normal neonate assessment and physical examination, diagnosis and management of ill babies as well as high-risk follow-up, transfer of babies and discharge planning. The ANNP also has a vital role in the education and training of junior doctors and midwifery/nursing students in the neonatal setting.

Neonatal midwife/nurse

These midwives and nurses specialise in caring for premature and ill babies in the neonatal setting. They will have undertaken additional education and learned new skills to enable them to practise at a higher level, utilising evidence-based care in order to provide the best possible outcome for vulnerable babies and their families. Some of these professionals will work in neonatal units, paediatric intensive care units or infant surgical units.

Paediatric nurse

Paediatric nurses are qualified in the children's branch of nursing and work with 0- to 16-year-olds in a variety of settings, from specialist baby care units to adolescent services. They also support, advise and educate parents and other close relatives. Once qualified, it is possible to specialise in hospital and community settings in areas such as burns and plastics, intensive care, child protection and cancer care.

Family-centred care

Family-centred care is a cornerstone of midwifery practice.

Midwives are responsible for providing comprehensive care to the pregnant woman, the newborn baby and family members; this approach is known as *family-centred care*. Understanding the makeup and function of the family is essential to delivering family-centred care.

Family ties

A family is a group of two or more persons who possibly live together in the same household, perform certain interrelated social tasks and share an emotional bond. Families can profoundly influence the individuals within them. Therefore, care that considers the family – not just the individual – has become the focus of modern nursing practice.

Changes such as the addition of a new family member alter the structure of the family. If one family member is ill or is going through a rough developmental period, other family members may feel tremendous strain. Family roles must be flexible enough to adjust to the myriad changes that occur with pregnancy and birth.

Family structures

Several different family structures exist today. These structures may change over the life cycle of the family because of such factors as work, birth, death and divorce. Family structures may also differ based on the family roles, generation issues, means of family support and sociocultural issues.

Types of family structures include:
- nuclear family
- cohabitation family
- extended or multigenerational family
- single-parent family
- blended family
- communal family
- gay or lesbian family
- foster family
- adoptive family.

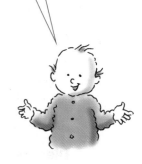

I may be small, but I have a big effect on my family's structure!

Nuclear family

A nuclear family is traditionally defined as a family consisting of a wife, a husband and a child or children. A nuclear family can provide support to and feel affection for family members because of its relatively small size; however, small family size may also be a weakness. For example, when a crisis arises, such as an illness, there are fewer family members to share the burden and provide support.

Cohabitation family

A cohabitation family is composed of a heterosexual couple who live together but aren't married. The living arrangement may be short or long term. A cohabitation family can offer psychological and financial support to its members in the same way as a traditional nuclear family.

Extended or multigenerational family

An extended or multigenerational family includes members of the nuclear family and other family members, such as grandparents, aunts, uncles, cousins and grandchildren. In this type of family, the main support person isn't necessarily a spouse or intimate partner. The primary caregiver may be a grandparent, an aunt or an uncle. This type of family typically has more members to share burdens and provide support but may experience financial problems because income must be stretched to accommodate more people.

Single-parent family

Today, single-parent families account for 23% of families with school-age children (www.statistics.gov.uk). Although in many of these families the mother is the single parent present, an increasing number of fathers are also rearing children alone. Single-parent families exist for many reasons, including divorce, death of a spouse and the decision to raise children outside of marriage.

Working hard for the money

Financial problems, such as low income, can be an issue for single parents. Even though an increasing number of single parents are fathers, most are mothers. Traditionally, the salaries of women have been lower than those of men. This situation poses a problem when a mother's salary is the only source of income for the family.

Flying solo

Another difficulty for the single-parent family is the lack of family support for childcare, which can be problematic if the single parent becomes ill. A single parent may also have difficulty fulfilling the multitude of parental roles that are required of her, such as being a mother and a 'father' in addition to being the sole income provider for the family.

> Sometimes, being a single parent means flying solo.

Blended family

In a blended family, two separate families join as one as a result of remarriage. Quite often (suggestion), conflicts and rivalries develop in these families when the children are exposed to new parenting methods. Jealousy and friction between family members may be an issue, especially when the newly formed family has children of its own. On the other hand, children of blended families may also be more adaptable to new situations.

Communal family

A communal family is a group of people who have chosen to live together but aren't necessarily related by marriage or blood; instead, they may be related by social or religious values. People in communal families may not adhere to traditional health care practices, but they may proactively participate in their health care and be receptive to client teaching.

> C'mon people now, smile on your brother. A communal family is a group of people who aren't related by blood or marriage but choose to live together. That's groovy!

Gay or lesbian family

Some gay and lesbian couples choose to include children in their families. These children may be adopted, or they may come from surrogate mothers, artificial insemination or previous unions or marriages.

Foster family

Foster parents provide care for children whose biological parents can no longer care for them. Foster family situations are usually temporary arrangements until the biological parents can resume care or until a family can adopt the foster child. Foster parents may or may not have children of their own.

Adoptive family

Families of all types can become adoptive families. Families adopt children for various reasons, which may include the inability to have children biologically. In some cases, families choose to adopt foster children whose parents are unable to provide care and are willing to have their children adopted. Sometimes, adoptive parents are the child's biological siblings or

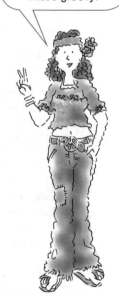

a relative of the parent. This type of family can be very rewarding but also poses many challenges to the family unit, especially if biological children also live in the family. Adoptions can be arranged through an agency, an international adoption programme or private resources.

Family tasks

A healthy family typically performs eight tasks to ensure its success as a working unit and the success of its members as individuals. These include:

- distribution of resources
- socialisation of family members
- division of labour
- physical maintenance
- maintenance of order
- reproduction, release and recruitment of family members
- placement of members into society
- safeguarding of motivation and morale.

Distribution of resources

Because each family has limited resources, the family needs to decide how those resources should be distributed. In some cases, certain family needs will be met and others won't. For example, one child may get new shoes, whereas another gets hand-me-down shoes.

Money isn't everything

Money isn't the only resource. Such resources as affection and space must also be distributed. For example, the eldest child may get his own room, whereas younger children may have to share a room. Most families can make these decisions well. Dysfunctional families or those with financial problems may have problems completing these tasks.

Socialisation of family members

Preparing children to live in society and to socialise with other individuals in their society is another important family task. If the culture of the family differs from the community in which it lives, this may be a difficult task.

Division of labour

Division of labour is the family task that involves assignment of responsibilities to each family member. For example, family members must decide who provides the family with monetary resources, who manages the home and who cares for the children. The division of labour may change within a family when a new baby arrives, especially if both parents work full-time.

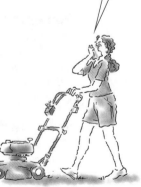

I could use some of that division of labour right about now!

Physical maintenance

The task of physical maintenance includes providing for basic needs, such as food, shelter, clothing and health care. The family fulfils these needs by finding and maintaining employment and securing housing. It's important to have enough resources to complete these tasks or the family may find itself in crisis. Improper distribution of resources can also lead to problems related to providing for basic needs. Physical maintenance also includes providing emotional support and caring for family members who are ill.

Maintenance of order

The task of maintenance of order includes communication among family members. It also involves setting rules for family members and defining each individual's place within the family. For example, when a new baby arrives, a family with a healthy maintenance of order and well-defined rules and roles knows where that new member belongs. Family members welcome the new baby as a part of the family unit and understand the baby's role as a family member. An unhealthy family may find this task difficult. Members of a family without a healthy maintenance of order may feel threatened that the baby will change their roles or take their places in the family. They may see the new baby as an intruder.

Reproduction, release and recruitment of family members

Reproduction, release and recruitment of family members can occur in several ways. For example:
- a new child is born (reproduction)
- a child leaves home for college (release)
- a child is adopted (recruitment)
- elderly parents come to live with the nuclear family (recruitment).

Even though family members don't always control reproduction, release and recruitment, accepting any of these life changes is a family task. A healthy family accepts the change and understands the effects that the change will have on family roles and functions.

Placement of members into society

Families also make decisions that define their place in society. In other words, when parents choose where to live and where to send their children to school, the family becomes part of a particular community within society. The activities they choose to participate in – such as after-school activities, church, sports or clubs – also define the family's place within the social community.

Safeguarding of motivation and morale

The task of safeguarding of motivation and morale is achieved through the development of family pride. Much of this is achieved through emotional encouragement and support. If family members are proud of their accomplishments, a sense of pride for each other and the family as a unit develops. This makes them more likely to care about one another and to defend the family and what the family does. They're also more likely to support one another during crises.

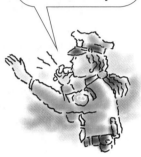

Hold it right there! Someone has to maintain order in the family, especially when a new member is on the way.

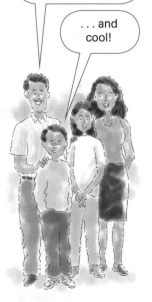

Change is a fact of life, and accepting and understanding that is part of what makes our family healthy . . .

. . . and cool!

The 'midwifery' process

When providing care, midwives follow 'the process steps', which are:
- assessment
- diagnosis
- planning
- implementation
- outcome evaluation.
These steps help to ensure quality and consistent care.

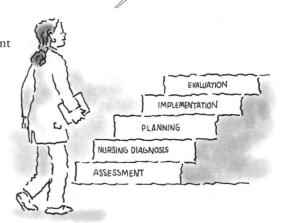

> The 'midwifery process' steps help to ensure high-quality, consistent care. They're also great for exercising my glutes!

Assessment

A midwifery assessment should include an assessment of the woman and her family. Assessment involves continually collecting data to identify a woman's actual and potential health needs. To plan appropriate care, data should accurately reflect the woman's life experiences and patterns of living. To accomplish this, adopt an objective and nonjudgemental approach when gathering data. Data can be obtained through a maternal history (medical and obstetric), physical examination and review of pertinent laboratory and medical information.

Maternal factors

During pregnancy, assess such maternal factors as:
- woman's age
- past medical history (family as well)
- menstrual history
- obstetric history
- present pregnancy
- reaction to fetal movement
- nutritional status.
Remember that the mother's health directly affects the well-being of the fetus.

Fetal factors

During pregnancy, assess such fetal factors as:
- ultrasound results – dates, normality
- movement
- heart rate
- growth/size

Baby factors

After birth, assess such neonatal factors as:
- Apgar scores
- gestational age
- weight in relation to gestational age
- vital signs
- feeding patterns/tolerance of feeds
- muscle tone
- characteristics of the baby's cry
- ability to pass urine and stools.

Family factors

Assessment should always reflect a family-centred approach. Be sure to assess family status, and note how it's affected by the pregnancy and birth. Be aware of how the family is coping with the new arrival and how parents, siblings and other family members are affected. Also, assess how the mother, father, siblings and other family members bond with the neonate.

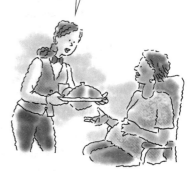

Here you go. It's our healthy mother–healthy fetus special, and it's just what the doctor ordered!

Diagnosis

Many women will have their pregnancy diagnosed, then book into a maternity unit for their care. There are various models of care available to women in the UK. These include:
- Hospital only care – the women attend the maternity unit for all their antenatal care
- Shared care – the women attend their general practitioner for some visits and the hospital for the remainder
- Midwife-led care – the women are cared for by a team of midwives who carry out all their antenatal and intranatal care and then care for them postnatally
- Independent midwives – these midwives have their own caseload of mothers and manage all their care – antenatally, intranatally and postnatally – if any complications arise the women are transferred to hospital right away.

It is important to know that all women must be assessed for their suitability for some of these models of care. For example, a woman classed as high-risk may not be suitable for midwife-led care as she is more likely to need medical intervention during her pregnancy or at delivery.

If a complication occurs during pregnancy, labour or postnatally, the midwife reports this to the obstetrician who makes a diagnosis and care is then planned accordingly.

Planning

After establishing whether the woman requires midwifery or medical management, you'll develop a care plan. A care plan serves as a communication tool among health care team members and helps ensure continuity of care. The plan consists of expected outcomes that describe behaviours or results to be achieved within a specified time, as well as the midwifery interventions needed to achieve these outcomes.

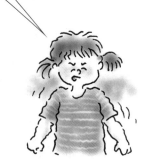

I'm supposed to express my feelings about the new baby? Well, get ready! You asked for it!

Keep it in the family

Be sure to include the woman and her family when planning and implementing the care plan. For example, an awareness of cultural differences is vital. Be aware of the family's changing needs, and be aware of the new mother's sensitivity and emotional concerns. (See *Ensuring a successful care plan*.) It is also important to know how much support the woman is getting from her family and friends.

Implementation

During the implementation phase of the midwifery process, you put your care plan into action. Implementation encompasses all midwifery interventions directed at managing the woman's condition and meeting her health care needs. When you're coordinating implementation, seek help from the woman as well as her family and friends.

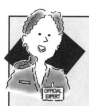

Advice from the experts

Ensuring a successful care plan

Your care plan must rest on a solid foundation of midwifery assessment and sound clinical judgements. It must also fit your client's needs when related to age, developmental level, culture and psychological as well as physiological requirements. Your plan should help the client attain the highest functional level possible, while posing minimal risk and not creating new problems.

At all stages of planning care, individualised needs, informed consent and evidence-based practice must be kept in mind.

Use the following guidelines to help ensure that your care plan is effective.

Be realistic

Avoid setting a goal that's too difficult for the client to achieve in a given time. For example, mothers stay in hospital for a very short period of time – your care plan needs to incorporate time as a factor.

Tailor your approach to each client's problem

Individualise your outcome statements and care interventions. Keep in mind that each client is different; no two client problems are alike.

Avoid vague terms

It's best to use precise, quantitative terms rather than vague ones. For example, if your client seems ambivalent towards her newborn infant, describe this behaviour: 'doesn't respond when the baby cries', 'watches television when changing the baby's nappy'. To indicate that the client's vital signs are stable, document specific measurements, such as 'heart rate less than 100 beats/minute' or 'systolic blood pressure greater than 100 mmHg'.

Review, revise, regroup

After implementing the care plan, continue to monitor the woman to gauge the effectiveness of interventions and to adjust them as her condition changes. Expect to review, revise and update the entire care plan regularly, according to unit policy.

Outcome evaluation

The outcome evaluation step of the midwifery process evaluates how well the woman met her care plan goals, or outcomes. It also evaluates the effectiveness of the care plan. To evaluate the plan effectively, you must establish criteria for measuring the goals and the outcomes of the plan. Then you must assess the woman's responses to these interventions. These responses help determine whether the care plan should be continued, discontinued or changed. Inevitably, this evaluation brings about new assessment information, which necessitates the creation of new obstetric/midwifery diagnoses and a modification of the plan.

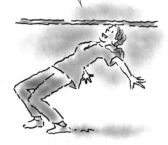

When it comes to care plans, remaining flexible is key. Be ready to monitor, review, revise and update.

Frequent follow-up plan

Evaluate the care plan frequently. This allows for changes and revisions as the needs of the woman and her family change, ensuring that the care plan accurately reflects the family's current needs.

Family response to pregnancy

Several factors can influence a family's response to pregnancy. These factors include:
- maternal age
- cultural beliefs
- whether the pregnancy was planned
- family dynamics
- social and economic resources
- age and health status of other family members
- mother's medical and obstetric history.

Maternal age

The mother's age can affect how family members respond to a pregnancy. If the mother is nearing menopause or is a teenager, then the family members may respond negatively to the pregnancy.

Waiting it out

Today, more families are waiting to have children until later in life. The number of women aged 40 and older having children has risen dramatically in the past 10 years. The number of women who have their first child after age 40 has also increased. If an older woman becomes pregnant, especially one who's already a mother, the family may react unfavourably. For example, older children may be disgusted by the idea that their parents are having sex, or by the pregnancy itself. Also, some family members may perceive pregnancy as the role of a young mother – not one nearing menopause.

Aren't you a little young?

Teenage pregnancy rates have also changed dramatically. The rates in the UK have decreased slightly, but they are still some of the highest in Europe. The government teenage pregnancy statistics from 1999 to 2006 published recently show the following.

Under-16 conceptions

The under-16 conception rate for England in 2005 was 7.7 per 1,000 girls aged 13–15. This is 13.0% lower than the Teenage Pregnancy Strategy's 1998 baseline rate of 8.8 conceptions per 1,000 girls aged 13–15.

Under-18 conceptions

The provisional 2006 under-18 conception rate for England of 40.4 per 1,000 girls aged 15–17 represents an overall decline of 13.3% since 1998 – the baseline year for the Teenage Pregnancy Strategy. The under-18 conception rate is now at its lowest level for over 20 years. The statistics can be accessed at http://www.everychildmatters.gov.uk/health/teenagepregnancy/statistics/

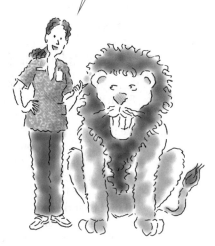

A lion-taming career and motherhood – not the best mix! No wonder so many women today are waiting to have children until later in life.

The teenage mother

If the mother is a young teenager who isn't married, the family may view the pregnancy unfavourably for several reasons. For example, family members may fear that the single mother won't be able to provide for her baby or that she won't finish her schooling. Family members may also be concerned about how their own roles will change as a result of the pregnancy. They may fear that they'll become full-time caregivers for the child. In addition, the family's religious beliefs may lead them to view the pregnancy as unacceptable or even sinful; they may reject the pregnant teenager as well as the child she carries.

Cultural beliefs

Cultural values can influence how a family plans for or reacts to childbearing. Some cultures view childbearing as something to be shared with others as soon as the pregnancy is known. Families in other cultures, such as the Jewish culture, shy away from being public about the pregnancy until it has reached a certain gestational stage.

Cultural norms affect family roles, behaviours and expectations. For example, culture may influence how a man participates in the pregnancy and childbirth. Some cultures allow only women in the birthing room during childbirth. In some cases, the birthing room is considered a woman's place – not a man's.

Cultural cues

Cultural values can also influence midwifery care. Acknowledging the cultural characteristics and beliefs of a woman and her family is an important part of family-centred care. To provide culturally competent care for women during pregnancy, the midwife needs to familiarise herself with the practices and customs of various cultures. In the UK many maternity units now print information leaflets in various languages and interpreters are provided when necessary.

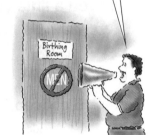

In some cultures, the birthing room is considered women-only territory. Push, dear, push!

Planned versus unplanned pregnancy

Some women view pregnancy as a natural and desired outcome of marriage. To them, having children is a natural progression after marriage. They may plan to have children, or they may not plan the pregnancy but are accepting when it happens. Women who are prepared to accept a pregnancy tend to seek medical validation when the first signs of pregnancy appear.

For other women, pregnancy may be unplanned; the woman may react with ambivalence, or she may deny her symptoms and postpone seeking medical validation. If the father doesn't want a child or the parents are having other difficulties in their relationship, family upheaval can result. In some cases, especially in some adolescents, pregnancy may be an unwanted result of sexual experimentation without contraception.

Expecting to be expecting

Just because a pregnancy is planned, however, doesn't mean that no family member will have trouble accepting it – possibly even the mother or father. The mother may initially want the pregnancy but may be ambivalent about how the pregnancy is changing her body. The parents as a unit may feel they aren't prepared to be parents or that they don't have enough experience around children. In addition, one family member may feel that the family's resources can't provide for a new addition. This too can lead to turmoil over the pregnancy.

Family dynamics

Family dynamics – including a family's structure and how it functions – also affect how a new pregnancy is perceived. Family members are influenced by their changing roles as well as by the physical and emotional changes the pregnant woman experiences. Some family members accept the pregnancy as a part of the family's growth. Other family members may view the pregnancy as a stressor and consider the new member an intruder.

For many families, pregnancy causes career and lifestyle changes that must be made to accommodate the new addition. The parents' ability to meet the physical and emotional needs of existing children in the family also changes.

Coping or moping?

The family support system may be affected as it attempts to cope with the pregnancy. Effective coping methods are demonstrated by the family's participation in parenting classes, childbirth education classes and antenatal care. Ineffective coping mechanisms are evidenced by delaying confirmation of the pregnancy, hiding the pregnancy or delaying antenatal care.

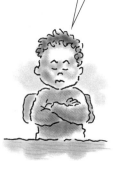

Some family members might be less than thrilled about a new baby. Not me! I'm ecstatic!

Social and economic resources

Economic status can also affect how a family responds to pregnancy. A pregnant woman living in a family whose financial responsibilities are stretched may delay antenatal care or choose not to take antenatal vitamins because of their cost. Many families are barely able to survive on two incomes; a pregnancy may reduce that income, which places emotional and financial strain on the family.

Age and health status of other family members

The health of other family members is another factor that can affect how a family views a pregnancy. If one family member is sick or has a long-term illness that requires a lot of family time and support, the addition of another family member may not be viewed favourably. It also affects the time family members have available to spend with the sick family member. As a result, family roles may have to change.

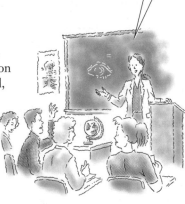

Because you're all participating in parenting and childbirth education classes, I can tell that you're coping well with pregnancy.

Sibling rivalry

Siblings may also be influenced by the arrival of a new family member. Some siblings may perceive the new addition as a threat to their position in the family and become jealous. Such threats can be real or perceived, especially when the sibling experiences separation from the mother when she's hospitalised.

What a difference a year makes

Sibling reaction depends on the child's age. For instance, toddlers are aware of the mother's changing appearance and may have difficulty with separation when the mother leaves. A toddler exhibits this stress by showing signs of regression. Nursery school children and school-age children are likely to be interested in the pregnancy and may ask a lot of questions. They may also express a willingness to participate in childcare. Adolescents, on the other hand, are more likely to be embarrassed by the mother's pregnancy because it represents sexual activity between their parents. However, they may also be very attentive to the needs of the mother.

Medical and obstetric history of the mother

Ideally, a woman should be in good health when she begins her pregnancy. Sometimes, however, a woman with an ongoing illness (such as cardiac disease) becomes pregnant. Such an illness can complicate the pregnancy and cause problems for the woman, affecting how the mother and other members of the family respond to the news. Family members may be concerned that a pregnancy could jeopardise the mother's health. Likewise, if a woman has an obstetric history that includes some difficult labours or births, the family may react unfavourably out of concern for the mother's health.

Ethical and legal issues

Some of the most difficult decisions made in the health care setting are those that involve children and their families. Because midwifery is so family-centred, conflicts commonly arise because family members don't agree on how a situation should be handled. In addition, the values of the health care provider may conflict with those of the family. Legal and ethical issues that may arise in midwifery/neonatal care include abortion, antenatal screening, conception issues, fetal tissue research, eugenics and gene manipulation and treatment of preterm and high-risk neonates. (See *Dealing with ethical and legal issues*.)

Dealing with ethical and legal issues

When you're faced with an ethical or a legal issue in your practice, such as abortion or in vitro fertilisation (IVF), be sure to follow these guidelines to ensure that you're providing the best care to your client and fulfilling your professional duties.

Inform and be informed

Midwives can help their clients make informed decisions by providing factual information, by practising supportive listening and by helping the family clarify its values.

Be self-aware

To reach your own resolutions about legal and ethical issues, you'll need to examine your views honestly and carefully. You'll want to periodically reevaluate your position in light of new medical information and your own experience. If you feel strongly about a particular issue, you should consider working in a practice that matches your views.

Remember your role

Every midwife has an ethical obligation to provide competent, compassionate care. Even if your views on a particular issue differ greatly from those of your client, don't allow your personal feelings to interfere with the quality of care you provide. Speak to your senior midwife or supervisor of midwives if you encounter a problem that is difficult to deal with. You may feel the need to consult your Royal College of Midwives representative if the issue has implications for your daily duties in that unit.

Abortion

In most instances, clients are more likely to be nursed in a gynae setting and so the midwife is less likely to be their carer. If this is not the case, abortion can pose a complex ethical dilemma for a midwife and her clients. A midwife who's ethically or morally opposed to abortion can't be forced to participate in the procedure. However, her employer can insist that she provide nursing care to all clients.

Nonjudgemental

No matter what your opinions are regarding abortion, don't allow personal feelings to interfere with your care for a post-abortion client and don't try to impose your values on the woman. A midwife's role is to provide the best possible care, not to judge or make comments about a client's personal decision.

Antenatal screening

Thanks to such diagnostic procedures as amniocentesis, ultrasound, alpha-fetoprotein screening and chorionic villi sampling, it's now possible to detect inherited and congenital abnormalities long before birth. In a few cases, the diagnosis has paved the way for repair of a defect in utero. However, because it's easier to detect genetic disorders than to treat them, antenatal screening commonly forces a client to choose between having an abortion and taking on the emotional and financial burden of raising a severely disabled child.

Benefits vs. risks

Antenatal diagnostic procedures involve some risk to the fetus. Amniocentesis, for example, causes serious complications or death in about 0.5% of fetuses. Some people feel that this risk creates a conflict between the rights of the fetus and the parents' right to know his health status.

Knowing is half the battle

If testing is to be considered ethical by clients and their families, the midwife must take steps to help the clients fully understand the procedure, comprehend what the test can and can't tell them and be informed about other available options. Thus, effective pre-test and post-test counselling sessions are essential parts of an ethical antenatal screening programme.

Conception issues

Infertility can have devastating effects on the emotional well-being of a couple who yearns for children. As a result, many couples spend time and money to conceive or adopt a child. When medical procedures (such as fertility medications, hysterosalpingostomy and artificial insemination) fail and adoption isn't an option, infertile couples may turn to IVF or surrogate motherhood.

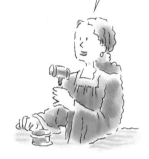

Regardless of our own views, it isn't a midwife's role to pass judgement on clients.

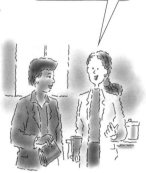

Counselling by the obstetrician, midwife and geneticist may support parents in making difficult decisions about antenatal screening.

In vitro fertilisation

In IVF, ova are removed from a woman's ovaries, placed in a petri dish filled with a sterilised growth medium, and covered with healthy motile spermatozoa for fertilisation. Three to five embryos are then implanted in the woman's uterus 10–14 days after fertilisation, and the remaining fertilised ova are frozen for future use or discarded. IVF can be performed using the partner's sperm (homologous) or a donor's sperm (heterologous).

What about the leftovers?

Some people hail the scientific manipulation of ova and sperm as a medical miracle. Others are concerned that IVF circumvents the natural process of procreation. Another IVF issue involves 'leftover' embryos. About 15–20 embryos may result from a single fertilisation effort, but only 2–3 of them are implanted in the woman's uterus. Some individuals question whether it's ethical to discard these 'leftover' embryos, destroy them or use them for scientific study.

No matter what your values are concerning IVF, keep in mind that your goal is to provide the best nursing care possible to your clients.

Surrogate motherhood

A surrogate mother is a woman who gives birth after carrying the fertilised ovum of another woman or, more commonly, after being artificially inseminated with sperm from the biological father. In the latter case, the biological father then legally adopts the infant.

Offering hope

Surrogate motherhood offers hope for infertile couples in which the woman is the infertile partner. It's also an option for a woman whose age or health makes pregnancy risky. A surrogate birth poses no greater risk to the fetus (or surrogate mother) than any average birth.

Whose rights are right?

One ethical concern about surrogate motherhood involves the potential conflicts concerning the rights of the surrogate mother, the infertile couple, the fetus and the society. The basic dispute involves who has the strongest claim to the child. Does the surrogate mother have rights by virtue of her biological connection? Does the surrogate contract guarantee the infertile couple the right to the child? Courts of law usually rule in favour of the infertile couple.

Support systems

In a surrogate mother situation, the midwife's role is to support her client. If the client she is caring for is a surrogate mother, collaboration with a social worker or a psychologist may be necessary.

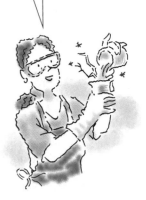

When it comes to modern treatments for infertility, one person's medical miracle is another person's controversy.

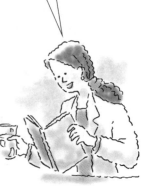

Staying in the research loop will help you provide the most up-to-date information to your clients.

Fetal tissue research

Transplants using stem cells from aborted fetuses offer hope for treating Parkinson's disease, Alzheimer's disease, diabetes and other degenerative disorders. Stem cells have the ability to become any body cell, but only for a short period of time before they become differentiated into specific cells. Stem cells also carry a reduced risk of rejection because of their immaturity.

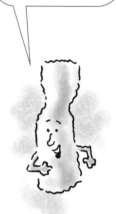

More and more scientists are using genes like me to screen for disease.

Stay in the loop

Such treatment is controversial and may conflict with your values or those of your client. As a midwife, you'll need to stay informed about developing research so that you can provide your clients with the most current information.

Eugenics and gene manipulation

Eugenics is the science of improving a species through control of hereditary factors – in other words, by manipulating the gene pool. In the past, medical research has been limited to efforts to repair or halt the damage caused by disease and injury. Today, however, genetic manipulation and engineering have tremendous potential for altering the course of human development.

It's all in the genes

Using current techniques, researchers can learn many things about a fetus before it's born, including its sex or whether it suffers from certain serious medical conditions. Deoxyribonucleic acid (DNA) can even tell parents what colour of hair their child will have or how tall he'll be.

Mr. Screen Genes

The identification of the genes responsible for inherited diseases and congenital malformations has spurred the development of new screening tests. Genetic testing is now a fairly common component of antenatal care, facilitating the identification of fetuses with such disorders as Down syndrome. The screening of neonates for phenylketonuria, cystic fibrosis, hypothyroidism, sickle cell Disease and others is routine now in most parts of the UK.

Harnessing the power of heredity

Many medical conditions don't have safe and effective treatments. In some cases, gene therapy can change that. Gene therapy using DNA can be used to:
- increase the activity of a gene in the body
- decrease the activity of a gene in the body
- introduce a new gene into the body.

Genetic engineering can even give science the ability to recreate the human body. Scientists frequently discover new ways to identify and manipulate the genetic material of everything from single-cell organisms to human beings.

Designer genes

There's little controversy about the ethics of gene therapy as it's currently practised. However, some groups express concerns about the future. Genetic engineering can potentially allow parents to choose what traits they want their child to have. These 'designer babies' may pose ethical dilemmas for some health care practitioners. Although enormous advances in technology are still needed before selecting such complicated traits as hair colour, intelligence and height becomes a reality, it's possible that these choices will be available to parents in the near future.

Keep informed

Genetic manipulation and gene therapy are still experimental in some cases. As a result, few nurses are directly involved in these aspects of genetic research. Nonetheless, you have an ethical obligation to stay informed and to support efforts to establish legal and technological safeguards.

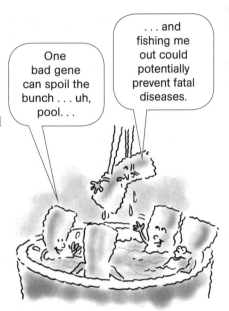

One bad gene can spoil the bunch . . . uh, pool. . .

. . . and fishing me out could potentially prevent fatal diseases.

Preterm and high-risk neonates

Twenty years ago, an infant born at 26 weeks' gestation had almost no chance of survival. This is no longer the case. Advances in neonatology, such as intrauterine surgery, synthetic lung surfactant and new antibiotics, help save increasingly smaller and sicker infants.

Matters of life and death

When you care for an extremely premature or a critically ill infant and his mother, family members look to you to assist them with life-and-death decisions. To help the parents of an extremely premature or critically ill neonate reach ethically sound decisions, you'll need to present all available options in a compassionate, unbiased manner using simple terms. By carefully helping family members consider the pros and cons of both initiating and withholding treatment, you can help them come to terms with the neonate's condition and reach a decision with which they'll be able to live.

Quick quiz

1. The intrapartum period starts:
   A. after delivery of the neonate and placenta.
   B. at the onset of contractions.
   C. at conception.
   D. during the second trimester.

Answer: B. The intrapartum period starts at the onset of contractions that cause cervical dilation and lasts through the first 1–4 hours after the birth of the neonate and delivery of the placenta.

2. A family that consists of parents, grandparents and grandchildren is known as:
    A. a cohabitation family.
    B. an extended family.
    C. a blended family.
    D. a communal family.

Answer: B. An extended or multigenerational family consists of the nuclear family as well as other family members, such as grandparents, aunts, uncles, cousins and grandchildren.

3. When a woman gives birth after carrying the fertilised ovum of another woman, it's called:
    A. in vitro fertilisation.
    B. caesarean birth.
    C. surrogate motherhood.
    D. gamete fertilisation.

Answer: C. Surrogate motherhood involves one woman giving birth after carrying the fertilised ovum of another woman or after being inseminated with sperm from the biological father.

4. The science of improving a species through control of hereditary factors by manipulation of the gene pool is called:
    A. eugenics.
    B. in vitro fertilisation.
    C. fetal tissue research.
    D. genealogy.

Answer: A. Eugenics is the science of improving a species through control of hereditary factors by manipulation of the gene pool.

Scoring

☆☆☆ If you answered all five questions correctly, fantastic! Your labour is paying off!

☆☆ If you answered four questions correctly, good work! You're sure to reproduce these results in later chapters!

☆ If you answered fewer than four questions correctly, don't worry! Just breathe, relax and push (through a review of the chapter, that is).

2 Conception and fetal development

Just the facts

In this chapter, you'll learn:

♦ anatomic structures and functions of the male and female reproductive systems

♦ effects of hormone production on sexual development

♦ the process of fertilisation

♦ stages of fetal development

♦ structural changes that result from pregnancy.

A look at conception and fetal development

Development of a functioning human being from a fertilised ovum involves a complex process of cell division, differentiation and organisation. Development begins with the union of spermatozoon and ovum (conception) to form a composite cell containing chromosomes from both parents. This composite cell (called a *zygote*) divides repeatedly. Finally, groups of differentiated cells organise into complex structures, such as the brain, spinal cord, liver, kidneys and other organs that function as integrated units.

To fully understand the dramatic physical changes that occur during pregnancy, you must be familiar with reproductive anatomy and physiology and the stages of fetal development. Let's start with the male reproductive system.

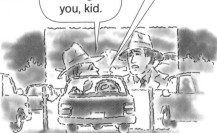

Male reproductive system

Anatomically, the main distinction between a male and a female is the presence of conspicuous external genitalia in the male. In contrast, the major reproductive organs of the female lie within the pelvic cavity.

Making introductions

The male reproductive system consists of the organs that produce, transfer and introduce mature sperm into the female reproductive tract, where fertilisation occurs. (See *Structures of the male reproductive system*, page 26.)

Multitasking

In addition to supplying male sex cells (spermatogenesis), the male reproductive system plays a part in the secretion of male sex hormones.

Penis

The organ of copulation, the penis deposits sperm in the female reproductive tract and acts as the terminal duct for the urinary tract. The penis also serves as the means for urine elimination. It consists of an attached root, a free shaft and an enlarged tip.

What's inside

Internally, the cylinder-shaped penile shaft consists of three columns of erectile tissue bound together by heavy fibrous tissue. Two corpora cavernosa form the major part of the penis. On the underside, the corpus spongiosum encases the urethra. Its enlarged proximal end forms the bulb of the penis.

The glans penis, at the distal end of the shaft, is a cone-shaped structure formed from the corpus spongiosum. Its lateral margin forms a ridge of tissue known as the *corona*. The glans penis is highly sensitive to sexual stimulation.

What's outside

Thin, loose skin covers the penile shaft. The urethral meatus opens through the glans to allow urination and ejaculation.

In a different vein

The penis receives blood through the internal pudendal artery. Blood then flows into the corpora cavernosa through the penile artery. Venous blood returns through the internal iliac vein to the vena cava.

Scrotum

The penis meets the scrotum, or scrotal sac, at the penoscrotal junction. Located posterior to the penis and anterior to the anus, the scrotum is an

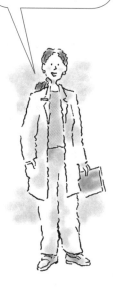

Here's the main difference – males have external genitalia, whereas most female reproductive organs are inside the pelvic cavity.

Structures of the male reproductive system

The male reproductive system consists of the penis, the scrotum and its contents, the prostate gland and the inguinal structures.

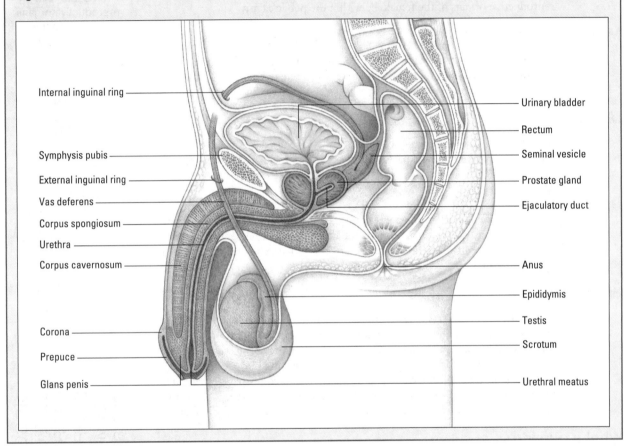

Internal inguinal ring

Symphysis pubis

External inguinal ring

Vas deferens

Corpus spongiosum

Urethra

Corpus cavernosum

Corona

Prepuce

Glans penis

Urinary bladder

Rectum

Seminal vesicle

Prostate gland

Ejaculatory duct

Anus

Epididymis

Testis

Scrotum

Urethral meatus

extra-abdominal pouch that consists of a thin layer of skin overlying a tighter, musclelike layer. This musclelike layer, in turn, overlies the tunica vaginalis, a serous membrane that covers the internal scrotal cavity.

Canals and rings

Internally, a septum divides the scrotum into two sacs, which each contains a testis, an epididymis and a spermatic cord. The spermatic cord is a connective tissue sheath that encases autonomic nerve fibres, blood vessels, lymph vessels and the vas deferens (also called the *ductus deferens*).

The spermatic cord travels from the testis through the inguinal canal, exiting the scrotum through the external inguinal ring and entering the abdominal cavity through the internal inguinal ring. The inguinal canal lies between the two rings.

Loads of nodes

Lymph nodes from the penis, scrotal surface and anus drain into the inguinal lymph nodes. Lymph nodes from the testes drain into the lateral aortic and preaortic lymph nodes in the abdomen.

Testes

The testes are enveloped in two layers of connective tissue called the *tunica vaginalis* (outer layer) and the *tunica albuginea* (inner layer). Extensions of the tunica albuginea separate the testes into lobules. Each lobule contains one to four seminiferous tubules, small tubes where spermatogenesis takes place.

Climate control

Spermatozoa development requires a temperature lower than that of the rest of the body. The dartos muscle, a smooth muscle in the superficial fasciae, causes scrotal skin to wrinkle, which helps regulate temperature. The cremaster muscle, rising from the internal oblique muscle, helps to govern temperature by elevating the testes.

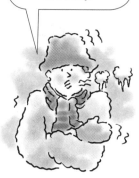

Brrrr! One of the jobs of the scrotum is to keep the testes cooler than the rest of the body.

Duct system

The male reproductive duct system, consisting of the epididymis, vas deferens and urethra, conveys sperm from the testes to the ejaculatory ducts near the bladder.

Swimmers, take your mark!

The epididymis is a coiled tube that's located superior to and along the posterior border of the testis. During ejaculation, smooth muscle in the epididymis contracts, ejecting spermatozoa into the vas deferens.

Descending tunnel

The vas deferens leads from the testes to the abdominal cavity, extends upward through the inguinal canal, arches over the urethra and descends behind the bladder. Its enlarged portion, called the *ampulla*, merges with the duct of the seminal vesicle to form the short ejaculatory duct. After passing through the prostate gland, the vas deferens joins with the urethra.

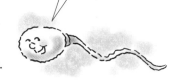

During ejaculation, smooth muscle in the epididymis contracts, sending spermatozoa into the vas deferens.

Tube to the outside

A small tube leading from the floor of the bladder to the exterior, the urethra consists of three parts:

prostatic urethra, which is surrounded by the prostate gland and drains the bladder membranous urethra, which passes through the urogenital diaphragm

 spongy urethra, which makes up about 75% of the entire urethra.

Accessory reproductive glands

The accessory reproductive glands, which produce most of the semen, include the seminal vesicles, bulbourethral glands (Cowper's glands) and prostate gland.

A pair of pairs

The seminal vesicles are paired sacs at the base of the bladder. The bulbourethral glands, also paired, are located inferior to the prostate.

Improving the odds

The walnut-size prostate gland lies under the bladder and surrounds the urethra. It consists of three lobes: the left and right lateral lobes and the median lobe.

The prostate gland continuously secretes prostatic fluid, a thin, milky, alkaline fluid. During sexual activity, prostatic fluid adds volume to semen. It also enhances sperm motility and improves the odds of conception by neutralising the acidity of the man's urethra and the woman's vagina.

Basically basic

Semen is a viscous, white secretion with a slightly alkaline pH (7.8–8) that consists of spermatozoa and accessory gland secretions. The seminal vesicles produce roughly 60% of the fluid portion of semen, whereas the prostate gland produces about 30%. A viscid fluid secreted by the bulbourethral glands also becomes part of semen.

Spermatogenesis

Sperm formation (also called *spermatogenesis*) begins when a male reaches puberty and usually continues throughout life.

Divide and conquer

Spermatogenesis occurs in four stages:

 In the first stage, the primary germinal epithelial cells, called *spermatogonia*, grow and develop into primary spermatocytes. Both spermatogonia and primary spermatocytes contain 46 chromosomes, consisting of 44 autosomes and the two sex chromosomes, X and Y.

 Next, primary spermatocytes divide to form secondary spermatocytes. No new chromosomes are formed in this stage; the pairs only divide. Each secondary spermatocyte contains one-half of the number of autosomes, 22; one secondary spermatocyte contains an X chromosome and the other, a Y chromosome.

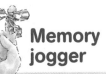

Memory jogger

To remember the meaning of spermatogenesis, keep in mind that genesis means 'beginning' or 'new'. Therefore, spermatogenesis means beginning of new sperm.

In the third stage, each secondary spermatocyte divides again to form spermatids (also called *spermatoblasts*).

Finally, the spermatids undergo a series of structural changes that transform them into mature spermatozoa, or sperm. Each spermatozoon has a head, neck, body and tail. The head contains the nucleus, and the tail, a large amount of adenosine triphosphate, which provides energy for sperm motility.

Queuing up

Newly mature sperm pass from the seminiferous tubules through the vasa recta into the epididymis. Only a small number of sperm can be stored in the epididymis. Most of them move into the vas deferens, where they're stored until sexual stimulation triggers emission.

Check the expiration date?

After ejaculation, sperm can survive for 24–72 hours at body temperature. Sperm cells retain their potency and can survive for up to 4 days in the female reproductive tract.

Hormonal control and sexual development

Androgens (male sex hormones) are produced in the testes and adrenal glands. Androgens are responsible for the development of male sex organs and secondary sex characteristics. One major androgen is testosterone.

Team captain

Leydig cells, located in the testes between the seminiferous tubules, secrete testosterone, the most significant male sex hormone. Testosterone is responsible for the development and maintenance of male sex organs and secondary sex characteristics, such as facial hair and vocal cord thickness. Testosterone is also required for spermatogenesis.

Calling the plays

Testosterone secretion begins approximately 2 months after conception, when the release of chorionic gonadotropins from the placenta stimulates Leydig cells in the male fetus. The presence of testosterone directly affects sexual differentiation in the fetus. With testosterone, fetal genitalia develop into penis, scrotum and testes; without testosterone, genitalia develop into clitoris, vagina and other female organs.

During the last 2 months of gestation, testosterone usually causes the testes to descend into the scrotum. If the testes don't descend after birth, exogenous testosterone may correct the problem.

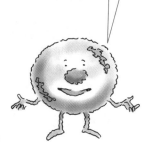

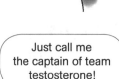

The number of sperm and their motility affect fertility. A low sperm count (less than 20 million per millilitre of semen) may be a cause of infertility.

Just call me the captain of team testosterone!

Other key players

Other hormones also affect male sexuality. Two of these, luteinising hormone (LH) – also called *interstitial cell-stimulating hormone* – and follicle-stimulating hormone (FSH), directly affect secretion of testosterone.

Waiting on the bench

During early childhood, a boy doesn't secrete gonadotropins and thus has little circulating testosterone. Secretion of gonadotropins from the pituitary gland, which usually occurs between ages 11 and 14, marks the onset of puberty. These pituitary gonadotropins stimulate testis functioning as well as testosterone secretion.

Put me in, coach!

During puberty, the penis and testes enlarge, and the male reaches full adult sexual and reproductive capability. Puberty also marks the development of male secondary sexual characteristics, including:

- distinct body hair distribution
- skin changes (such as increased secretion by sweat and sebaceous glands)
- deepening of the voice (from laryngeal enlargement)
- increased musculoskeletal development
- other intracellular and extracellular changes.

Star player

After a male achieves full physical maturity, usually by age 20, sexual and reproductive functions remain fairly consistent throughout life.

Subtle changes

With ageing, a man may experience subtle changes in sexual function, but he doesn't lose the ability to reproduce. For example, an elderly man may require more time to achieve an erection, experience less firm erections and have reduced ejaculatory volume. After ejaculation, he may take longer to regain an erection.

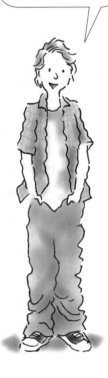

Hey, I've almost reached full physical maturity. Now can I borrow the car?

Female reproductive system

Unlike the male reproductive system, the female system is largely internal, housed within the pelvic cavity.

External genitalia

The external female genitalia, or vulva, include the mons pubis, labia majora, labia minora, clitoris and adjacent structures. These structures are visible on inspection. (See *Structures of the female reproductive system*, pages 32 and 33.)

Mons pubis

The mons pubis is a rounded cushion of fatty and connective tissue covered by skin and coarse, curly hair in a triangular pattern over the symphysis pubis (the joint formed by the union of the pubic bones anteriorly).

Labia majora

The labia majora are two raised folds of adipose and connective tissue that border the vulva on either side, extending from the mons pubis to the perineum. After onset of the first menses (called *menarche*), the outer surface of the labia is covered with pubic hair. The inner surface is pink and moist.

Labia minora

The labia minora are two moist folds of mucosal tissue, dark pink to red in colour, that lie within and alongside the labia majora. Each upper section divides into an upper and lower lamella. The two upper lamellae join to form the prepuce, a hoodlike covering over the clitoris. The two lower lamellae form the frenulum, the posterior portion of the clitoris.

The lower labial sections taper down and back from the clitoris to the perineum, where they join to form the fourchette, a thin tissue fold along the anterior edge of the perineum.

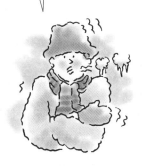

The labia are highly vascular and have many nerve endings – making them sensitive to pain, pressure, touch, sexual stimulation and temperature extremes.

Minor in name only

The labia minora contain sebaceous glands, which secrete a lubricant that also acts as a bactericide. Like the labia majora, they're rich in blood vessels and nerve endings, making them highly responsive to stimulation. They swell in response to sexual stimulation, a reaction that triggers other changes that prepare the genitalia for coitus.

Clitoris

The clitoris is the small, protuberant organ just beneath the arch of the mons pubis. It contains erectile tissue, venous cavernous spaces and specialized sensory corpuscles, which are stimulated during sexual activity.

Adjacent structures

The vestibule is an oval area bounded anteriorly by the clitoris, laterally by the labia minora and posteriorly by the fourchette.

Featuring glands

The mucus-producing Skene's glands are found on both sides of the urethral opening. Openings of the two mucus-producing Bartholin's glands are located laterally and posteriorly on either side of the inner vaginal orifice.

The urethral meatus is the slitlike opening below the clitoris through which urine leaves the body. In the centre of the vestibule is the vaginal orifice. It may be completely or partially covered by the hymen, a tissue membrane.

Structures of the female reproductive system

The female reproductive system consists of external and internal genitalia. These structures include the vagina, cervix, uterus, fallopian tubes, ovaries and other structures. Reproductive, urinary and GI structures are housed in the female pelvis. These include the bladder, anus and rectum.

View of external genitalia in lithotomy position

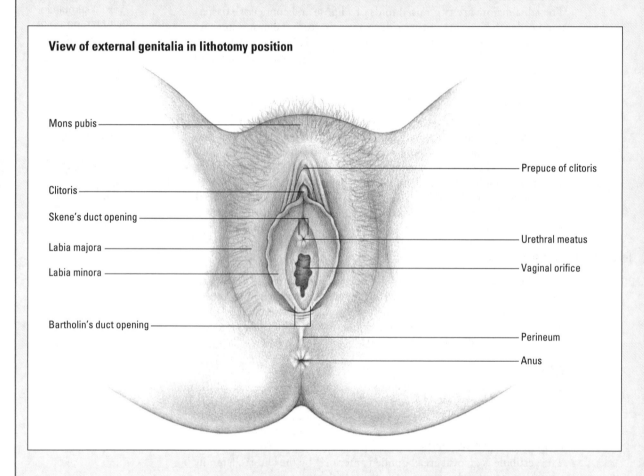

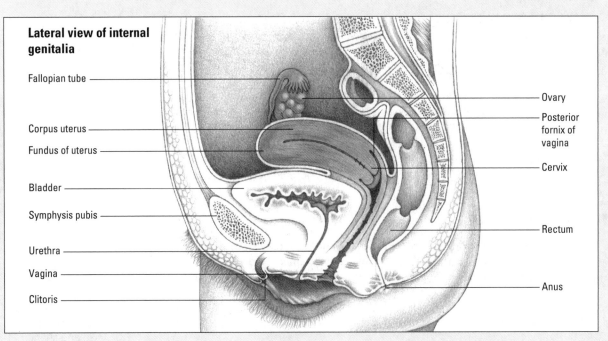

Lateral view of internal genitalia

- Fallopian tube
- Corpus uterus
- Fundus of uterus
- Bladder
- Symphysis pubis
- Urethra
- Vagina
- Clitoris
- Ovary
- Posterior fornix of vagina
- Cervix
- Rectum
- Anus

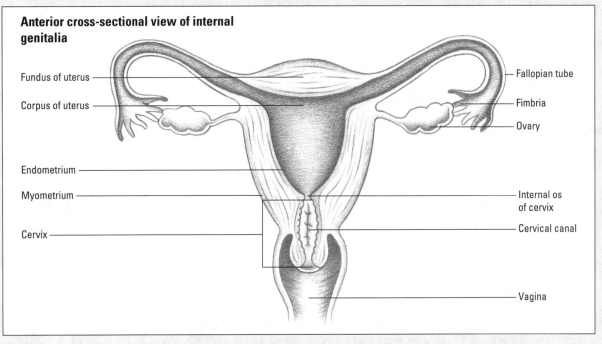

Anterior cross-sectional view of internal genitalia

- Fundus of uterus
- Corpus of uterus
- Endometrium
- Myometrium
- Cervix
- Fallopian tube
- Fimbria
- Ovary
- Internal os of cervix
- Cervical canal
- Vagina

Not too simple

Located between the lower vagina and the anal canal, the perineum is a complex structure of muscles, blood vessels, fasciae, nerves and lymphatics.

Internal genitalia

The female internal genitalia include the vagina, cervix, uterus, fallopian tubes, ovaries and mammary glands. The main function of these specialised organs is reproduction.

Vagina

The vagina, a highly elastic muscular tube, is located between the urethra and the rectum.

Three layers . . .

The vaginal wall has three tissue layers: epithelial tissue, loose connective tissue and muscle tissue. The uterine cervix connects the uterus to the vaginal vault. Four fornices, recesses in the vaginal wall, surround the cervix.

. . . three functions

The vagina has three main functions:

to accommodate the penis during coitus

to channel blood discharged from the uterus during menstruation

to serve as the birth canal during childbirth.

Separate but equal

The upper, middle and lower vaginal sections have separate blood supplies. Branches of the uterine arteries supply blood to the upper vagina, the inferior vesical arteries supply blood to the middle vagina and the haemorrhoidal and internal pudendal arteries feed into the lower vagina.

Blood returns through a vast venous plexus to the haemorrhoidal, pudendal and uterine veins, and then to the hypogastric veins. This plexus merges with the vertebral venous plexus.

Cervix

The cervix is the lowest portion of the uterus. It projects into the upper portion of the vagina. The end that opens into the vagina is called the *external os*, and the end that opens into the uterus, the *internal os*. The cervix is sealed with thick mucus. This prevents sperm from entering except for a few days around ovulation when the plug becomes thinner.

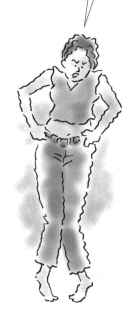

Over time, everything changes – the size and shape of the cervix, and the size and shape of my hips!

Kids change everything!

Childbirth permanently alters the cervix. In a female who hasn't delivered a child, the external os is a round opening about 3 mm in diameter; after the first childbirth, it becomes a small transverse slit with irregular edges.

Uterus

The uterus is a small, firm, pear-shaped, muscular organ situated between the bladder and the rectum. It typically lies at almost 90° to the vagina. The mucous membrane lining of the uterus is called the *endometrium*, and the muscular layer of the uterus is called the *myometrium*.

Fundamental fundus

During pregnancy, the elastic, upper portion of the uterus, called the *fundus*, accommodates most of the growing fetus until 32 weeks when the lower segment stretches, giving the fetus a bit more room to grow. The uterus, as it expands during pregnancy, has two main segments – the upper segment, which forms most of the body of the gravid uterus, and the lower segment, which forms in the third trimester to become the inferior portion and joins with the cervical canal, and expands so that it extends into the vagina.

Fallopian tubes

Two fallopian tubes attach to the uterus at the upper angles of the fundus. These narrow cylinders of muscle fibres are where fertilisation occurs.

Riding the wave

The curved portion of the fallopian tube, called the *ampulla*, ends in the funnel-shaped infundibulum. Fingerlike projections in the infundibulum, called *fimbriae*, move in waves that sweep the mature ovum (female gamete, or sex cell) from the ovary into the fallopian tube.

Ovaries

The ovaries are located on either side of the uterus. The size, shape and position of the ovaries vary with age. Round, smooth and pink at birth, they grow larger, flatten and turn greyish by puberty. During the childbearing years, they take on an almond shape and a rough, pitted surface; after menopause, they shrink and turn white.

Swept away

The ovaries' main function is to produce mature ova. At birth, each ovary contains approximately 400,000 graafian follicles. During the childbearing years, one graafian follicle produces a mature ovum during the first half of each menstrual cycle. As the ovum matures, the follicle ruptures and the ovum is swept into the fallopian tube.

The ovaries also produce oestrogen and progesterone as well as a small amount of androgens.

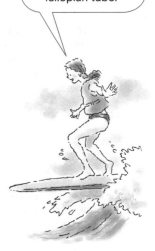

Fingerlike projections called *fimbriae* move in waves, sweeping the ovum from the ovary to the fallopian tube.

Mammary glands

The mammary glands, located in the breast, are specialised accessory glands that secrete milk. Although present in both sexes, they typically function only in the female.

Each mammary gland contains 15–20 lobes that are separated by fibrous connective tissue and fat. Within the lobes are clustered acini – tiny, saclike duct terminals that secrete milk during lactation.

The ducts draining the lobules converge to form excretory (*lactiferous*) ducts and sinuses (*ampullae*), which store milk during lactation. These ducts drain onto the nipple surface through 15–20 openings. (See *The female breast*.)

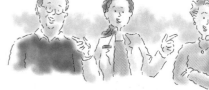

Both males and females have mammary glands – but they typically function only in the female.

Hormonal function and the menstrual cycle

Like the male body, the female body changes as it ages in response to hormonal control. When a female reaches the age of menstruation, the

---

The female breast

The breasts are located on either side of the anterior chest wall over the greater pectoral and the anterior serratus muscles. Within the areola, the pigmented area in the centre of the breast, lies the nipple. Erectile tissue in the nipple responds to cold, friction and sexual stimulation.

Support and separate

Each breast is composed of glandular, fibrous and adipose tissue. Glandular tissue contains 15–20 lobes made up of clustered acini, tiny saclike duct terminals that secrete milk. Fibrous Cooper's ligaments support the breasts; adipose tissue separates the two breasts.

Produce and drain

Milk glands in each breast produce milk by acini cells and then deliver it to the nipple by a lactiferous duct.

Sebaceous glands on the areolar surface, called Montgomery's tubercles, produce sebum, which lubricates the areola and nipple during breastfeeding.

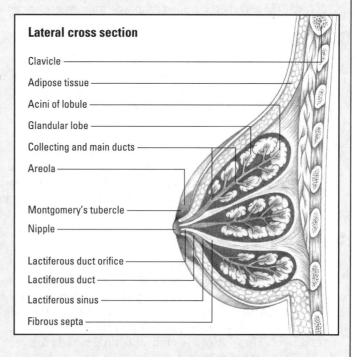

Lateral cross section

- Clavicle
- Adipose tissue
- Acini of lobule
- Glandular lobe
- Collecting and main ducts
- Areola
- Montgomery's tubercle
- Nipple
- Lactiferous duct orifice
- Lactiferous duct
- Lactiferous sinus
- Fibrous septa

hypothalamus, ovaries and pituitary gland secrete hormones – oestrogen, progesterone, FSH and LH – that affect the build-up and shedding of the endometrium during the menstrual cycle. (See *Events in the female reproductive cycle*, pages 38 and 39.)

A spurt of growth

During adolescence, the release of hormones causes a rapid increase in physical growth and spurs the development of secondary sex characteristics. This growth spurt begins at approximately age 11 and continues until early adolescence, or about 3 years later.

Irregularity of the menstrual cycle is common during this time because of failure of the female to ovulate. With menarche, the uterine body flexes on the cervix and the ovaries are situated in the pelvic cavity.

A monthly thing

The menstrual cycle is a complex process that involves both the reproductive and endocrine systems. The cycle averages 28 days.

Supply exhausted

In contrast to the slowly declining hormones of the ageing male, the ageing female's hormones decline rapidly in a process called *menopause*. Although the pituitary gland still releases FSH and LH, the body has exhausted its supply of ovarian follicles that respond to these hormones, and menstruation no longer occurs.

Cessation of menses usually occurs between ages 45 and 55. Some women experience menopause early, possibly as a result of genetics, ovarian damage, autoimmune disorders or surgical interventions such as hysterectomy. When menopause occurs before age 45, it's known as *premature menopause*.

Menopause can be broken down into three stages: perimenopause, menopause and postmenopause.

Climactic climacteric

Perimenopause consists of the 8–10 years (called the *climacteric years*) of declining ovarian function that occurs before menopause. During this time, the ovaries gradually begin to produce less oestrogen, and the woman may experience irregular menses that become further apart and produce a lighter flow. As menopause progresses, the ovaries stop producing progesterone and oestrogen altogether.

Out of eggs

A woman is considered to have reached the menopause stage after menses are absent for 1 year. At this stage, the ovaries have stopped producing eggs and have almost completely stopped producing oestrogen.

Signs and symptoms of menopause include:
• hot flashes (sudden feelings of warmth that spread throughout the upper body and may be accompanied by blushing or sweating)

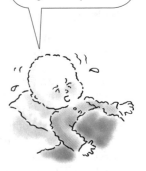

Are you telling me I have to wait until I'm 11 before I'll have my growth spurt?

Events in the female reproductive cycle

The female reproductive cycle usually lasts 28 days. During this cycle, three major types of changes occur simultaneously: ovulatory, hormonal and endometrial (involving the lining [endometrium] of the uterus).

Ovulatory

- Ovulatory changes, which usually last 5 days, begin on day 1 of the menstrual cycle.
- As the cycle begins, low oestrogen and progesterone levels in the bloodstream stimulate the hypothalamus to secrete gonadotropin-releasing hormone (Gn-RH). In turn, Gn-RH stimulates the anterior pituitary gland to secrete follicle-stimulating hormone (FSH) and luteinising hormone (LH).
- Follicle development within the ovary (in the follicular phase) is spurred by increased levels of FSH and, to a lesser extent, LH.
- When the follicle matures, a spike in the LH level occurs, causing the follicle to rupture and release the ovum, thus initiating ovulation.
- After ovulation (in the luteal phase), the collapsed follicle forms the corpus luteum, which degenerates if fertilisation doesn't occur.

Hormonal

- During the follicular phase of the ovarian cycle, the increasing FSH and LH levels that stimulate follicle growth also stimulate increased secretion of the hormone oestrogen.
- Oestrogen secretion peaks just before ovulation. This peak sets in motion the spike in LH levels, which causes ovulation.
- After ovulation (about day 14), oestrogen levels decline rapidly. In the luteal phase of the ovarian cycle, the corpus luteum is formed and begins to release progesterone and oestrogen.
- As the corpus luteum degenerates, levels of both of these ovarian hormones decline.

Endometrial

- The endometrium is receptive to implantation of an embryo for only a short time in the reproductive cycle. Thus, it's no accident that its most receptive phase occurs about 7 days after the ovarian cycle's release of an ovum – just in time to receive a fertilised ovum.
- In the first 5 days of the reproductive cycle, the endometrium sheds its functional layer, leaving the basal layer (the deepest layer) intact. Menstrual flow consists of this detached layer and accompanying blood from the detachment process.
- The endometrium begins regenerating its functional layer at about day 6 (the proliferative phase), spurred by rising oestrogen levels.
- After ovulation, increased progesterone secretion stimulates conversion of the functional layer into a secretory mucosa (secretory phase), which is more receptive to implantation of the fertilised ovum.
- If implantation doesn't occur, the corpus luteum degenerates, progesterone levels drop and the endometrium again sheds its functional layer.

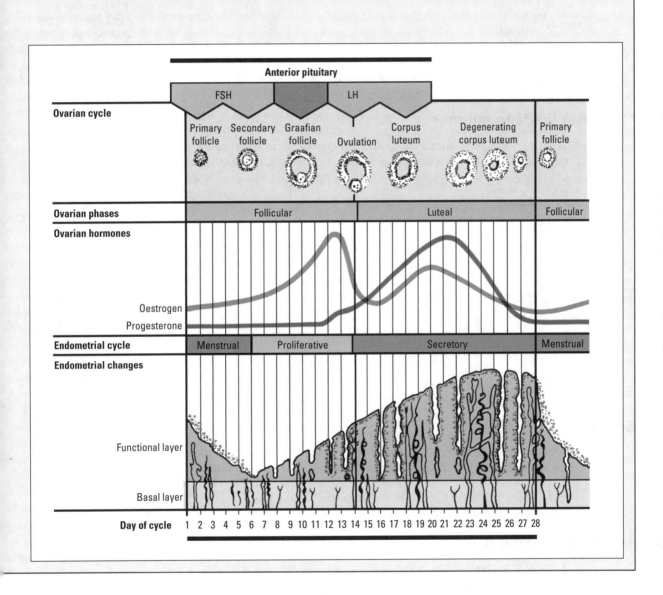

- irregular or skipped menses
- mood swings and irritability
- fatigue
- insomnia
- headaches
- changes in sex drive
- vaginal dryness.

Menopause can be confirmed through analysis of FSH levels or a Pap-like test that assesses for vaginal atrophy.

One thing leads to another

Postmenopause refers to the years after menopause. During this stage, the symptoms of menopause cease for most women. However, the risk of other health problems increases as a result of declining oestrogen levels. These problems include:

- osteoporosis
- heart disease
- decreased skin elasticity
- vision deterioration.

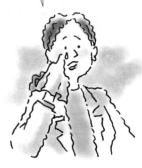

Mood swings – just one of the possible signs and symptoms of menopause (sniff).

Fertilisation

Production of a new human being begins with *fertilisation*, the union of a spermatozoon and an ovum to form a single new cell. After fertilisation occurs, dramatic changes begin inside a woman's body. The cells of the fertilised ovum begin dividing as the ovum travels to the uterine cavity, where it implants itself in the uterine lining. (See *How fertilisation occurs*, page 41.)

Survivial of the fittest

For fertilisation to take place, however, the spermatozoon must first reach the ovum. Although a single ejaculation deposits several hundred million spermatozoa, many are destroyed by acidic vaginal secretions. The only spermatozoa that survive are those that enter the cervical canal, where cervical mucus protects them.

Timing is everything

The ability of spermatozoa to penetrate the cervical mucus depends on the phase of the menstrual cycle at the time of transit:
- Early in the cycle, oestrogen and progesterone levels cause the mucus to thicken, making it more difficult for spermatozoa to pass through the cervix.
- During midcycle, however, when the mucus is relatively thin, spermatozoa can pass readily through the cervix.
- Later in the cycle, the cervical mucus thickens again, hindering spermatozoa passage.

It's a lot of work for one sperm! After I make my way through the cervical mucus, uterine contractions help me to penetrate the fallopian tubes.

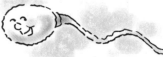

How fertilisation occurs

Fertilisation begins when the spermatozoon is activated upon contact with the ovum. Here's what happens.

The spermatozoon, which has a covering called the *acrosome*, approaches the ovum.

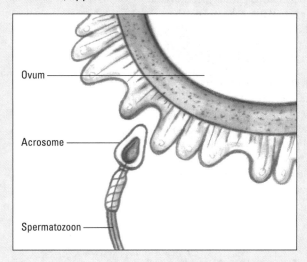

The acrosome develops small perforations through which it releases enzymes necessary for the sperm to penetrate the protective layers of the ovum before fertilisation.

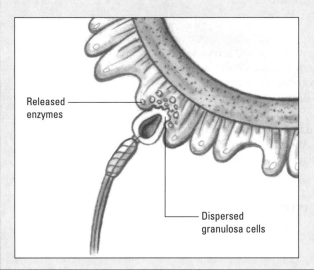

The spermatozoon then penetrates the zona pellucida (the inner membrane of the ovum). This triggers the ovum's second meiotic division (following meiosis), making the zona pellucida impenetrable to other spermatozoa.

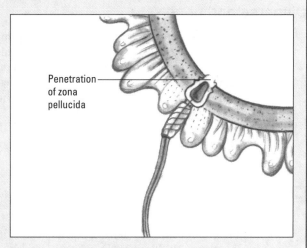

After the spermatozoon penetrates the ovum, its nucleus is released into the ovum, its tail degenerates and its head enlarges and fuses with the ovum's nucleus. This fusion provides the fertilised ovum, called a *zygote*, with 46 chromosomes.

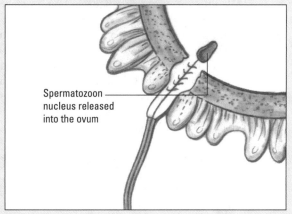

Help along the way

Spermatozoa travel through the female reproductive tract by means of flagellar movements (whiplike movements of the tail). After spermatozoa pass through the cervical mucus, however, the female reproductive system assists them on their journey with rhythmic contractions of the uterus that help the spermatozoa to penetrate the fallopian tubes. Spermatozoa are typically viable (able to fertilise the ovum) for up to 2 days after ejaculation; however, they can survive in the reproductive tract for up to 4 days.

Disperse and penetrate

Before a spermatozoon can penetrate the ovum, it must disperse the granulosa cells and penetrate the zona pellucida, the thick, transparent layer surrounding the incompletely developed ovum. Enzymes in the acrosome (head cap) of the spermatozoon permit this penetration. After penetration, the ovum completes its second meiotic division and the zona pellucida prevents penetration by other spermatozoa.

The spermatozoon's head then fuses with the ovum nucleus, creating a cell nucleus with 46 chromosomes. The fertilised ovum is called a *zygote*.

Pregnancy

Pregnancy starts with fertilisation and ends with childbirth; on average, its duration is 38–40 weeks. During this period (called *gestation*), the zygote divides as it passes through the fallopian tube and attaches to the uterine lining by implantation. A complex sequence of preembryonic, embryonic and fetal developments transforms the zygote into a full-term fetus.

Making predictions

Because the uterus grows throughout pregnancy, uterine size serves as a rough estimate of gestation. The fertilisation date is rarely known, so the woman's expected delivery date is typically calculated from the beginning of her last menses. The tool used for calculating delivery dates is known as *Nägele's rule*.

Here's how it works: if you know the 1st day of the last menstrual cycle, simply count back 3 months from that date and then add 7 days. For example, let's say that the 1st day of the last menses was April 29. Count back 3 months, which gets you to January 29, and then add 7 days for an approximate due date of February 6.

Stages of fetal development

During pregnancy, the fetus undergoes three major stages of development:

 preembryonic period (fertilisation to week 3)

embryonic period (weeks 4 through 7)

 fetal period (week 8 through birth).

It all starts here

The preembryonic phase starts with ovum fertilisation and lasts 3 weeks. As the zygote passes through the fallopian tube, it undergoes a series of mitotic divisions, or cleavage. (See *Preembryonic development*, page 44.)

Zygote to embryo

During the embryonic period (the 4th through to the 7th week of gestation), the developing zygote starts to take on a human shape and is now called an *embryo*. Each germ layer – the ectoderm, mesoderm and endoderm – eventually forms specific tissues in the embryo. (See *Embryonic development*, page 45.)

Organ systems form during the embryonic period. During this time, the embryo is particularly vulnerable to injury by maternal drug use, certain maternal infections and other factors.

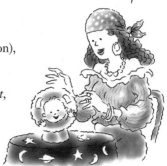

Nägele's rule can't predict the future, but it can provide a good estimation of when a baby will be born.

Baby on the way!

During the fetal stage of development, which extends from the 8th week until birth, the maturing fetus enlarges and grows heavier. (See *From embryo to fetus*, page 46.)

Two unusual features appear during this stage:

 The fetus's head is disproportionately large compared to its body. (This feature changes after birth as the infant grows.)

 The fetus lacks subcutaneous fat. (Fat starts to accumulate shortly before birth.)

Structural changes in the ovaries and uterus

During pregnancy, the reproductive system undergoes a number of changes.

Corpus luteum

Pregnancy changes the usual development of the corpus luteum and results in the development of the following structures:
- decidua
- amniotic sac and fluid
- yolk sac
- placenta.

Preembryonic development

The preembryonic phase lasts from conception until approximately the end of week 3 of development.

Zygote . . .

As the fertilised ovum advances through the fallopian tube towards the uterus, it undergoes mitotic division, forming daughter cells, initially called *blastomeres*, that each contains the same number of chromosomes as the parent cell. The first cell division ends about 30 hours after fertilisation; subsequent divisions occur rapidly.

The *zygote*, as it's now called, develops into a small mass of cells called a *morula*, which reaches the uterus at about day 3 after fertilisation. Fluid that amasses in the centre of the morula forms a central cavity.

. . . into blastocyst

The structure is now called a *blastocyst*. The blastocyst consists of a thin trophoblast layer, which includes the blastocyst cavity, and the inner cell mass. The trophoblast develops into fetal membranes and the placenta. The inner cell mass later forms the embryo (late blastocyst).

Getting attached: Blastocyst and endometrium

During the next phase, the blastocyst stays within the zona pellucida, unattached to the uterus. The zona pellucida degenerates and, by the end of week 1 after fertilisation, the blastocyst attaches to the endometrium. The part of the blastocyst adjacent to the inner cell mass is the first part to become attached.

The trophoblast, in contact with the endometrial lining, proliferates and invades the underlying endometrium by separating and dissolving endometrial cells.

Letting it all sink in

During the next week, the invading blastocyst sinks below the endometrium's surface. The penetration site seals, restoring the continuity of the endometrial surface.

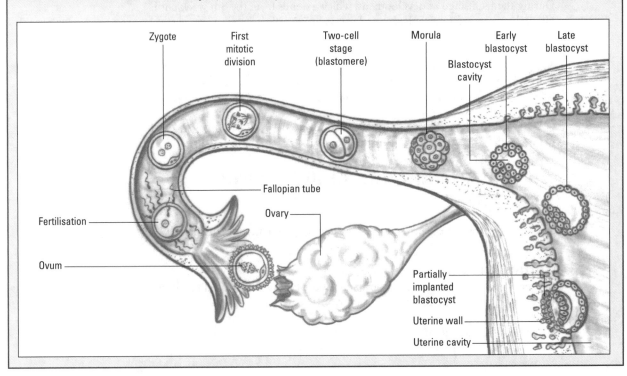

Embryonic development

Each of the three germ layers – ectoderm, mesoderm and endoderm – forms specific tissues and organs in the developing embryo.

Ectoderm

The ectoderm, the outermost layer, develops into the:

- epidermis
- nervous system
- pituitary gland
- tooth enamel
- salivary glands
- optic lens
- lining of lower portion of anal canal
- hair.

Mesoderm

The mesoderm, the middle layer, develops into:

- connective and supporting tissue
- the blood and vascular system
- musculature
- teeth (except enamel)
- the mesothelial lining of pericardial, pleural and peritoneal cavities
- the kidneys and ureters.

Endoderm

The endoderm, the innermost layer, becomes the epithelial lining of the:

- pharynx and trachea
- auditory canal
- alimentary canal
- liver
- pancreas
- bladder and urethra
- prostate.

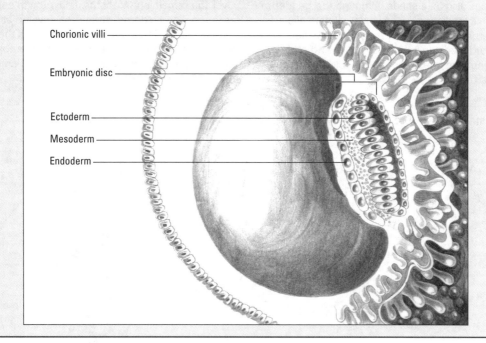

Chorionic villi
Embryonic disc
Ectoderm
Mesoderm
Endoderm

Normal functioning of the corpus luteum requires continuous stimulation by LH. Progesterone produced by the corpus luteum suppresses LH release by the pituitary gland. If pregnancy occurs, the corpus luteum continues to produce progesterone until the placenta takes over. Otherwise, the corpus luteum atrophies 3 days before menstrual flow begins.

From embryo to fetus

Significant growth and development take place within the first 3 months following conception, as the embryo develops into a fetus that nearly resembles a full-term infant.

Month 1

At the end of the first month, the embryo has a definite form. The head, the trunk and the tiny buds that will become the arms and the legs are discernible. The cardiovascular system has begun to function, and the umbilical cord is visible in its most primitive form.

Month 2

During the second month, the embryo – called a *fetus* from week 8 – grows to 1" (2.5 cm) and weighs 1 g (1/30 oz). The head and facial features develop as the eyes, ears, nose, lips, tongue and tooth buds form. The arms and legs also take shape. Although the gender of the fetus isn't yet discernible, all external genitalia are present. Cardiovascular function is complete, and the umbilical cord has a definite form. At the end of the second month, the fetus resembles a full-term infant except for size.

Month 3

During the third month, the fetus grows to 7.6 cm (3") and weighs 28.3 g (1 oz). Teeth and bones begin to appear, and the kidneys start to function. The fetus opens its mouth to swallow, grasps with its fully developed hands and prepares for breathing by inhaling and exhaling (although its lungs aren't functioning). At the end of the first *trimester* (the 3-month periods into which pregnancy is divided), its gender is distinguishable.

Months 3–9

Over the remaining 6 months, fetal growth continues as internal and external structures develop at a rapid rate. In the third trimester, the fetus stores the fats and minerals it will need to live outside the womb. At birth, the average full-term fetus measures 50.1 cm (20") and weighs 3–3.5 kg (7–7½ lb).

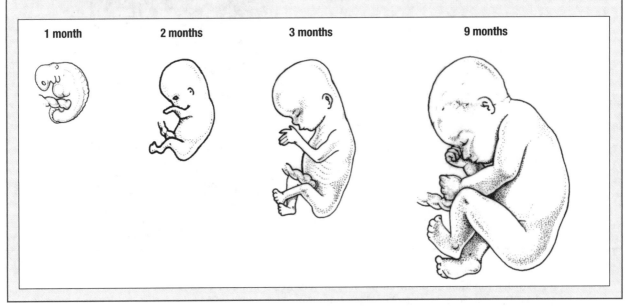

1 month   2 months   3 months   9 months

Hormone soup

With age, the corpus luteum grows less responsive to LH. Therefore, the mature corpus luteum degenerates unless stimulated by progressively increasing amounts of LH.

Pregnancy stimulates the placental tissue to secrete large amounts of human chorionic gonadotropin (HCG), which resembles LH and FSH. HCG prevents corpus luteum degeneration, stimulating the corpus luteum to produce large amounts of oestrogen and progesterone.

Ups and downs of HCG

The corpus luteum, stimulated by the hormone HCG, produces the oestrogen and the progesterone needed to maintain the pregnancy during the first 3 months. HCG can be detected as early as 9 days after fertilisation and can provide confirmation of pregnancy even before the woman has missed her first menses.

The HCG level gradually increases during this time, peaks at about 10 weeks of gestation and then gradually declines.

Decidua

The decidua is the endometrial lining of the uterus that undergoes hormone-induced changes during pregnancy. Decidual cells secrete the following three substances:
* the hormone *prolactin*, which promotes lactation
* a peptide hormone, *relaxin*, which induces relaxation of the connective tissue of the symphysis pubis and pelvic ligaments and promotes cervical dilation
* a potent hormonelike fatty acid, *prostaglandin*, which mediates several physiological functions. (See *Development of the decidua and fetal membranes*, page 48.)

Amniotic sac and fluid

The amniotic sac, enclosed within the chorion, gradually grows and surrounds the embryo. As it enlarges, the amniotic sac expands into the chorionic cavity, eventually filling the cavity and fusing with the chorion by the 8th week of gestation.

A warm, protective sea

The amniotic sac and amniotic fluid serve the fetus in two important ways, one during gestation and the other during delivery. During gestation, the fluid gives the fetus a buoyant, temperature-controlled environment. Later, amniotic fluid serves as a fluid wedge that helps to open the cervix during birth.

Some from mum, some from baby

Early in pregnancy, amniotic fluid comes chiefly from three sources:

    fluid filtering into the amniotic sac from maternal blood as it passes through the uterus

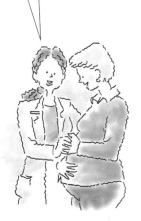

The fetus isn't the only changing feature during pregnancy – the mother's reproductive system undergoes changes as well.

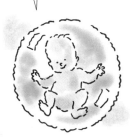

Amniotic fluid protects me during pregnancy – and later helps open the cervix for delivery.

Development of the decidua and fetal membranes

Specialised tissues support, protect and nurture the embryo and fetus throughout its development. Among these tissues, the decidua and fetal membranes begin to develop shortly after conception.

Decidua

During pregnancy, the endometrial lining is called the *decidua*. It provides a nesting place for the developing ovum and has some endocrine functions.

Based primarily on its position relative to the embryo, the decidua may be known as the *decidua basalis*, which lies beneath the chorionic vesicle; the *decidua capsularis*, which stretches over the vesicle; or the *decidua parietalis*, which lines the remainder of the endometrial cavity.

Fetal membranes

The *chorion* is a membrane that forms the outer wall of the blastocyst. Vascular projections, called *chorionic villi*, arise from its periphery. As the chorionic vesicle enlarges, villi arising from the superficial portion of the chorion, called the *chorion laeve*, atrophy, leaving this surface smooth. Villi arising from the deeper part of the chorion, called the *chorion frondosum*, proliferate, projecting into the large blood vessels within the decidua basalis through which the maternal blood flows.

Blood vessels that form within the growing villi become connected with blood vessels that form in the chorion, in the body stalk and within the body of the embryo. Blood begins to flow through this developing network of vessels as soon as the embryo's heart starts to beat.

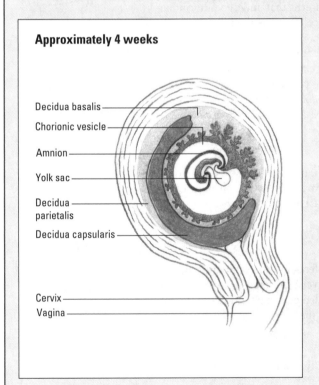

Approximately 4 weeks

Decidua basalis
Chorionic vesicle
Amnion
Yolk sac
Decidua parietalis
Decidua capsularis
Cervix
Vagina

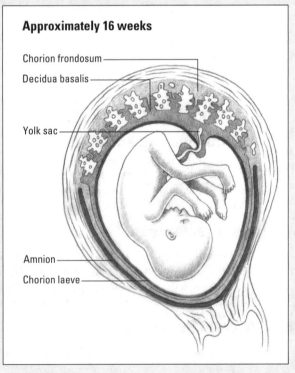

Approximately 16 weeks

Chorion frondosum
Decidua basalis
Yolk sac
Amnion
Chorion laeve

fluid filtering into the amniotic sac from fetal blood passing through the placenta

fluid diffusing into the amniotic sac from the fetal skin and respiratory tract.

Later in pregnancy, when the fetal kidneys begin to function, the fetus urinates into the amniotic fluid. Fetal urine then becomes the major source of amniotic fluid.

Production of amniotic fluid from maternal and fetal sources balances amniotic fluid that's lost through the fetal GI tract. Typically, the fetus swallows up to several hundred millilitres of amniotic fluid each day. The fluid is absorbed into the fetal circulation from the fetal GI tract; some is transferred from the fetal circulation to the maternal circulation and excreted in maternal urine.

Yolk sac

The yolk sac forms next to the endoderm of the germ disc; a portion of it is incorporated into the developing embryo and forms the GI tract. Another portion of the sac develops into primitive germ cells, which travel to the developing gonads and eventually form *oocytes* (the precursor of the ovum) or *spermatocytes* (the precursor of the spermatozoon) after gender has been determined.

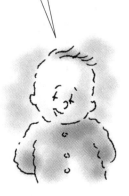

I've always had a good appetite – even as a fetus, when I slurped down lots of amniotic fluid each day! (Frankly, I prefer milk.)

Here today, gone tomorrow

During early embryonic development, the yolk sac also forms blood cells. Eventually, it undergoes atrophy and disintegrates.

Placenta

Using the umbilical cord as its conduit, the flattened, disc-shaped placenta provides nutrients to and removes wastes from the fetus from the third month of pregnancy until birth. The placenta is formed from the chorion, its chorionic villi and the adjacent decidua basalis.

A fetal lifeline

The umbilical cord contains two arteries and one vein and links the fetus to the placenta. The umbilical arteries, which transport blood from the fetus to the placenta, take a spiral course on the cord, divide on the placental surface and branch off to the chorionic villi. (See *Picturing the placenta*, page 50.)

In a helpful vein

The placenta is a highly vascular organ. Large veins on its surface gather blood returning from the villi and join to form the single umbilical vein, which enters the cord, returning blood to the fetus.

Specialists on the job

The placenta contains two highly specialised circulatory systems:
• The *uteroplacental* circulation carries oxygenated arterial blood from the maternal circulation to the intervillous spaces – large spaces separating

Picturing the placenta

At term, the placenta (the spongy structure within the uterus from which the fetus derives nourishment) is flat, cakelike and round or oval. It measures 15–19.5 cm (6–7¾) in diameter and 2–3 cm in breadth at its thickest part. The maternal side is lobulated; the fetal side is shiny.

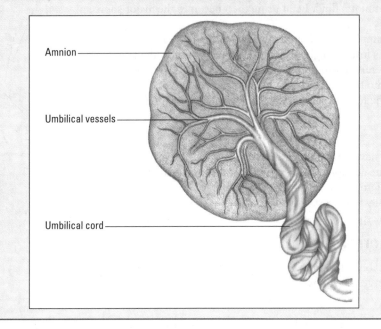

Amnion

Umbilical vessels

Umbilical cord

chorionic villi in the placenta. Blood enters the intervillous spaces from uterine arteries that penetrate the basal part of the placenta; it leaves the intervillous spaces and flows back into the maternal circulation through veins in the basal part of the placenta near the arteries.

• The *fetoplacental* circulation transports oxygen-depleted blood from the fetus to the chorionic villi by the umbilical arteries and returns oxygenated blood to the fetus through the umbilical vein.

Placenta takes charge

For the first 3 months of pregnancy, the corpus luteum is the main source of oestrogen and progesterone – hormones required during pregnancy. By the end of the third month, however, the placenta produces most of the hormones; the corpus luteum persists but is no longer needed to maintain the pregnancy.

Hormones on the rise

The levels of oestrogen and progesterone, two steroid hormones, increase progressively throughout pregnancy. Oestrogen stimulates uterine development to provide a suitable environment for the fetus.

The placenta has two circulation systems – one involving maternal blood and another transporting fetal blood.

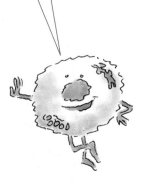

Progesterone, synthesised by the placenta from maternal cholesterol, reduces uterine muscle irritability and prevents spontaneous abortion of the fetus.

Keep those acids coming

The placenta also produces human placental lactogen (HPL), which resembles growth hormone. HPL stimulates maternal protein and fat metabolism to ensure a sufficient supply of amino acids and fatty acids for the mother and the fetus. HPL also stimulates breast growth in preparation for lactation. Throughout pregnancy, HPL levels rise progressively.

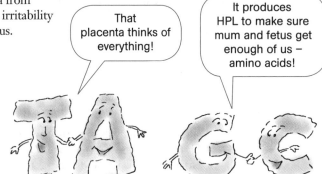

Quick quiz

1. Spermatogenesis is:
   A. the growth and development of sperm into primary spermatocytes.
   B. the division of spermatocytes to form secondary spermatocytes.
   C. the structural changing of spermatids.
   D. the entire process of sperm formation.

Answer: D. Spermatogenesis refers to the entire process of sperm formation – from the development of primary spermatocytes to the formation of fully functional spermatozoa.

2. The primary function of the scrotum is to:
   A. provide storage for newly developed sperm.
   B. maintain a cool temperature for the testes.
   C. deposit sperm in the female reproductive tract.
   D. provide a place for spermatogenesis to take place.

Answer: B. The function of the scrotum is to maintain a cool temperature for the testes, which is necessary for spermatozoa formation.

3. The main function of the ovaries is to:
   A. secrete hormones that affect the build-up and shedding of the endometrium during the menstrual cycle.
   B. accommodate a growing fetus during pregnancy.
   C. produce mature ova.
   D. channel blood discharged from the uterus during menstruation.

Answer: C. The main function of the ovaries is to produce mature ova.

4. The corpus luteum degenerates in which phase of the female reproductive cycle?
 A. Luteal
 B. Follicular
 C. Proliferative
 D. Ovarian

Answer: A. The corpus luteum degenerates in the luteal phase of the ovarian cycle of reproduction.

5. The four hormones involved in the menstrual cycle are:
 A. LH, progesterone, oestrogen and testosterone.
 B. oestrogen, FSH, LH and androgens.
 C. oestrogen, progesterone, LH and FSH.
 D. LH, oestrogen, testosterone and androgens.

Answer: C. The four hormones involved in the menstrual cycle are oestrogen, progesterone, LH and FSH.

6. Each of the three germ layers forms specific tissues and organs in the developing:
 A. zygote.
 B. ovum.
 C. embryo.
 D. fetus.

Answer: C. Each of the three germ layers (ectoderm, mesoderm and endoderm) forms specific tissues and organs in the developing embryo.

7. The structure that guards the fetus is the:
 A. decidua.
 B. amniotic sac.
 C. corpus luteum.
 D. yolk sac.

Answer: B. The structure that guards the fetus by producing a buoyant, temperature-controlled environment is the amniotic sac.

Scoring

☆☆☆ If you answered all seven questions correctly, fantastic! You're fertilisation-friendly!

☆☆ If you answered five or six questions correctly, excellent! Now reproduce that success in the chapters ahead!

☆ If you answered fewer than five questions correctly, don't fear! Your concept of conception will improve after a little review.

③ Family planning, contraception and infertility

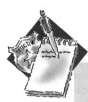

Just the facts

In this chapter, you'll learn:

♦ goals of family planning

♦ various methods of contraception, including the advantages and disadvantages of each

♦ surgical methods of family planning

♦ issues related to elective termination of pregnancy

♦ causes of infertility

♦ treatments and procedures used to correct infertility.

A look at family planning

Family planning involves the decisions couples or individuals make regarding when (and if) they should have children, how many children to have and how long to wait between pregnancies. Family planning also consists of choices to prevent or achieve pregnancy and to control the timing and number of pregnancies. Family planning is a personal topic that has many ethical, physical, emotional, religious and legal implications. Effectiveness, cost, contraindications and adverse effects for all contraceptives should be presented to the woman and her partner so that they can make an informed decision.

More information about contraception and where it's available can be obtained from the Brook Centre at admin@brookcentres.org.uk or the Family Planning Association at www.fpa.org.uk

> Information is power. Keep couples informed so they can make the family planning decisions that are best for them.

A look at contraception

Contraception is the deliberate prevention of conception, using a method or device to avert fertilisation of an ovum.

Choosing a contraceptive

When discussing with a client the contraceptive methods that are most appropriate for her and her partner, remember that a contraceptive should be safe, easily obtained, free from adverse effects, affordable, acceptable to the user and her partner and free from effects on future pregnancies. In addition, couples should use a contraceptive that's as close as possible to being 100% effective.

History lesson

Information from the client's menstrual and obstetric history should be used to determine which contraceptive method is best for her. The client's history is also used to plan appropriate client teaching.

An assessment for family planning involves collecting a reproductive history, including:
- interval between menses
- duration and amount of flow
- problems that occur during menses
- number of previous pregnancies
- number of previous births (and date of each)
- duration of each pregnancy
- type of each delivery
- gender and weight of children when delivered
- problems during previous pregnancies
- problems after delivery.

Identify potential complications

The woman's health history may also identify potential risks of complications and help to determine whether hormonal contraceptives are safe for her to use. For example, a breastfeeding mother may be prescribed the progesterone only pill, which may cause her milk supply to decrease.

Factor in the partner

In some cases, the health of the client's sexual partner influences which contraception method is used. For example, if the client's sexual partner is infected with human immunodeficiency virus (HIV), ideally, she should practise abstinence. If this isn't an option for your client, encourage her to use a condom to prevent conception as well as infection transmission.

Implementing the chosen contraceptive

The effectiveness and safety of any contraceptive depends greatly on the client's knowledge of and compliance with the chosen method. The client's inability to

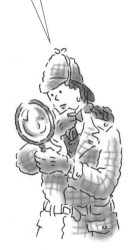

It's elementary, my dear Watson! A client's health history will provide clues about which contraceptive method is best for her.

Education edge

Teaching tips on contraception

Here are some points you should cover when teaching a client about contraception:

- Teach proper use of the selected contraceptive, and describe the procedure for the chosen method accurately.
- Discuss possible adverse reactions. Direct the client to report adverse reactions to her health care provider.
- Stress the importance of keeping follow-up appointments. During follow-up visits, contraceptive use and adverse reactions are evaluated and a repeat Papanicolaou test (Pap test or smear) is performed. Follow-up visits also provide an opportunity to address any questions the client may have.
- Answer all questions in a manner that's easily understood by the client.

understand proper use of the contraceptive device or an unwillingness to use it correctly or consistently may result in pregnancy. That's why teaching is such an important component of family planning. (See *Teaching tips on contraception*.)

With proper instruction and information, the client should be able to:
- describe the use of the selected contraceptive correctly
- describe adverse reactions to the selected contraceptive and state her responsibility to report any that occur
- state that she'll make an appointment for her next visit (if indicated)
- express that the current method of birth control is an acceptable method for her.

> Where are those instructions? Having the right information and instructions is key to the proper use of contraceptives – and to fixing this bike!

Methods of contraception

Contraceptive methods include abstinence, natural family planning methods, oral contraceptives, the morning-after pill (MAP), the intravaginal method, transdermal contraceptive patches, I.M. injections, intrauterine contraceptive devices and mechanical and chemical barrier methods.

Abstinence

Abstinence, or refraining from having sexual intercourse, has a 0% failure rate. It's also the most effective way to prevent the transmission of sexually transmitted diseases (STDs). However, most individuals – especially adolescents – don't consider it an option or a form of contraception. Abstinence should always be presented as an option to the client in addition to information about other forms of contraception.

The plus side

Here are the advantages of abstinence:
- It's the only method that's 100% effective against pregnancy and sexually transmitted infections (STIs).

- It's free.
- There are no contraindications.

The minus side

Here are the disadvantages of abstinence:
- Partners and peers may have negative reactions to it.
- It requires commitment and self-control from both partners.

Natural family planning methods

Natural family planning methods are contraceptive methods that don't use chemicals or foreign material or devices to prevent pregnancy. Religious beliefs may prevent some individuals from using hormonal or internal contraceptive devices. Others just prefer a more natural method of planning or preventing pregnancy. Natural family planning methods include the rhythm (calendar) method, basal body temperature (BBT) method, cervical mucus (Billings) method, symptothermal method, ovulation awareness and coitus interruptus.

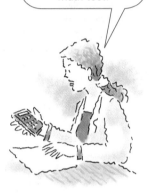

Calculate the woman's fertile days? Nobody told me there would be a math test!

Keeping count

For most natural family planning methods, the woman's fertile days must be calculated so that she can abstain from intercourse on those days. Various methods are used to determine the woman's fertile period. The effectiveness of these methods depends on the couples' willingness to refrain from sex on the female partner's fertile days. Failure rates vary from 10% to 20%.

Rhythm method

The rhythm, or calendar, method requires that the couple refrain from intercourse on the days that the woman is most likely to conceive based on her menstrual cycle. This fertile period usually lasts from 3 or 4 days before until 3 or 4 days after ovulation.

Dear diary

Teach the woman to keep a diary of her menstrual cycle to determine when ovulation is most likely to occur. She should do this for six consecutive cycles. To calculate her safe periods, tell her to subtract 18 from the shortest cycle and 11 from the longest cycle that she has documented. For instance, if she had six menstrual cycles that lasted 26–30 days, her fertile period would be from the 8th day (26 minus 18) to the 19th day (30 minus 11). To ensure that pregnancy doesn't occur, she and her partner should abstain from intercourse during days 8 to 19 of her menstrual cycle. During those fertile days, she and her partner may also choose to use contraceptive foam. (See *Using the calendar method*, page 57.)

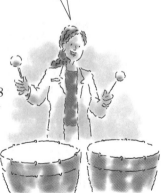

I've got rhythm, I've got music . . . but that won't necessarily keep me from getting pregnant. The rhythm method requires meticulous record keeping and the ability to monitor body changes.

The plus side

Here are the advantages of the rhythm method:
- No drugs or devices are needed.
- It's free.

Using the calendar method

This illustration demonstrates how the calendar method would be used to determine the woman's fertile period (ovulation) and when she should abstain from coitus.

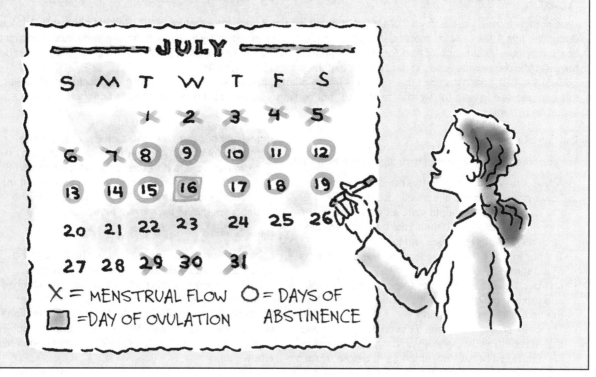

- It may be acceptable to members of religious groups that oppose birth control.
- It encourages couples to learn more about how the female body functions.
- It encourages communication between partners.
- It can also be used to plan a pregnancy.

The minus side

Here are the disadvantages of the rhythm method:
- It requires meticulous record keeping as well as an ability and willingness for the woman to monitor her body changes.
- It restricts sexual spontaneity during the woman's fertile period.
- It requires extended periods of abstinence from intercourse.
- It's only reliable for women with regular menstrual cycles.
- It may be unreliable during periods of illness, infection or stress.

Education edge

Teaching a client how to take BBT

Here are tips to help you teach your client about recording basal body temperature (BBT). Remind her that BBT is lower during the first 2 weeks of the menstrual cycle, before ovulation. Immediately after ovulation, the temperature begins to rise. It continues to rise until it's time for the next menses. This rise in temperature indicates that progesterone has been released into the system, which, in turn, means that the woman has ovulated.

Charting BBT doesn't predict the exact day of ovulation; it just indicates that ovulation has occurred. However, this can be used to help the woman to monitor her ovulatory pattern and give her a time frame during which ovulation occurs.

Getting started

Tell your client to follow these instructions for taking BBT:

- Advise the woman to chart the days of menstrual flow by darkening the squares above the 98°F (36.7°C) mark. She should start with the first day of her menses (day 1) and then take her temperature each day after her menses ends.
- Tell her to use a thermometer that measures tenths of a degree.
- Instruct the client to take her temperature as soon as she wakes up. Tell her that it's important to do this at the same time each morning.
- The client should then place a dot on the graph's line that matches the temperature reading. (Tell her not to be surprised if her waking temperature before ovulation is 35.6 or 36.1°C.) If she forgets to take her temperature on one day, instruct her to leave that day blank on the graph and not to connect the dots.

- Instruct her to make notes on the graph if she misses taking her temperature, feels sick, can't sleep or wakes up at a different time. Advise her also that if she's taking any medicine – even aspirin – it may affect her temperature. Remind her to mark the dates when she has sexual intercourse.

Sample chart

Look over the sample temperature chart, recorded by 'Susan Jones'. Ms Jones used an S to record sexual intercourse and made notes showing she had insomnia on September 27. She forgot to take her temperature on September 19. Notice that she didn't connect the dots on this day. Her temperature dipped on September 24 (day 15 of the cycle) and began rising afterwards.

Of course, your client's chart will be larger and will probably include temperatures over 37.4°C and under 36.1°C

Basal body temperature

Just before the day of ovulation, a woman's BBT falls about one-half of a degree. At the time of ovulation, her BBT rises a full degree because of progesterone influence.

Ups and downs, highs and lows

To use the BBT method of contraception, a woman must take her temperature every morning before sitting up, getting out of bed or beginning her morning activity. (See *Teaching a client how to take BBT.*) By recording this daily temperature, she can see a slight dip and then an increase in body temperature. The increase in temperature indicates that she has ovulated. She should refrain from intercourse for the next 3 days. Three days is significant because this is

Sample temperature chart

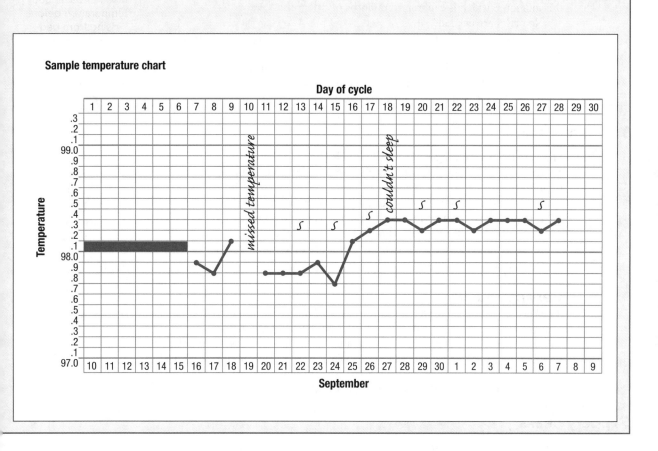

the lifespan of a discharged ovum. Because sperm can survive in the female reproductive tract for 4 days, the BBT method of contraception is typically combined with the calendar method so that the couple can abstain from intercourse a few days before ovulation as well.

Various variables

One problem with this method is that many things can affect BBT. The woman may forget and take her temperature after rising out of bed or she may have a slight illness. These situations cause a rise in temperature. If the woman changes her daily routine, the change in activity could also affect her body temperature, which may lead her to mistakenly interpret a fertile day as a safe day and vice versa.

The plus side

Here are the advantages of the BBT method:
• It's inexpensive. The only expense involved is the cost of a BBT thermometer, which is calibrated in tenths of a degree.
• No drugs are needed.
• It may be acceptable to members of religious groups that oppose birth control.
• It encourages couples to learn more about how the female body functions.
• It encourages communication between partners.
• It can also be used to plan a pregnancy.

The minus side

Here are the disadvantages of the BBT method:
• It requires meticulous record keeping and an ability and willingness to monitor the woman's body changes.
• It restricts sexual spontaneity during the woman's fertile period.
• It requires extended periods of abstinence from intercourse.
• It's reliable only for women with regular menstrual cycles.
• It may be unreliable during periods of illness, infection or stress.
• It's contraindicated in women who have irregular menses.

Cervical mucus

The cervical mucus method (also known as the *Billings method*) predicts changes in the cervical mucus during ovulation. Each month, before a woman's menses, the cervical mucus becomes thick and stretches when pulled between the thumb and forefinger. The normal stretchable amount of cervical mucus (also known as *spinnbarkeit*) is 8–10 cm. Just before ovulation, the cervical mucus becomes thin, watery, transparent and copious.

Slippery peaks

During the peak of ovulation, the cervical mucus becomes slippery and stretches at least 2.5 cm before the strand breaks. Breast tenderness and anterior tilt of the cervix also occur with ovulation. The fertile period consists of all the days that the cervical mucus is copious and the 3 days after the peak date. During these days, the woman and her partner should abstain from intercourse to avoid conception.

Consistently checking consistency

Cervical mucus must be assessed every day for changes in consistency and amounts to be sure that those changes signify ovulation. Assessing cervical mucus after intercourse is unreliable because seminal fluid has a watery, postovulatory consistency, which can be confused with ovulatory mucus.

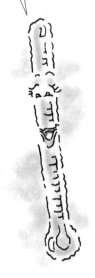

To get an accurate reading, a woman should take her basal body temperature before rising from bed.

The plus side

Here are the advantages of the cervical mucus method:
- No drugs or devices are needed.
- It's free.
- It may be acceptable to members of religious groups that oppose birth control.
- It encourages couples to learn more about how the female body functions.
- It encourages communication between partners.
- It can also be used to plan a pregnancy.
- There are no contraindications.

The minus side

Here are the disadvantages of the cervical mucus method:
- It requires meticulous record keeping and an ability and willingness to monitor the woman's body changes.
- It restricts sexual spontaneity during the woman's fertile period.
- It requires extended periods of abstinence from intercourse.
- It's reliable only for women with regular menstrual cycles.
- It may be unreliable during periods of illness, infection or stress.

Symptothermal method

The symptothermal method combines the BBT method with the cervical mucus method. The woman takes her daily temperature and watches for the rise in temperature that signals the onset of ovulation. She also assesses her cervical mucus every day. The couple abstains from intercourse until 3 days after the rise in basal temperature or the fourth day after the peak day (indicating ovulation) of cervical mucus because these signs signify the woman's fertile period. Combining these two methods is more effective than using either method alone.

The plus side

Here are the advantages of the symptothermal method:
- It's inexpensive. The only expense involved is the cost of a BBT thermometer, which is calibrated in tenths of a degree.
- No drugs are needed.
- It may be acceptable to members of religious groups that oppose birth control.
- It encourages women and their partners to learn more about how the female body functions.
- It encourages communication between partners.
- It can also be used to plan a pregnancy.

The minus side

Here are the disadvantages of the symptothermal method:
- It requires meticulous record keeping and ability and willingness of a woman to monitor body changes.

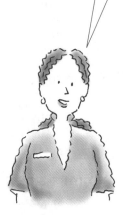

Combining the BBT and cervical mucus methods is more effective than using just one method.

- It restricts sexual spontaneity during the woman's fertile period.
- It requires extended periods of abstinence from intercourse.
- It's reliable only for women with regular menstrual cycles.
- It may be unreliable during periods of illness, infection or stress.

Coitus interruptus

Coitus interruptus, one of the oldest known methods of contraception, involves withdrawal of the penis from the vagina during intercourse before ejaculation. However, because preejaculation fluid that's deposited outside the vagina may contain spermatozoa, fertilisation can occur.

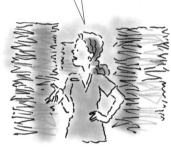

Phew! The symptothermal method certainly requires meticulous record keeping!

The plus side

Here are the advantages of the coitus interruptus method:
- It's free.
- It doesn't involve record keeping.
- There are no contraindications.

The minus side

Here are the disadvantages of the coitus interruptus method:
- It isn't reliable.
- It restricts sexual spontaneity.

Oral contraceptives

Oral contraceptives (birth control pills) are hormonal contraceptives that consist of synthetic oestrogen and progesterone. The oestrogen suppresses production of follicle-stimulating hormone (FSH) and LH, which, in turn, suppresses ovulation. The progesterone complements the oestrogen's action by causing a decrease in cervical mucus permeability, which limits sperm's access to the ova. Progesterone also decreases the possibility of implantation by interfering with endometrial proliferation.

Double dosage

There are three types of oral contraceptives:

Monophasic oral contraceptives provide fixed doses of oestrogen and progesterone throughout a 21-day cycle. These preparations provide a steady dose of oestrogen but an increased amount of progestin during the last 11 days of the menstrual cycle.

Triphasic oral contraceptives maintain a cycle more like a woman's natural menstrual cycle because they vary the amount of oestrogen and progestin throughout the cycle. Triphasic oral contraceptives have a lower incidence of breakthrough bleeding than monophasic oral contraceptives. These are more widely prescribed in Australia.

Education edge

Performing a home ovulation test

A home ovulation test helps the woman determine the best time to try to become pregnant or to prevent pregnancy by monitoring the amount of luteinising hormone (LH) that's found in her urine. These test kits can be purchased over the counter.

Normally, during each menstrual cycle, levels of LH rise suddenly, causing an egg to be released from the ovary 24–36 hours later.

Getting ready

Tell your client to follow these instructions before performing a home ovulation test:

- Read the kit's directions thoroughly before performing the test.
- Before testing, calculate the length of the menstrual cycle. Count from the beginning of one menses to the beginning of the next menses. (The woman should count her first day of bleeding as day 1. She can use a chart such as the one shown at right to determine when to begin testing.)
- This test can be performed any time of the day or night, but it should be performed at the same time every day.
- Don't urinate for at least 4 hours before taking the test, and don't drink a lot of fluids for several hours before the test.

Taking the test

Tell your client to follow these instructions for performing a home ovulation test:

- Remove the test stick from the packet.
- Sit on the toilet and direct the absorbent tip of the test stick downward and directly into the urine stream for at least 5 seconds or until it's thoroughly wet.
- Be careful not to urinate on the window of the stick.
- Alternatively, urinate in a clean, dry cup or container and then dip the test stick (absorbent tip only) into the urine for at least 5 seconds.
- Place the stick on a clean, flat, dry surface.

Reading the results

Explain to your client the following instructions for reading home ovulation test results:

- Wait at least 5 minutes before reading the results. When the test is finished, a line appears in the small window (control window).
- If there's no line in the large rectangular window (test window) or if the line is lighter than the line in the small rectangular window (control window), the client hasn't

begun an LH surge. She should continue testing daily.

- If she sees one line in the large rectangular window that's similar to or darker than the line in the small window, she's experiencing an LH surge. This means that ovulation should occur within the next 24–36 hours.
- Once the woman has determined that she's about to ovulate, she'll know she's at the start of the most fertile time of her cycle and should use this information to plan accordingly.

Length of cycle	Start test this many days after last menses begins	Length of cycle	Start test this many days after last menses begins
21	5	31	14
22	5	32	15
23	6	33	16
24	7	34	17
25	8	34	18
26	9	36	19
27	10	37	20
28	11	38	21
29	12	39	22
30	13	40	23

Small but powerful

A mini pill (progesterone only) is available for women who can't take oestrogen-based pills because of a history of thrombophlebitis. This type of pill is taken every day – even when the woman has her menses. Progestins in the pill inhibit the development of the endometrium, thus preventing implantation.

21- or 28-day package deals

Monophasic and triphasic oral contraceptives are dispensed in either 21- or 28-day packs. The first pill is usually taken, for example, on the first Sunday or Monday following the start of a woman's menses, but it's possible to start oral contraceptives on any day. For a woman who has recently given birth, oral contraceptives can be started on the first Sunday or Monday 2 weeks after delivery. Clients should be advised to use an additional form of contraception for the first week after starting an oral contraceptive because the drug doesn't take effect for 7 days. (See *Teaching tips on oral contraceptives*.)

Birth control pills that are prescribed in a 21-day dispenser allow the woman to take a pill every day for 3 weeks. She should expect to start her menstrual flow about 4 days after she takes a cycle of pills. The 28-day pills are packaged with 21 days of birth control pills and 7 days of placebos. The woman starts the new pack of pills when she finishes the last pack, eliminating the risk of forgetting to start a new pack.

> What a team! The oestrogen in oral contraceptives suppresses ovulation and the progesterone decreases the permeability of cervical mucus.

The plus side

Here are the advantages of oral contraceptives:
• Monophasic and triphasic oral contraceptives are 99.5% effective. The failure rate is about 3%; failure usually occurs because the woman

Education edge
Teaching tips on oral contraceptives

Be sure to include these tips when teaching clients about oral contraceptives:

• Inform the client about possible adverse reactions, such as fluid retention, weight gain, breast tenderness, headache, breakthrough bleeding, chloasma, acne, yeast infection, nausea and fatigue. It may be necessary to change the type or dosage of the contraceptive to relieve these adverse reactions.
• Instruct the client on the dietary needs of a woman who's taking an oral contraceptive. Tell her to increase her intake of foods high in vitamin B_6 (wheat, corn, liver, meat) and folic acid (liver; green, leafy vegetables). About 20–30% of oral contraceptive users have dietary deficiencies of vitamin B_6 and folic acid. Moreover, health care professionals speculate that oral contraceptive users should also increase their intake of vitamins A, B_2, B_{12}, C and niacin.
• Advise the client to use an additional form of contraception for the first 7 days after starting the drug because it doesn't take effect for 7 days.
• Advise the client to use an additional form of contraception when taking antibiotics.

forgets to take the pill or because of other individual differences in the woman's physiology.

• They don't inhibit sexual spontaneity.

• They may reduce the risk of endometrial and ovarian cancer, ectopic pregnancy, ovarian cysts and noncancerous breast tumours.

• They decrease the risk of pelvic inflammatory disease (PID) and dysmenorrhoea.

• They regulate the menstrual cycle and may diminish or eliminate premenstrual tension.

• They are free on the NHS.

The minus side

Here are the disadvantages of oral contraceptives:

• They don't protect the woman or her partner from STIs.

• They must be taken daily.

• Illnesses that cause vomiting may reduce their effectiveness.

• Some antibiotics reduce their effectiveness.

• Contraindicated in women who have a family history of stroke, coronary artery disease, thromboembolic disease or liver disease; and those who have undiagnosed vaginal bleeding, malignancy of the reproductive system, malignant cell growth or hypertension.

• Women who are older than age 40, and those who have a history of or have been diagnosed with diabetes mellitus, elevated triglyceride or cholesterol level, breast or reproductive tract malignancy, high blood pressure, obesity, seizure disorder, sickle cell disease, mental depression and migraines or other vascular-type headaches, should be strongly cautioned about taking oral contraceptives for birth control. The possible side effects of oral contraceptives may be more severe in women who fall under these categories.

• A woman older than age 35 is at increased risk for a fatal heart attack if she smokes more than 15 cigarettes per day and takes oral contraceptives.

• Adverse effects include nausea, headache, weight gain, depression, mild hypertension, breast tenderness, breakthrough bleeding and monilial vaginal infections.

• When a woman wants to conceive, she may not be able to for up to 8 months after stopping oral contraceptives. The pituitary gland requires a recovery period to begin the stimulation of cyclic gonadotropins, such as FSH and LH, which help regulate ovulation. In addition, many practitioners recommend that women not become pregnant within 2 months of stopping oral contraceptives.

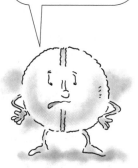

Oral contraceptives can help to regulate the menstrual cycle and decrease premenstrual symptoms. However, they need to be taken daily and they don't protect against STDs.

Morning-after pill

Also called *emergency contraception*, the MAP prevents pregnancy in the event of unprotected sexual intercourse or failure of a birth control method (such as a broken condom). It may be obtained from general practitioners (GPs), family planning clinics and genitourinary medicine

(GUM) clinics/walk-in centres. It can also be bought from chemists without prescription for about £20. The MAP is a pregnancy prevention measure, not an abortion pill.

The MAP is given as two doses of hormones: progesterone alone, oestrogen alone or a combination of both. The first dose must be taken within 72 hours of sexual intercourse; a second dose is taken 12 hours later. A woman may be prescribed a certain number of oral hormonal contraceptive pills from a birth control pack (oestrogen and progesterone combination) or she may be prescribed a 'plan B' pack, which contains 0.75 mg of levonorgestrel.

Medications for nausea may also be prescribed, and the woman is instructed to return to the office or clinic in 3 weeks. She must also be instructed to use a birth control method consistently until her menstrual period begins.

The plus side

Here are the advantages of the MAP:
• It's 75–95% effective, depending on which product is used, when in the cycle intercourse occurred, how soon the woman uses the method and whether she has had unprotected intercourse within the past 72 hours.
• It doesn't inhibit sexual spontaneity.
• It's readily available when unforeseen circumstances occur.

The minus side

Here are the disadvantages of the MAP:
• It doesn't offer protection from STDs.
• It must be taken within a 72-hour period after intercourse, and again 12 hours later.
• The hormone dosage is larger than that of oral hormonal contraceptives and commonly causes nausea, vomiting and malaise.
• It can be expensive.
• Contraindications and precautions are similar to those for other oral hormonal contraceptives.

Intravaginal method

Another method of introducing hormones into the woman's circulation is the intravaginal route by a cervical ring that slowly releases contraceptive hormones. Called the NuvaRing, the woman inserts it into her vagina, where it stays held in by the vaginal walls, for 3 weeks. She then removes it, allowing her menstruation to occur, and then reinserts it after 1 week.

The plus side

Here are the advantages of the intravaginal method:
• It's inserted only every 3 weeks.
• The woman doesn't have to remember to take a pill every day.
• The woman has fewer hormonal peaks and decreases because of the slow but steady release.

- It's 99% effective.
- It allows sexual spontaneity.
- It's discreet.
- It's easy to insert.

The minus side

Here are the disadvantages of the intravaginal method:
- It doesn't protect the woman or her partner from STIs.
- It's contraindicated in women who are pregnant or may become pregnant; those who are breastfeeding; those who have a family history of stroke, coronary artery disease, thrombohaemolytic disease or liver disease; those who have undiagnosed vaginal bleeding and those who are sensitive to the material in the ring.
- Women who are over age 40; women who have a history of or have been diagnosed with diabetes mellitus, elevated triglycerides or cholesterol level, breast or reproductive tact malignancy, high blood pressure, obesity, seizure disorder, sickle cell disease, mental depression and migraines or other vascular-type headaches and women who smoke should be strongly cautioned about using a hormonal contraceptive ring. The possible side effects of hormonal contraceptives may be greater in women with a history of these disorders.

The NuvaRing is still not licensed for use in the UK but is undergoing trials at present.

Transdermal contraceptive patches

The transdermal contraceptive patch is a highly effective, weekly hormonal birth control patch that's worn on the skin. A combination of oestrogen and progestin is integrated into the patch. The hormones are absorbed into the skin and then transferred into the bloodstream.

Patchwork

The patch is very thin, beige and smooth, and measures 4.4 cm^2. It can be worn on the upper outer arm, buttocks, abdomen or upper torso. The patch is worn for 1 week and replaced on the same day of the week for 3 consecutive weeks. No patch is worn during the fourth week. Studies have shown that the patch remains attached and effective when the client bathes, swims, exercises or wears it in humid weather.

What a trooper! The transdermal contraceptive patch remains attached to the skin, even when the woman bathes, swims or exercises.

The plus side

Here are the advantages of the transdermal contraceptive patch:
- It's 99% effective in preventing pregnancy if used exactly as directed.
- It's convenient. No preparation is needed before intercourse.
- It's a good alternative for clients who commonly forget to take oral contraceptives.

The minus side

Here are the disadvantages of the transdermal patch:
• It doesn't protect the woman or her partner from STDs.
• It's contraindicated in women who are breastfeeding; those who have a family history of stroke, coronary artery disease, thrombohaemolytic disease or liver disease; those who have undiagnosed vaginal bleeding and those who are sensitive to the adhesive used on the patch.
• Women who are over age 40; women who have a history of or have been diagnosed with diabetes mellitus, elevated triglycerides or cholesterol level, breast or reproductive tract malignancy, high blood pressure, obesity, seizure disorder, sickle cell disease, mental depression and migraines or other vascular-type headaches and women who smoke should be strongly cautioned about using a transdermal contraceptive patch for birth control. The possible side effects of hormonal contraceptives may be more severe in women who fall under these categories.
• It has been found to be slightly less effective in women who weigh more than 89.8 kg. These women may need to consider another form of contraception.
• Some antibiotics reduce its effectiveness.

I.M. injections

I.M. injections of medroxyprogesterone (Depo-Provera) are administered every 12 weeks. Depo-Provera stops ovulation from occurring by suppressing the release of gonadotropic hormones. It also changes the cervical mucosa to prevent sperm from entering the uterus.

The plus side

Here are the advantages of I.M. Depo-Provera:
• It doesn't inhibit sexual response.
• Except for abstinence, it's more effective than other birth control methods.
• It helps prevent endometrial cancer.
• Its free on the NHS.

The minus side

Here are the disadvantages of I.M. Depo-Provera:
• It requires an injection every 12 weeks.
• If the woman wants to become pregnant, it may take 9–24 months after the last injection to conceive.
• It doesn't protect against STIs.
• Its effects can't be reversed after it's injected.
• It may cause changes in the menstrual cycle.
• It may cause weight gain because of an increase in appetite.
• It may cause headache, fatigue and nervousness.

- It's contraindicated if the woman is pregnant or has liver disease, undiagnosed vaginal bleeding, breast cancer, blood clotting disorders or cardiovascular disease.
- It is discouraged in young women in some regions of the UK due to the increased risk of brittle bone disease.

Intrauterine contraceptive device

The intrauterine contraceptive device (IUCD) is a plastic contraceptive device that's inserted into the uterus through the cervical canal. (See *IUCD insertion*, page 70.) The IUCD is inserted into and removed from the uterus most easily during the woman's menses, when the cervical canal is slightly dilated. Inserting the device during menses also reduces the likelihood of inserting an IUCD into a woman who's pregnant.

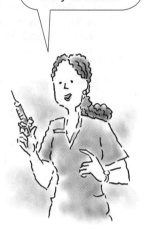

Depo-Provera is highly effective, but it does require a bit of an "Ouch!" every 12 weeks.

Copper interference

One type of IUCD, the Flexi-T 300, is a T-shaped, polyethylene device with copper wrapped around its vertical stem. The copper interferes with sperm mobility, decreasing the possibility of sperm crossing the uterine space. A knotted monofilament retrieval string is attached through a hole in the stem.

Progesterone reserve

Another type of IUCD, the Progestasert IUCD system, is a T-shaped device made of an ethylene vinyl acetate copolymer with a knotted monofilament retrieval string attached through a hole in the vertical stem. Progesterone is stored in the hollow vertical stem, suspended in an oil base. The drug gradually diffuses into the uterus and prevents endometrium proliferation. This IUCD must be replaced annually to replenish the progesterone. The Progestasert system may relieve excessive menstrual blood loss and dysmenorrhoea.

If a woman becomes pregnant with an IUCD in place, the device can be left; however, it's usually removed to prevent spontaneous abortion and infection.

The plus side

Here are the advantages of an IUCD:
- It doesn't inhibit sexual spontaneity.
- Neither partner feels the device during intercourse.
- It's free on the NHS.

The minus side

Here are the disadvantages of an IUCD:
- It may cause uterine cramping on insertion.
- It may cause infection, especially in the initial weeks after insertion.
- It can be spontaneously expelled in the first year by 5–20% of women.

IUCD insertion

An intrauterine contraceptive device (IUCD) is a plastic contraceptive device that's inserted into a woman's uterus through the cervical canal. This is performed most easily during menses. A bimanual examination is performed to determine uterine position, shape and size.

Before IUCD insertion, make sure that the procedure has been explained to the client and that her questions have been addressed. Also, be sure to obtain informed consent.

How it's done

Here's how the device is inserted.

1 The movable flange on the inserter barrel of the IUCD is set to the depth of the uterus (measured in centimetres). The loaded inserter tube is introduced through the cervical canal and into the uterus.

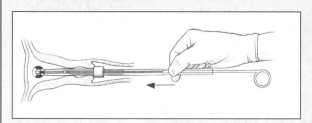

3 The plunger is gently advanced until resistance is felt. This action ensures high fundal placement of the IUCD and may reduce the potential for expulsion.

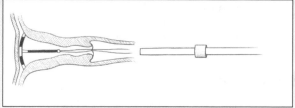

2 The IUCD is inserted by retracting the inserter slowly about 1.3 cm over the plunger while the plunger is held still. This allows the arms to open.

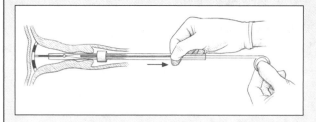

4 The solid rod is withdrawn while the inserting barrel is held stationary. The insertion barrel is then withdrawn from the cervix. The strings are clipped about 2.5–7.5 cm from the cervical os. This action leaves sufficient string for checking the placement of and removing the IUCD.

- It doesn't protect against STIs.
- The incidence of PID increases with IUCD use. Most cases of PID occur during the first 3 months after insertion. After 3 months, the risk of PID is lower unless preinsertion screening failed to identify a person at risk for STIs. The woman should be instructed to watch for signs of PID. (See *Signs of PID*, page 71.)
- It increases the risk of ectopic pregnancy.

- It's contraindicated in women who have Wilson's disease (because of the inability to metabolise copper properly).
- It's contraindicated in women who have active, recent or recurrent PID; infection or inflammation of the genital tract; STIs; diseases that suppress immune function, including HIV; unexplained cervical or vaginal bleeding; previous problems with IUCDs; cancer of the reproductive organs or a history of ectopic pregnancy. Insertion is also contraindicated in women who have severe vasovagal reactivity, difficulty obtaining emergency care, valvular heart disease, anatomic uterine deformities, anaemia or nulliparity.

Commonly used IUCD devices are Flext-T®, Gynefix®, Nova-T® 380, TT380®, UT380®, Multiload CU375®, amongst others.

Intrauterine systems

IUCD devices like the Mirena IUS are very effective, not only as a method of contraceptive but also, because it releases progesterone, in making periods less heavy or painful.

Barrier methods

In the barrier methods of contraception, a chemical or mechanical barrier is inserted between the cervix and the sperm to prevent the sperm from entering the uterus, travelling to the fallopian tubes and fertilising the ovum. Because barrier methods don't use hormones, they're sometimes favoured over hormonal contraceptives, which can cause many adverse effects. However, failure rates for barrier methods are higher than that for hormonal contraceptives.

Barrier methods include spermicidal products, diaphragms, cervical caps, vaginal rings and male and female condoms.

Spermicidal products

Before intercourse, spermicidal products are inserted into the vagina. Their goal is to kill sperms before the sperms enter the cervix. Spermicides also change the pH of the vaginal fluid to a strong acid, which isn't conducive to sperm survival. Vaginally inserted spermicides are available in gels, creams, films, foams and suppositories.

The gels, foams and creams are inserted using an applicator and should be inserted at least 1 hour before intercourse. The woman should be instructed not to douche for 6 hours after intercourse to ensure that the agent has completed its spermicidal action in the vagina and cervix.

Spermicidal films are made of glycerine that's impregnated with nonoxynol 9. The film is folded and then inserted into the vagina. When the film makes contact with vaginal secretions or precoital penile emissions, it dissolves and carbon dioxide foam forms to protect the cervix against invading spermatozoa.

Spermicidal suppositories consist of cocoa butter and glycerine and are filled with nonoxynol 9. The suppositories are inserted into the

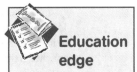

Education edge

Signs of PID

If your client has an intrauterine contraceptive device, tell her that untreated vaginal infections can progress to pelvic inflammatory disease (PID). Instruct the client to watch for signs and symptoms of PID, such as:

- fever of 38.3°C
- purulent vaginal discharge
- painful intercourse
- abdominal or pelvic pain
- suprapubic tenderness or guarding
- tenderness on bimanual examination.

Barrier methods block us from entering the uterus and fertilising the ovum.

That doesn't seem fair!

DO NOT ENTER

vagina, where they dissolve to release the spermicide. The suppository takes 15 minutes to dissolve, so women should be instructed to insert it 15 minutes before intercourse. Spermicides should always be used in conjunction with another barrier method e.g. condoms.

The plus side

Here are the advantages of spermicidal products:
- They're inexpensive.
- They may be purchased over the counter, which makes them easily accessible.
- They don't require a visit to a health care provider.
- They can be obtained free from family planning clinics.
- Spermicidal films wash away with natural body fluids.
- Nonoxynol 9, one of the most preferred spermicides, may also help prevent the spread of STIs.
- Vaginally inserted spermicides may be used in combination with other birth control methods to increase their effectiveness.
- They're useful in emergency situations such as when a condom breaks.

The minus side

Here are the disadvantages of spermicidal products:
- They need to be inserted from 15 minutes to 1 hour before intercourse, so they may interfere with sexual spontaneity.
- Some spermicides may be irritating to the vagina and penile tissue.
- Some women are bothered by the vaginal leakage that can occur, especially after using cocoa- and glycerine-based suppositories.
- The film foam's effectiveness depends on vaginal secretions; therefore, it isn't recommended for women who are nearing menopause because decreased vaginal secretions make the film less effective.
- Spermicidal products may be contraindicated in women who have acute cervicitis because of the risk of further irritation.

Diaphragm

The diaphragm is another barrier-type contraceptive that mechanically blocks sperm from entering the cervix. It's composed of a soft, latex dome that's supported by a round, metal spring on the outside. A diaphragm can be inserted up to 2 hours before intercourse. Optimum effectiveness is achieved by using it in combination with spermicidal jelly that's applied to the rim of the diaphragm before it's inserted. Diaphragms are available in various sizes and must be fitted to the individual. (See *Inserting a diaphragm*, page 73.)

The plus side

Here are the advantages of the diaphragm:
- It's a good choice for women who choose not to use hormonal contraceptives or don't feel that they can use natural family planning methods effectively.

Education edge

Inserting a diaphragm

As you insert a diaphragm, instruct the woman to prepare her for inserting the diaphragm herself. Identify structures and the feelings associated with proper insertion. Follow these steps for insertion.

After putting on gloves, lubricate the rim or dome of the fitting ring or diaphragm to lessen the discomfort of insertion.

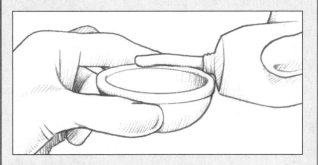

Fold the diaphragm in half with one hand by pressing the opposite sides together. Hold the vulva open with your other hand.

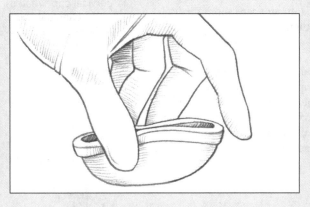

Slide the folded diaphragm into the vagina and towards the posterior cervicovaginal fornix.

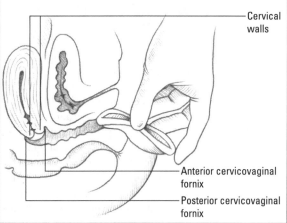

Cervical walls

Anterior cervicovaginal fornix

Posterior cervicovaginal fornix

The diaphragm should fit below the symphysis and cover the cervix. The proximal ring should fit behind the pubic arch with minimal pressure. Note that the cervix is palpable behind the diaphragm. The cervix feels like a 'nose'.

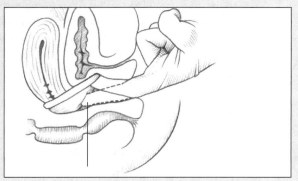

- When combined with spermicidal jelly, its effectiveness ranges from 80% to 93% for new users and increases to 97% for long-term users.
- It causes few adverse reactions.
- It helps protect against STIs when used with spermicide.
- It doesn't alter the body's metabolic or physiological processes.
- It can be inserted up to 2 hours before intercourse.
- If it's correctly fitted and inserted, neither partner can feel it during intercourse.

The minus side

Here are the disadvantages of the diaphragm:
- It must be inserted before intercourse and may interfere with spontaneity.
- Although it can be left in place for up to 24 hours, if intercourse is repeated before 6 hours (which is how long the diaphragm must be left in place after intercourse) more spermicidal gel must be inserted. The diaphragm can't be removed and replaced because this could cause sperm to bypass the spermicidal gel and fertilisation could occur.
- The pressure it creates on the urethra may cause a higher incidence of upper urinary tract infections (UTIs).
- It must be refitted after birth, cervical surgery, miscarriage, dilatation and curettage (D&C), therapeutic abortion or weight gain or loss of more than 6.8 kg because of cervical shape changes.
- It's contraindicated in women who have a history of cystocele, rectocele, uterine retroversion, prolapse, retroflexion or anteflexion because the cervix position may be displaced, making insertion and proper fit questionable.
- It's contraindicated in clients with a history of toxic shock syndrome or repeated UTIs, vaginal stenosis, pelvic abnormalities or allergy to spermicidal jellies or rubber. It's also contraindicated in women who show an unwillingness to learn proper techniques for diaphragm care and insertion.
- It can't be used in the first 6 weeks postpartum.

Cervical cap

The cervical cap is another barrier-type method of contraception. It's similar to the diaphragm but smaller. It's a thimble-shaped, soft rubber cup that the woman places over the cervix. The cap is held in place by suction. The addition of a spermicide creates a chemical barrier as well. Women who aren't suited for diaphragms may use cervical caps. Failure of the cervical cap is commonly due to failure to use the device or inappropriate use of the device. (See *Recognising a correct fit*, page 75.)

The plus side

Here are the advantages of the cervical cap:
- It requires less spermicide, and is less likely to become dislodged during intercourse.
- It's 85% effective for nulliparous women and 70% effective for parous women when used correctly and consistently.

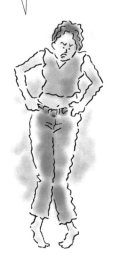

Size really does matter when it comes to diaphragms – not to mention jeans!

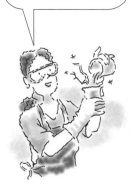

Along with a spermicide, a cervical cap creates a mechanical and chemical barrier.

Advice from the experts

Recognising a correct fit

With the proper fit, the gap or space between the base of the cervix and the inside of the cervical cap ring should be 1–2 mm (to reduce the possibility of dislodgement), and the rim should fill the cervicovaginal fornix.

To verify a good fit, leave the cervical cap in place for 1–2 minutes. Then, with the cap in place, pinch the dome until there's a dimple. A dimple that takes about 30 seconds to resume a domed appearance indicates good suction and a good fit. If the cap is too small, the rim leaves a gap where the cervix remains exposed. If the cap is too large, it isn't snug against the cervix and is more easily dislodged.

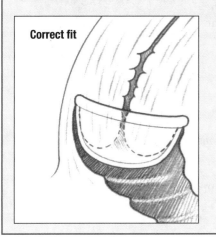

Correct fit

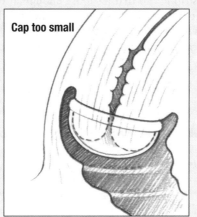

Cap too small

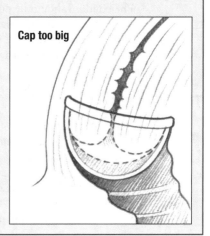

Cap too big

- It doesn't alter hormones.
- It can be inserted up to 8 hours before intercourse.
- It doesn't require reapplication of spermicide before repeated intercourse.
- It can remain in place longer than a diaphragm because it doesn't exert pressure on the vaginal walls or urethra.

The minus side

Here are the disadvantages of the cervical cap:
- It requires possible refitting after weight gain or loss of 6.8 kg or more, recent pregnancy, recent pelvic surgery or cap slippage.
- It may be difficult to insert or remove.
- It may cause an allergic reaction or vaginal lacerations and thickening of the vaginal mucosa.
- It may cause a foul odour if left in place for more than 36 hours.
- It can't be used during menstruation or during the first 6 postpartum weeks.

- It shouldn't be left in place longer than 24 hours.
- It's contraindicated in women with a history of toxic shock syndrome, a previously abnormal cervical smear test, allergy to latex or spermicide, an abnormally short or long cervix, history of PID, cervicitis, papillomavirus infection, cervical cancer or undiagnosed vaginal bleeding.

Male condom

A male condom is a latex or synthetic sheath that's placed over the erect penis before intercourse. It prevents pregnancy by collecting spermatozoa in the tip of the condom, preventing them from entering the vagina.

Position is important

The condom should be positioned so that it's loose enough at the penis tip to collect ejaculate but not so loose that it comes off the penis. The penis must be withdrawn before it becomes flaccid after ejaculation or sperm can escape from the condom into the vagina.

> In ballet as well as condom usage, exact position is critical.

The plus side

Here are the advantages of the male condom:
- Many women favour male condoms because they put the responsibility of birth control on the male.
- No health care visit is needed.
- It's available over the counter in pharmacies and grocery shops.
- It's easy to carry.
- It prevents the spread of STIs.

The minus side

Here are the disadvantages of the male condom:
- It must be applied before any vulvar penile contact takes place because preejaculation fluid may contain sperm.
- It may cause an allergic reaction if the product contains latex and either partner is allergic.
- It may break during use if it's used incorrectly or is of poor quality.
- It can't be reused.
- Sexual pleasure may be affected.
- It may interfere with spontaneity.

> A female condom? What's good for the goose is 95% effective for the gander!

Female condom

A female condom is made of latex and lubricated with nonoxynol 9. The inner ring (closed end) covers the cervix. The outer ring (open end) rests against the vaginal opening. Female condoms are intended for one-time use and shouldn't be used in combination with male condoms. (See *Inserting a female condom*, page 77.)

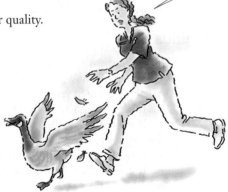

Education edge

Inserting a female condom

A female condom is made of latex and lubricated with nonoxynol 9. It has an inner ring that covers the cervix and an outer ring that rests against the vaginal opening, as shown below.

Fold the inner ring in half with one hand by pressing the opposite sides together, as shown below. When inserted, the inner ring covers the cervix.

After the condom is inserted, the outer ring (open end) rests against the vaginal opening.

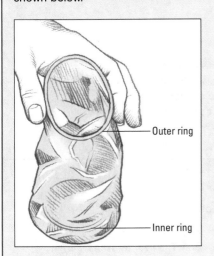

Outer ring

Inner ring

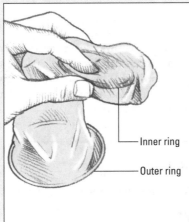

Inner ring

Outer ring

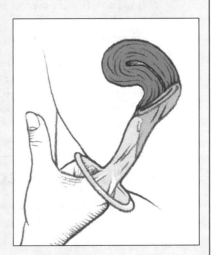

The plus side

Here are the advantages of the female condom:
- It's 95% effective.
- It helps prevent the spread of STIs.
- It can be purchased over the counter.

The minus side

Here are the disadvantages of the female condom:
- It's more expensive than the male condom.
- It's difficult to use and hasn't gained as much acceptance as a male condom.
- Pregnancy can occur as a result of failure to use or incorrect use.
- It may break or become dislodged.
- It's contraindicated in clients or partners with latex allergies.
- It may interfere with spontaneity.

Surgical methods of family planning

Surgical methods of family planning include vasectomy (for men) and tubal ligation (for women). These procedures are the most commonly chosen contraceptive methods for couples over age 30.

Reversal reality

It's possible to reverse these procedures, but it's expensive and isn't always effective. Therefore, surgical sterilisation should be chosen only when the woman and her partner, if applicable, have thoroughly discussed the options and know that these procedures are for permanent contraception.

Vasectomy

Vasectomy is a procedure in which the pathway for spermatozoa is surgically severed. Incisions are made on each side of the scrotum, and the vas deferens is cut and tied, then plugged or cauterised. This blocks the passage of sperm. The testes continue to produce sperm as usual, but the sperm can't pass the severed vas deferens. (See *A closer look at vasectomy*.)

A closer look at vasectomy

In a vasectomy, the vas deferens is surgically altered to prohibit the passage of sperm. Here's how.

The surgeon makes two small incisions, one on each side of the scrotum.

He then cuts the vas deferens with scissors.

The vas deferens is then cauterised or plugged to block the passage of sperm.

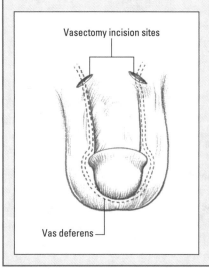

Vasectomy incision sites

Vas deferens

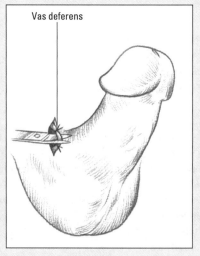

Vas deferens

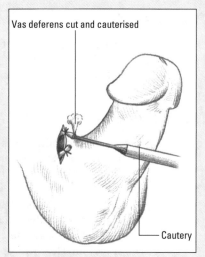

Vas deferens cut and cauterised

Cautery

Lying in wait

The man should be cautioned that sperm remaining in the vas deferens at the time of surgery may remain viable for as long as 6 months. An additional form of contraception should be used until two negative sperm reports have been obtained. These reports confirm that all of the remaining sperm in the vas deferens has been ejaculated.

To prevent clients from making a rash decision regarding vasectomy, explain that this procedure should be viewed as irreversible, although reversal is possible in 95% of cases.

> Vasectomy is 99.6% effective, and it can be done as an outpatient procedure with little or no pain.

The plus side

Here are the advantages of vasectomy:
• It can be done as an outpatient procedure, with little anaesthesia and minimal pain.
• It's 99.6% effective.
• It doesn't interfere with male erection, and the male still produces seminal fluid – it just doesn't contain sperm.

The minus side

Here are the disadvantages of vasectomy:
• Misconceptions about the procedure may lead some men to resist it.
• Some reports indicate that vasectomy may be associated with the development of kidney stones.
• It's contraindicated in individuals who aren't entirely certain of their decision to choose permanent sterilisation, and in those with specific surgical risks such as an anaesthesia allergy.

Tubal sterilisation (Ligation)

In tubal sterilisation, a laparoscope is used to cauterise, crush, clamp or block the fallopian tubes, thus preventing pregnancy by blocking the passage of ova and sperm. The procedure is performed after menses and before ovulation. It can be performed following caesarean section but most doctors advise women to wait for at least several weeks after the birth in case complications arise during pregnancy or afterwards, in the baby's condition (tubes may be swollen after and clips may dislodge).

Here's how it works:

A small incision is made in the abdomen.

Carbon dioxide is pumped into the abdominal cavity to lift the abdominal wall, providing an easier view of the surgical area.

A lighted laparoscope is inserted, and the fallopian tubes are located.

An electric current is then used to cauterise the tubes, or the tubes are clamped and cut.

A closer look at tubal sterilisation

In a laparoscopic tubal sterilisation, the surgeon inserts a laparoscope and occludes the fallopian tube by cauterising, crushing, clamping or blocking. This prevents the passage of ova and sperm.

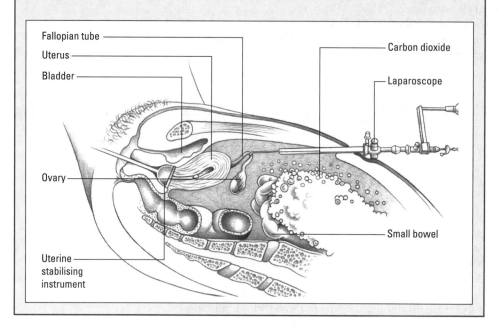

Fallopian tube
Uterus
Bladder
Carbon dioxide
Laparoscope
Ovary
Small bowel
Uterine stabilising instrument

After surgery, the woman may notice some abdominal bloating from the carbon dioxide, but this subsides. (See *A closer look at tubal sterilisation*.)

Sneak attack

Women should be cautioned to not have unprotected intercourse before the procedure because sperm that can become trapped in the tube could fertilise an ovum, resulting in an ectopic pregnancy.

This procedure should be viewed as irreversible. Although reversal is successful in 40–75% of women, this process is difficult and could cause an ectopic pregnancy.

The plus side

Here are the advantages of tubal sterilisation:
- It can be performed on an outpatient basis, and the woman is usually discharged within a few hours after the procedure.
- It's 99.6% effective.
- It's been associated with a decreased incidence of ovarian cancer.
- A woman can resume intercourse 2–3 days after having the procedure.

Women should protect themselves from unwanted pregnancy before undergoing tubal sterilisation. Trapped sperm could launch a sneak attack, resulting in an ectopic pregnancy.

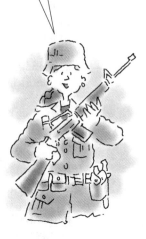

The minus side

Here are the disadvantages of tubal sterilisation:
• Some women may be reluctant to choose it because it requires a small surgical incision and general anaesthesia.
• Complications include a risk of bowel perforation and haemorrhage and the typical risks of general anaesthesia (allergy, arrhythmia) during the procedure.
• Contraindications include umbilical hernia and obesity.
• Post-tubal ligation syndrome may occur. This includes vaginal spotting and intermittent vaginal bleeding as well as severe lower abdominal cramping.
• It isn't recommended for individuals who aren't certain of their decision to choose permanent sterilisation.

Alternatives to tubal ligation?

A microinsert called Essure has been licensed in the USA and Europe. The tiny, coiled devices are inserted into the fallopian tubes and within 3 months, they cause the tissue to grow and thicken until it blocks the tubes, preventing the sperm getting in. No hormones are involved and the procedure only takes 45 minutes to perform. (Not yet licensed in the UK.)

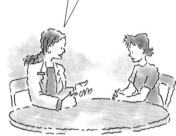

Tubal sterilisation is 99.6% effective and can be performed on an outpatient basis.

Elective termination of pregnancy

A procedure that's performed to deliberately end a pregnancy is known as an *elective termination of pregnancy*. Also known as an *induced abortion*, elective termination of pregnancy can be performed for many reasons, some of which involve:
• pregnancy that threatens a woman's life
• pregnancy in which amniocentesis identifies a chromosomal defect in the fetus
• pregnancy that results from rape or incest
• pregnancy in which the woman chooses not to have a child.
  Abortion is a pretty emotive subject and one that most midwives find challenging in their practice. It involves ethical, moral and religious issues which the midwife has to address on behalf of her client. In Northern Ireland, abortion is still illegal except in exceptional circumstances when it is necessary to preserve the life of the mother.
  Elective terminations of pregnancy can be medically or surgically induced.

Medically induced abortion

In the medically induced method of abortion, a progesterone antagonist called *mifepristone* (Mifeprex [RU-486]) is taken to block the effect of progesterone and prevent implantation of the fertilised ovum. The drug is taken as a single dose at any time within 28 days' gestation. If a spontaneous abortion doesn't occur, *misoprostol* ([Cytotec], a prostaglandin E1 analogue) is administered 3 days later.

Uterine contractions occur with mild cramping, and the products of conception are expelled. One advantage to using this method is that it decreases the risk of damage to the uterus that can occur from instruments used in surgically induced abortions.

Consider this

Disadvantages of medically induced elective termination include the possibility of incomplete abortion as well as prolonged bleeding. Medically induced abortion is contraindicated in women with suspected or confirmed ectopic pregnancy (unless she is closely monitored and the pregnancy is at fewer than 6 weeks' gestation); haemorrhagic disorders; current long-term systemic corticosteroid therapy; history of allergy to mifepristone, misoprostol or other prostaglandins; an IUCD or chronic adrenal failure.

Surgically induced abortions

Depending on the gestation at the time of the abortion, surgical abortion can be performed in several ways. These include D&C, dilatation and vacuum extraction (D&E), saline induction and hysterotomy.

Dilatation and vacuum extraction

D&E uses the same technique as D&C except that the products of conception are removed by vacuum extraction. Some facilities admit the woman the day before the procedure to begin cervical dilation. This can be achieved by inserting into the cervix a laminaria tent made of seaweed that has been dried and sterilised. This helps maintain the integrity of the cervix so that future pregnancies aren't threatened. As the seaweed from the laminaria tent absorbs the moisture from the cervix and vagina, it begins to swell and dilate the cervix. Then a small catheter is inserted, and the products of conception are extracted by the vacuum over a 5-minute period.

This procedure can be performed between 12 and 16 weeks' gestation as either an outpatient or inpatient procedure. Complications such as uterine puncture and infections can occur.

Saline induction

Saline induction can be performed to terminate pregnancy if gestation is between 16 and 24 weeks. In saline induction, hypertonic saline solution is inserted through the uterine cavity into the amniotic fluid, which forces fluid to shift, causing the placenta and endometrium to slough.

Infertility

Infertility is defined as the inability to conceive after 1 year of consistent attempts without using contraception. As many as 10–15% of couples who desire children experience infertility. (See *What's behind rising infertility rates?*, page 83.)

What's behind rising infertility rates?

Childless couples need to feel that they aren't alone. Let them know that the number of couples dealing with infertility has doubled in recent years. Factors that may contribute to rising infertility rates include:

- ageing – more and more couples postpone childbearing until age 30 or older, allowing age and concomitant disease processes to affect fertility
- sexually transmitted diseases, which may be responsible for up to 20% of infertility cases

- intrauterine contraceptive devices, which can cause pelvic inflammatory disease and consequent infertility
- environmental factors such as toxins
- complications of abortion or childbirth.

There's also a higher incidence of infertility in females who:

- have irregular or absent periods
- experience pain during sexual intercourse
- have had ruptured appendices or other abdominal surgeries.

Infertility can be considered primary or secondary:
- *Primary infertility* refers to infertility that occurs in couples who have not previously conceived.
- *Secondary infertility* refers to infertility that occurs in couples who have previously conceived.

Skilful and sensitive

Talking to a couple about infertility and its treatment requires many skills. For instance, you need to guide them sensitively through rigorous tests and treatments – some of which may be painful and embarrassing. At the same time, you need to help them deal with their own emotions.

Bittersweet emotions

A diagnosis of infertility may stir up many feelings and conflicts, such as anger, guilt and blame, which may disrupt relationships and alter self-esteem. What's more, although treatment heightens the hope of conception, it can also lead to deep disappointment if fertility measures fail. (See *Infertility teaching topics*, page 84.)

Infertile couples need open communication to help build their trust and confidence in the health care team. Understandably, many couples feel uncomfortable discussing their sex life, let alone having intercourse assigned on a rigid schedule that's designed to take advantage of peak fertile days.

> Infertility can be an emotional tug of war for many couples. You'll need to guide them sensitively through many tests and treatments.

Conditions for conception

Many couples think that conception occurs easily when, in fact, certain conditions must be present for conception to occur. These include:
- sufficient and motile sperm
- mucus secretions that promote sperm movement in the reproductive tract

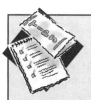

Education edge

Infertility teaching topics

When teaching clients about infertility, be sure to cover these topics.

- Definition of infertility
- Possible causes, such as ovulatory dysfunction and structural abnormalities
- Fertility drugs, including menotropins (Pergonal) and clomiphene (Clomid)
- Explanation of in vitro fertilisation–embryo transfer (IVF-ET) and gamete intrafallopian transfer (GIFT), if appropriate
- Artificial insemination
- Surgery to promote fertility, including varicocelectomy, hysteroscopy, laparoscopy and laparotomy
- Psychological counselling

- unobstructed uterus and open fallopian tubes that allow sperm-free passage
- regular ovulation and healthy ova
- hormonal sufficiency and balance that support implantation of the embryo in the uterus
- sexual intercourse timed so that sperm fertilise the ovum within 24 hours of the ovum's release.

Sex-specific causes of infertility

Many conditions can cause infertility in men and women.

Just for him

Some causes of male infertility remain unknown, but factors that have been identified include:
- structural abnormalities, such as varicoceles (enlarged, varicose veins in the scrotum that can affect sperm number and motility) and hypospadias
- infection, possibly from an STI
- hormonal imbalances that reduce the amount of spermatozoa produced or disrupt their ability to travel effectively in the female reproductive tract
- heat (produced by wearing tight-fitting underwear or jeans, sitting in a hot tub or hot bath water or driving long distances) that adversely affects sperm number and motility
- fever-producing illnesses that adversely affect sperm number and motility
- penile or testicular injury or congenital anomalies that diminish sperm
- certain prescription drugs known to affect sperm quality
- use of substances such as alcohol, marijuana, cocaine and tobacco that are suspected of affecting sperm quality

- coital frequency – either too often or too seldom – which may decrease sperm number and motility
- environmental agents, such as exposure to radiation or other industrial and environmental toxins
- psychological and emotional stress.

Just for her

Female infertility usually stems from anovulation (ovulatory dysfunction), fallopian tube obstruction, uterine conditions or pelvic abnormalities caused by one or more of the following factors:
- hormonal imbalances that prevent the ovary from releasing ova regularly (or at all) or from producing enough progesterone to support growth and maintain the uterine lining needed for implantation of the embryo
- infection or inflammation (past, chronic or current) that damages the ovaries and fallopian tubes, such as from PID, STDs, appendicitis, childhood disease or surgical trauma
- structural abnormalities, such as a uterus scarred by infection or one that's abnormally shaped or positioned since birth, deformed by fibroid tumours, exposed to diethylstilbestrol or injured by conisation
- mucosal abnormalities caused by infection, inadequate hormone levels or antibodies to sperm, which may create a hostile environment that prevents sperm from entering the uterus and continuing to the fallopian tubes
- endometriosis (in some women), in which the endometrial tissue – usually confined to the inner lining of the uterine cavity – is deposited outside the uterus on such structures as the ovaries or fallopian tubes, causing inflammation and scarring
- endocrine abnormalities, such as elevated prolactin levels and pituitary, thyroid or adrenal dysfunction
- recreational drug use (including tobacco, marijuana and cocaine) and environmental and occupational factors (exposure to heat and chemicals).

Normogonadotrophic anovulation

Normogonadotrophic anovulation is usually seen in women with polycystic ovary syndrome and in those who are overweight. Women with normogonadotrophic anovulation have normal FSH levels but elevated LH levels. They may also bleed in response to a progesterone withdrawal test.

Hyperprolactinaemic anovulation

In hyperprolactinaemic anovulation, excessive prolactin secretion impairs ovarian function. Elevated levels of prolactin in the blood are normal during lactation but are otherwise pathological. Hyperprolactinaemic anovulation may also be caused by physical or emotional stress, rapid weight loss or a pituitary adenoma.

Hypogonadotrophic anovulation

Hypogonadotrophic anovulation may be caused by stress, weight loss or excessive exercise. In many cases, this type of anovulation is functional and transient. An organic cause should be excluded, however, particularly if the woman displays neurological symptoms. Women with hypogonadotrophic anovulation typically have low levels of FSH, LH and oestrogen and an absence of withdrawal bleeding after a progesterone challenge test.

Hypergonadotrophic anovulation
Hypergonadotrophic anovulation results from ovarian resistance or failure. It's commonly diagnosed when repeated measurements show plasma levels of FSH are higher than 20 mIU/ml.

Treatment options

Infertility can be treated with drugs, special procedures or various types of surgery.

Medications
Drugs can be used in several ways to help treat infertility. They may be prescribed to treat certain conditions that inhibit fertility. For example, antibiotics may be prescribed for infections or danazol (Danocrine) may be ordered for a woman with endometriosis. Drugs designed to initiate ovulation, improve cervical mucus or stimulate sperm production may also be prescribed.

Just for him

For men whose infertility is caused by hypogonadism secondary to pituitary or hypothalamic failure, treatment may include human menopausal gonadotropins (hMGs), human chorionic gonadotropin (HCG) or pulsatile gonadotropin-releasing hormone (Gn-RH). These medications are highly effective in achieving sperm quality that's sufficient to induce pregnancy.

Just for her

For women, the type of fertility drug prescribed depends on the type of anovulation.

Normogonadotrophic anovulation
Recommended treatments for normogonadotrophic anovulation include clomiphene (Clomid) or tamoxifen (Nolvadex) combined with weight reduction.

Invigorating the ovaries

Clomiphene (Clomid) is an oestrogen agonist used to stimulate the ovaries. The drug binds to oestrogen receptors, decreasing the number available, and falsely signals the hypothalamus to increase FSH and LH, resulting in the release of more ova.

The drug is taken on cycle days 5 through to 10 and may produce ovulation 6–11 days after the last dose. The woman needs to have intercourse every other day for 1 week beginning 5 days after she takes her last dose. The initial dose may not cause ovulation and the dosage may be adjusted later. The

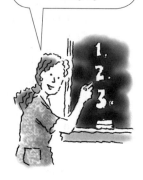

Infertility can be treated with drugs, special procedures or surgery.

hMGs, HCG and Gn-RH all help to achieve sperm quality that's sufficient to induce pregnancy.

woman should document the ovulatory process by keeping a BBT chart or by using an ovulation prediction kit (or both).

Additional effects

The drug may trigger multiple ova development and release, but the incidence of multiple births (mostly twins) stays near 5%. The drug may also make her feel moody from fluctuating hormone levels. If the woman fails to have a normal menses, she should contact her doctor, who may withhold the drug and order a pregnancy test.

The woman may experience slight bloating and hot flashes (caused by the release of an LH, which indicates that the drug is working). She may also experience dysmenorrhoea as a result of the drug triggering the ovulatory cycle (the first cycle she has had in a while).

Instruct the woman to report blurred vision; other visual changes, such as spots or flashing lights and severe headaches that are unrelieved by analgesics. Additionally, instruct the woman to tell her doctor if abdominal distention, bloating, pain or weight gain occurs. These effects may signal ovarian enlargement or ovarian cysts, and treatment may need to be discontinued.

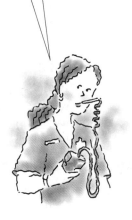

Is it hot in here? Clomiphene may cause hot flushes in some women.

And another thing

Another therapy for normogonadotrophic anovulation is the administration of pulsatile Gn-RH or FSH to induce multiple follicular growth, followed by HCG and timed intercourse or assisted reproductive techniques.

Hyperprolactinaemic anovulation

Treatment for hyperprolactinaemic anovulation includes bromocriptine (Parlodel) or chemically related dopamine agonists, such as cabergoline (Dostinex). If pituitary function is normal, these drugs can be combined with clomiphene or tamoxifen to induce ovulation.

Hypogonadotrophic anovulation

Treatment of hypogonadotrophic anovulation varies depending on the cause. In the presence of primary pituitary failure, ovulation can be induced with pulsatile Gn-RH. In women with suspected luteal phase defects, progesterone may be administered during the luteal phase for three to six cycles.

Hypergonadotrophic anovulation

No current drug therapy has restored ovulation in patients with hypergonadotrophic anovulation. Adoption or ova donation may be recommended.

Infertility procedures

Such procedures as IVF-ET, GIFT, zygote intrafallopian transfer (ZIFT), intracytoplasmic sperm injection (ICSI), embryo donation and intrauterine insemination (sometimes called artificial insemination) may be recommended to help treat infertility.

In vitro fertilisation–embryo transfer

IVF-ET refers to the removal of one or more mature oocytes from a woman's ovary by laparoscopy. After removal, these oocytes are fertilised by exposing them to sperm under laboratory conditions outside the woman's body. Embryo transfer (ET) is the insertion of these laboratory-grown fertilised ova (zygotes) into the woman's uterus. This is performed approximately 40 hours after fertilisation. Ideally, one or more of the zygotes implant. IVF-ET circumvents the need for a fallopian tube to pick up an ovum or to propel a fertilised ovum to the uterus.

The perfect candidates

IVF-ET is performed for couples who haven't been able to conceive as a result of damaged or blocked fallopian tubes. It can also be used if the man has oligospermia (low sperm count) or if the woman lacks the cervical mucus that enables sperm to travel from the vagina into the cervix.

Agents of ovulation

The woman is given an ovulation drug, such as clomiphene or menotropins (Pergonal). On about the tenth day of her menstrual cycle, the ovaries are examined; when the size of the follicles appears to be mature, the woman is given an injection of HCG hormone. This causes ovulation to occur within 38–42 hours. Then the IVF-ET procedure is performed. (See *How IVF works*, page 89.)

Ova donation

Donor ovum may be used in IVF-ET instead of the woman's ovum if the woman doesn't ovulate or if she carries a sex-linked disease that she doesn't want to pass on to her offspring.

Alternate eggs

In ova donation, ova that are retrieved from a well-screened and hormonally stimulated donor are fertilised in a Petri dish by sperm from the recipient's partner or a sperm donor. After an incubation period, the best embryos are transferred into the recipient's uterus. The rest may be frozen for possible use in a second transfer if necessary or if the recipient desires a second child genetically related to the first. Ova donation is an emotional, expensive and time-intensive experience. However, it offers a realistic, successful option for clients who otherwise have no way to have a child. Experienced programmes report clinical pregnancy rates of 50% per ova donation cycle. These success rates are better than pregnancy rates with IVF cycles using a woman's own ova.

Meet the candidates

Good recipient candidates for ova donation include women who:
- have never had a spontaneous menses
- stopped menstruating at an early age

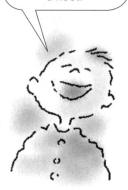

Can you believe it? I started life as a laboratory-grown zygote, transferred into my mum's uterus. What a hoot!

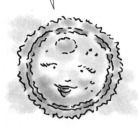

Although it can be expensive, ova donation may be a good alternative for a woman who doesn't ovulate.

Female pelvic organs

The female pelvis includes reproductive, urinary and GI structures. Reproductive structures include the internal and external genitalia. Hormonal influences determine the development and function of these structures and affect fertility and childbearing.

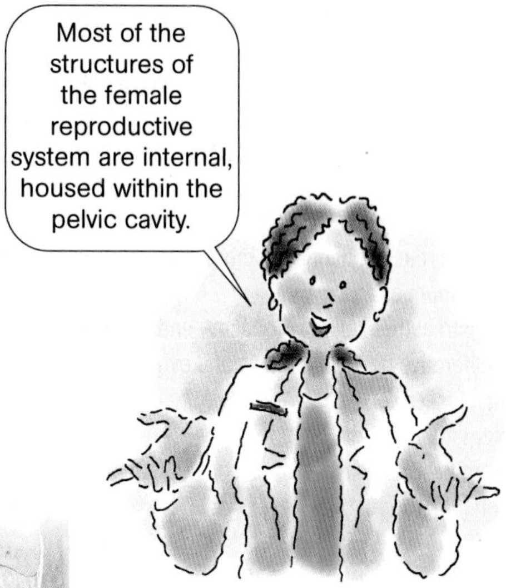

> Most of the structures of the female reproductive system are internal, housed within the pelvic cavity.

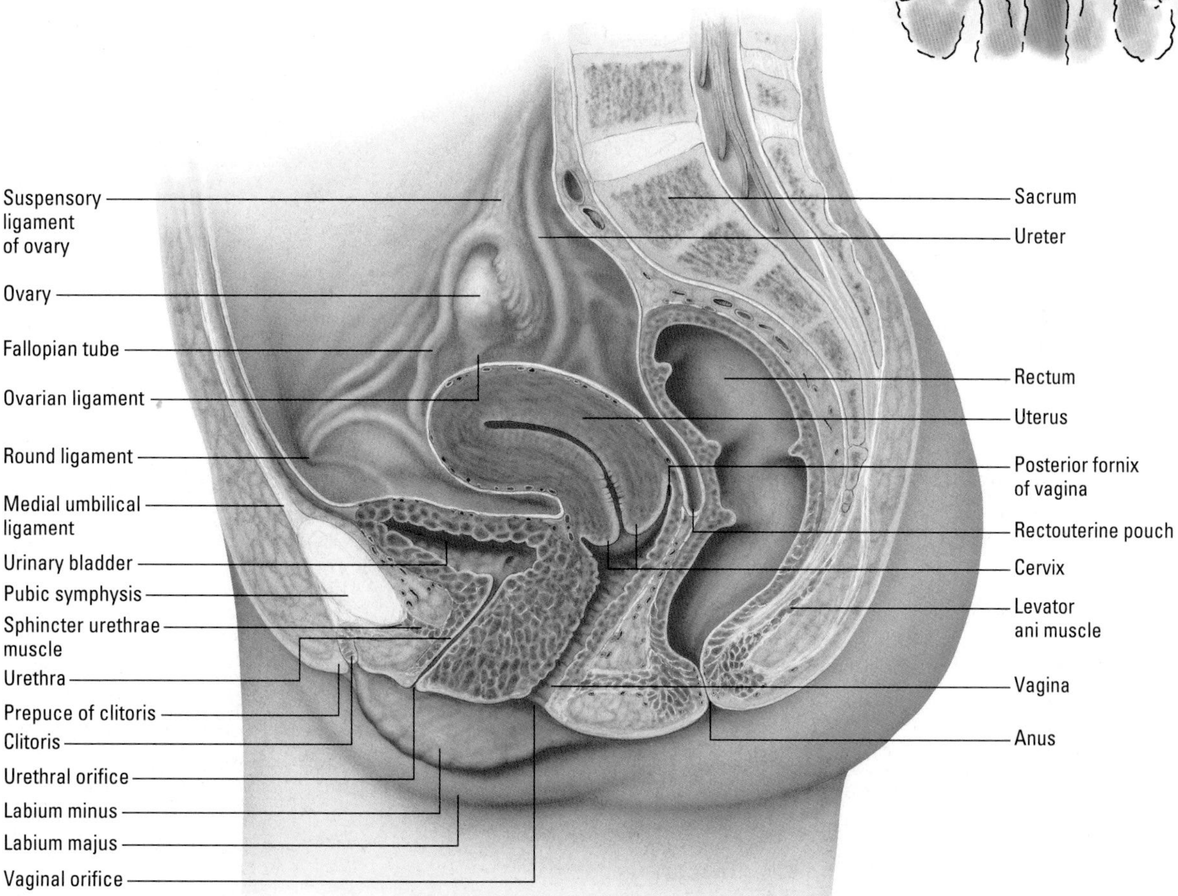

Suspensory ligament of ovary

Ovary

Fallopian tube

Ovarian ligament

Round ligament

Medial umbilical ligament

Urinary bladder

Pubic symphysis

Sphincter urethrae muscle

Urethra

Prepuce of clitoris

Clitoris

Urethral orifice

Labium minus

Labium majus

Vaginal orifice

Sacrum

Ureter

Rectum

Uterus

Posterior fornix of vagina

Rectouterine pouch

Cervix

Levator ani muscle

Vagina

Anus

Ovarian and uterine changes during the menstrual cycle

The hypothalamus, ovaries and pituitary gland secrete hormones that affect the build-up and shedding of the endometrium during the menstrual cycle. The menstrual cycle normally occurs over 28 days, although it may range from 22 to 34 days. The cycle is regulated by fluctuating hormone levels that, in turn, are regulated by negative and positive feedback mechanisms involving the hypothalamus, pituitary glands and ovaries.

The hormonal changes of the menstrual cycle trigger a series of changes in the uterine endometrium as follows:
• menstrual (preovulatory) phase—endometrium exfoliates and sheds
• proliferative (follicular) phase and ovulation—endometrium proliferates
• luteal (secretory) phase—endometrium becomes thick and secretory to prepare for the implantation of a fertilised ovum
• premenstrual phase—in absence of fertilisation, oestrogen and progesterone levels drop and the endometrium sheds.

These illustrations show the relationship between ovarian changes and uterine changes during the menstrual cycle.

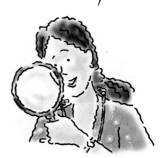

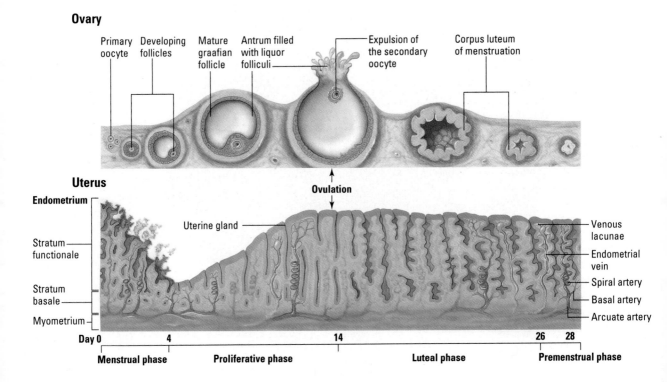

Ovary

Primary oocyte | Developing follicles | Mature graafian follicle | Antrum filled with liquor folliculi | Expulsion of the secondary oocyte | Corpus luteum of menstruation

Uterus — Ovulation

Endometrium

Uterine gland — Venous lacunae

Stratum functionale — Endometrial vein

Stratum basale — Spiral artery / Basal artery

Myometrium — Arcuate artery

Day 0 — 4 — 14 — 26 — 28

Menstrual phase | Proliferative phase | Luteal phase | Premenstrual phase

Fertilisation and implantation

During monthly ovulation, an ovum is released from the ovary into the fallopian tube, where it travels towards the uterus. If present, sperm from the male move through the fallopian tube, where they meet the ovum.

If a sperm penetrates the ovum, fertilisation occurs and the ovum is called a *zygote.* The zygote continues to travel towards the uterus, dividing many times until it becomes a blastocyst. When the blastocyst reaches the uterus, it implants in the uterine wall and continues to develop over the next 9 months.

Ovum (Egg)

Spermatozoon (Sperm)

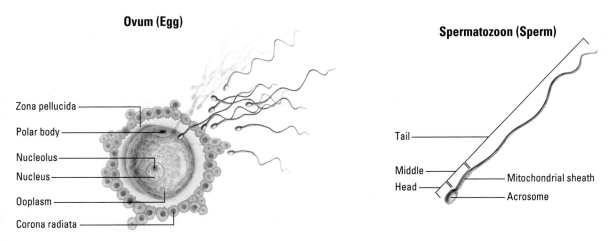

Zona pellucida
Polar body
Nucleolus
Nucleus
Ooplasm
Corona radiata

Tail
Middle
Head
Mitochondrial sheath
Acrosome

Fertilisation and implantation

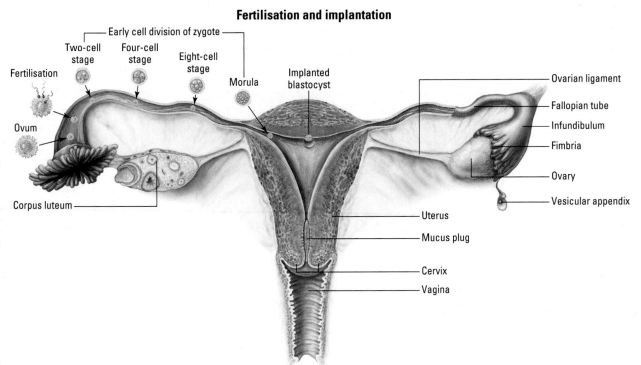

Early cell division of zygote
Two-cell stage
Four-cell stage
Eight-cell stage
Morula
Implanted blastocyst
Fertilisation
Ovum
Corpus luteum

Ovarian ligament
Fallopian tube
Infundibulum
Fimbria
Ovary
Vesicular appendix
Uterus
Mucus plug
Cervix
Vagina

Male pelvic structures

In the male, pelvic structures include GI, reproductive and urinary organs. These structures are illustrated below.

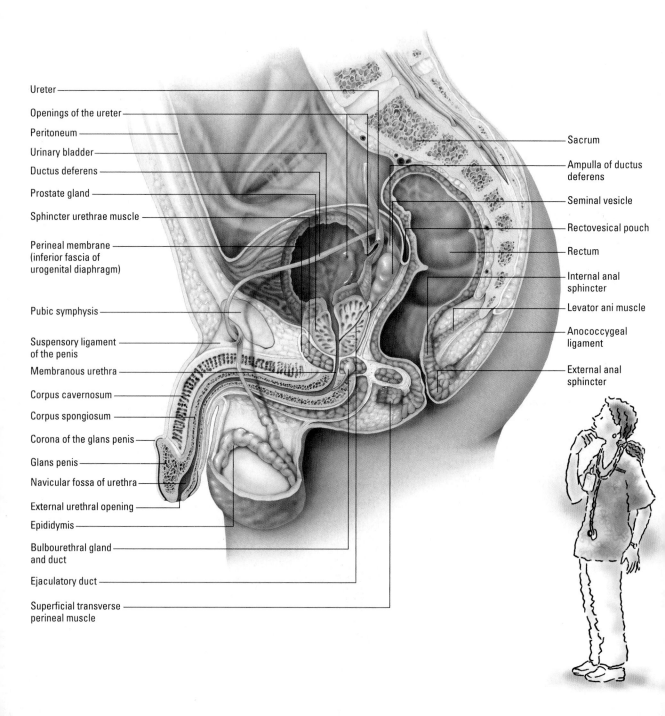

Ureter

Openings of the ureter

Peritoneum

Urinary bladder

Ductus deferens

Prostate gland

Sphincter urethrae muscle

Perineal membrane
(inferior fascia of
urogenital diaphragm)

Pubic symphysis

Suspensory ligament
of the penis

Membranous urethra

Corpus cavernosum

Corpus spongiosum

Corona of the glans penis

Glans penis

Navicular fossa of urethra

External urethral opening

Epididymis

Bulbourethral gland
and duct

Ejaculatory duct

Superficial transverse
perineal muscle

Sacrum

Ampulla of ductus
deferens

Seminal vesicle

Rectovesical pouch

Rectum

Internal anal
sphincter

Levator ani muscle

Anococcygeal
ligament

External anal
sphincter

How IVF works

For clients who meet the necessary criteria, in vitro fertilisation–embryo transfer (IVF-ET) bypasses the barriers to in vivo fertilisation.

In IVF-ET, after the ovaries receive hormonal stimulation, laparoscopy may be used to visualise and aspirate fluid (containing eggs) from the ovarian follicles. (To avoid using laparoscopy and a general anaesthetic, an ultrasound technique may be used, first to visualise the ovarian follicles and then to guide a needle through the back of the vagina to retrieve fluid and eggs from the ovarian follicles.) The eggs are then placed in a test tube or a laboratory dish containing a culture medium for 3–6 hours.

Next, sperm from the woman's partner (or a donor) is added to the dish. Two days after insemination, the now-fertilised egg or embryo is transferred into the woman's uterus, where it may implant and establish a pregnancy.

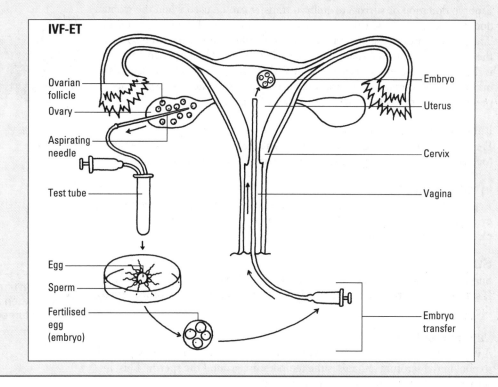

IVF-ET

Labels: Ovarian follicle, Ovary, Aspirating needle, Test tube, Egg, Sperm, Fertilised egg (embryo), Embryo, Uterus, Cervix, Vagina, Embryo transfer

- produced few or no eggs, or an elevated FSH level, in a previous IVF cycle
- have stopped menstruating (usually in their 40s) or don't respond well to fertility drugs
- have an FSH level of 15 or more on day 3 of a Clomiphene Challenge Test (research suggests these women won't be successful with IVF using their own eggs)
- have had multiple IVF cycles and failed to achieve a pregnancy.

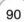

Second surprise

In addition to the usual risks of IVF, approximately 15–20% of ova donation pregnancies result in miscarriage and 20–25% result in multiple births.

Gamete intrafallopian transfer
In GIFT, the ovaries are stimulated with fertility drugs and the results are monitored. Next, ova are collected from the ovaries transvaginally by needle aspiration. They're placed in a catheter with sperm and then transferred into the fallopian tube, allowing fertilisation and implantation to occur naturally from that point.

Embryo donation or surrogate embryo transfer
Embryo donation or surrogate embryo transfer can be used when the woman doesn't ovulate or if the woman has ovarian failure but a functioning uterus. The partner or donor sperm can be used to fertilise a donated ovum so that the embryo contains one-half of the pair's gene pool. The fertilised oocyte is then placed in the woman's uterus by ET or GIFT. Some clients see this option as an advantage over adoption because it allows them to experience pregnancy and they may have a shorter wait for a child.

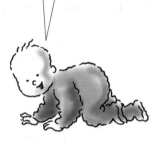

Ova donation pregnancies can result in twins, triplets or even more! Stock up on those nappies!

Intrauterine insemination
Healthy sperm are inserted into the womb at the woman's most fertile time (ovulation time) in the hope that the ovum will be fertilised successfully.

In vitro maturation
Eggs are taken from the ovaries before maturation, reducing the need for ovary-stimulating hormones. They are matured in an incubator and then placed in the womb ready to be fertilised by the sperm.

Surgery
Surgeries for infertility include varicocelectomy, laparoscopy and laparotomy. If surgery is required to enhance fertility, be sure to explain the procedure to the client.

Varicocelectomy
A varicocele is a varicosity (abnormality) of the spermatic vein. It allows blood to pool in the scrotum and raises the temperature around the sperm. This, in turn, may reduce sperm production and motility.

A surgery called varicocelectomy can be performed to repair or remove a varicocele. A small incision is made in the scrotum, and the enlarged, varicose-like vein that causes this condition is tied off.

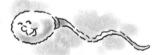

I don't function well when the heat is turned up.

Laparoscopy
A female client may need surgery to treat tubal disease, endometriosis or such pelvic conditions as adhesions. A laparoscopy is used to visualise the pelvic and upper abdominal organs and peritoneal surfaces. It can also be used to visualise the distance between the fallopian tubes and the ovaries. If this distance is too

large, the discharged ovum can't enter the tube. Dye can be injected into the uterus to assess tubal patency. The laparoscope can also be used to examine the fimbria (the fingerlike projections in the fallopian tubes that accept the ovum as it's released from the ovary and heads towards the fallopian tubes). If PID has damaged them, normal conception is unlikely.

Complications of laparoscopy include excessive bleeding, abdominal cramps and shoulder pain resulting from the abdomen being inflated with carbon dioxide.

Hysteroscopy

A hysteroscopy is the visualisation of the uterus through insertion of a hysteroscope. A hysteroscope is a thin, hollow, fibre-optic tube that's inserted through the vagina and cervix into the uterus. This procedure is done to remove uterine polyps and small fibroid tumours.

Further information about infertility, investigations and treatment can be obtained from the Human Fertilisation and Embryology Authority at admin@hfea.gov.uk

Quick quiz

1. Which family planning method requires assessment of the quality of cervical mucus throughout the menstrual cycle?
    A.   Rhythm method
    B.   Coitus interruptus
    C.   Billings method
    D.   Basal body temperature

Answer: C. The Billings method requires assessment of cervical mucus, which is minimal and not stretchy until ovulation occurs. At the time of ovulation, the cervical mucus is present in greater quantity, is stretchy and is more favourable to penetration by sperm.

2. A vasectomy is considered 100% effective after:
    A.   approximately 2 weeks.
    B.   approximately 4 weeks.
    C.   two consecutive sperm counts show zero sperm.
    D.   six consecutive sperm counts show zero sperm.

Answer: C. A vasectomy is considered 100% effective after two consecutive sperm counts show zero sperm. Some sperm remain in the proximal vas deferens after vasectomy. It may take up to several months to clear the proximal ducts of sperm.

3. Which woman is the best candidate for using an IUCD?
    A.   A woman with Wilson's disease.
    B.   A mother of two with no history of PID.
    C.   A mother of one who has a history of severe dysmenorrhoea.
    D.   A 35-year-old woman with recent PID.

Answer: B. An IUCD is an optimal contraceptive for a woman who has no history of PID, dysmenorrhoea or previous IUCD failures.

4. A 20-year-old woman arrives at a family planning clinic seeking emergency contraception 48 hours after she had unprotected sexual intercourse. The nurse correctly responds by saying:

    A.   'Come right in so we can get you started'.

    B.   'You must wait 72 hours before the pill will work'.

    C.   'You need to wait until you have missed your period'.

    D.   'The pills must be started the morning after intercourse'.

Answer: A. The first dose of hormones must be taken within 72 hours of sexual intercourse.

5. A 38-year-old woman asks about IVF-ET. Which statement about IVF-ET is correct ?

    A.   Oocytes are retrieved from the ovary, placed in a catheter with washed motile sperm and transferred into the fallopian tube.

    B.   An indication for this procedure would be unexplained infertility with normal tubal anatomy and patency and absence of previous tubal disease.

    C.   The woman's ova are collected from the ovaries, fertilised in the laboratory with sperm and transferred to her uterus after normal embryo development has occurred.

    D.   Blastocytes are retrieved from the ovary and transferred into the fallopian tube.

Answer: C. IVF-ET refers to fertilisation of the ovum in a laboratory. The woman's ova are collected from the ovaries, fertilised in the laboratory with sperm and transferred to her uterus after normal embryo development has occurred.

Scoring

☆☆☆   If you answered all five questions correctly, super! Your conception of the material is right on target!

☆☆   If you answered three or four questions correctly, smile! Your planning method seems to work!

☆   If you answered fewer than three questions correctly, don't worry. Just make plans to do some extra family planning review.

4 Physiological and psychosocial adaptations to pregnancy

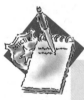

Just the facts

In this chapter, you'll learn:

♦ presumptive, probable and positive signs of pregnancy
♦ ways in which the major body systems are affected by pregnancy
♦ methods of promoting acceptance of pregnancy
♦ psychosocial changes that occur during each trimester.

A look at pregnancy changes

During pregnancy, a woman undergoes many physiological and psychosocial changes. Her body adapts in response to the demands of the growing fetus while her mind prepares for the responsibilities that come with becoming a parent. Physiological changes initially indicate pregnancy; these changes continue to affect the body throughout pregnancy as the fetus grows and develops. Psychosocial changes occur in both the mother and father and may vary from trimester to trimester.

Physiological signs of pregnancy

Pregnancy produces several types of physiological changes that must be evaluated before a definitive diagnosis of pregnancy is made. The changes can be:
- presumptive (subjective)
- probable (objective)
- positive.

Neither presumptive nor probable signs confirm pregnancy because both can be caused by other medical conditions; they simply suggest pregnancy, especially when several are present at the same time. (See *Making sense out of pregnancy signs*, pages 95 and 96.)

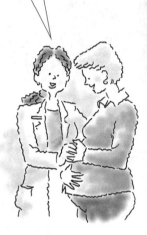

Women can expect a wide range of changes during pregnancy – good practice for all those nappy changes once the baby is born!

Presumptive signs of pregnancy

Presumptive signs of pregnancy are those that can be assumed to indicate pregnancy until more concrete signs develop. These signs include breast changes, nausea and vomiting, amenorrhoea, urinary frequency, fatigue, uterine enlargement, quickening and skin changes. A pregnant woman typically reports some presumptive signs.

Breast changes
Tingling, tender or swollen breasts can occur as early as a few days after conception. The areola may darken and tiny glands around the nipple, called *Montgomery's tubercles*, may become elevated.

Nausea and vomiting
At least 50% of pregnant women experience nausea and vomiting early in pregnancy (commonly called *morning sickness*). These symptoms are typically the first sensations experienced during pregnancy. Nausea and vomiting

Memory jogger

To remember the three categories of pregnancy signs, think of the three **Ps:**

Presumptive – Think of a presumptive sign as one that suggests, 'If I had to guess, I'd say yes!'

Probable – Think of a probable sign as one that means, this lady is most likely going to give birth!

Positive – Think of a positive sign as one that confirms, in about 9 months, this woman is going to have a baby!

Making sense out of pregnancy signs

This chart classifies the signs of pregnancy into three categories: presumptive, probable and positive.

Sign	Weeks from implantation	Other possible causes
Presumptive		
Breast changes, including feelings of tenderness, fullness or tingling, and enlargement or darkening of areola	2	• Hormonal contraceptives • Hyperprolactinaemia induced by tranquillisers • Infection • Prolactin-secreting pituitary tumour • Pseudocyesis • Premenstrual syndrome
Feeling of nausea or vomiting upon arising	2	• Gastric disorders • Infections • Psychological disorders, such as pseudocyesis and anorexia nervosa
Amenorrhoea	2	• Anovulation • Blocked endometrial cavity • Endocrine changes • Illness • Medications (phenothiazines, Depo-Provera) • Metabolic changes • Stress
Frequent urination	3	• Emotional stress • Pelvic tumour • Renal disease • Urinary tract infection
Fatigue	12	• Anaemia • Chronic illness • Depression • Stress
Uterine enlargement in which the uterus can be palpated over the symphysis pubis	12	• Ascites • Obesity • Uterine or pelvic tumour
Quickening (fetal movement felt by the woman)	18	• Excessive flatus • Increased peristalsis
Linea nigra (line of dark pigment on the abdomen)	24	• Cardiopulmonary disorders • Oestrogen–progestin hormonal contraceptives • Obesity • Pelvic tumour
Melasma or chloasma (dark pigment on the face)	24	• Cardiopulmonary disorders • Oestrogen–progestin hormonal contraceptives • Obesity • Pelvic tumour

(continued)

Making sense out of pregnancy signs *(continued)*

Sign	Weeks from implantation	Other possible causes
Presumptive (continued)		
Striae gravidarum (red streaks/stretch marks on the abdomen)	24	• Cardiopulmonary disorders • Oestrogen–progestin hormonal contraceptives • Obesity • Pelvic tumour
Probable		
Serum laboratory tests revealing the presence of human chorionic gonadotropin (hCG) hormone	1	• Cross-reaction of luteinising hormone (similar to hCG) • Hydatidiform mole
Chadwick's sign (vagina changes colour from pink to violet)	6	• Hyperaemia of cervix, vagina or vulva
Goodell's sign (cervix softens)	6	• Oestrogen–progestin hormonal contraceptives
Hegar's sign (lower uterine segment softens)	6	• Excessively soft uterine walls
Sonographic evidence of gestational sac in which characteristic ring is evident	6	None
Ballottement (fetus can be felt to rise against abdominal wall when lower uterine segment is tapped on during bimanual examination)	16	• Ascites • Uterine tumour or polyps
Braxton Hicks contractions (periodic uterine tightening)	20	• GI distress • Haematometra • Uterine tumour
Palpation of fetal outline through abdomen	20	• Subserous uterine myoma
Positive		
Sonographic evidence of fetal outline	8	None
Fetal heart audible by Doppler ultrasound	10–12	None
Palpation of fetal movement through abdomen	20	None

usually begin at 4–6 weeks' gestation. These symptoms usually stop at the end of the first trimester, but they may last slightly longer in some women.

Amenorrhoea

Amenorrhoea is the cessation of menses. For a woman who has regular menses, this may be the first indication that she's pregnant.

Urinary frequency

A pregnant woman may notice an increase in urinary frequency during the first 3 months of pregnancy. This symptom continues until the uterus rises out of the pelvis and relieves pressure on the bladder. Urinary frequency may return at the end of pregnancy as lightening occurs (the fetal head exerts renewed pressure on the bladder).

Fatigue

A pregnant woman may report that she's often fatigued. During the first trimester, the woman's body works hard to manufacture the placenta and to adjust to the many other physical demands of pregnancy, while she mentally and emotionally prepares for motherhood. Around 16 weeks' gestation, the body has adjusted to the pregnancy, the placenta's development is complete and the woman should start to have more energy.

Uterine enlargement

Softening of the uterus and fetal growth cause the uterus to enlarge and stretch the abdominal wall.

Quickening

Quickening is recognisable movements of the fetus. It can occur anywhere between the 14th and 26th weeks of pregnancy, but typically it is noticed between weeks 18 and 22.

Fluttering flutterflies

To the woman, quickening may feel like fluttering movements in her lower abdomen.

Skin changes

Numerous skin changes occur during pregnancy, including those listed here:
* *Linea nigra* refers to a dark line that extends from the umbilicus or above to the mons pubis. In the primigravida, this line develops at approximately the third month of pregnancy. In the multiparous woman, linea nigra typically appears before the third month. (See *Skin changes during pregnancy*, page 98.)
* *Melasma*, also known as *chloasma* or the 'mask of pregnancy', refers to darkened areas that may appear on the face, especially on the cheeks and across the nose. Melasma appears after the 16th week of pregnancy and gradually becomes more pronounced. After childbirth, it typically fades.
* *Striae gravidarum* refers to red or pinkish streaks that appear on the sides of the abdominal wall and sometimes on the thighs. In the multiparous woman, these striae are more sliver in colour.

Probable signs of pregnancy

Probable signs of pregnancy strongly suggest pregnancy. They're more reliable indicators of pregnancy than presumptive signs, but they can also be explained by other medical conditions. Probable signs include positive laboratory tests, such as serum and urine tests; positive results on a home pregnancy test; Chadwick's sign; Goodell's sign; Hegar's sign; sonographic evidence of a gestational sac; ballottement and Braxton Hicks contractions.

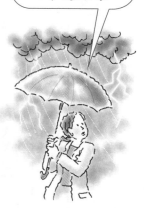

When it rains, it pours! Urinary frequency may increase during the first 3 months of pregnancy – and again at the end of pregnancy.

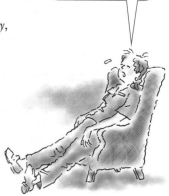

Pregnancy can be tiring – especially during the first 16 weeks.

Skin changes during pregnancy

Linea nigra and striae gravidarum are two skin changes that occur during pregnancy. Both fade after pregnancy, with striae gravidarum fading to glistening silvery lines.

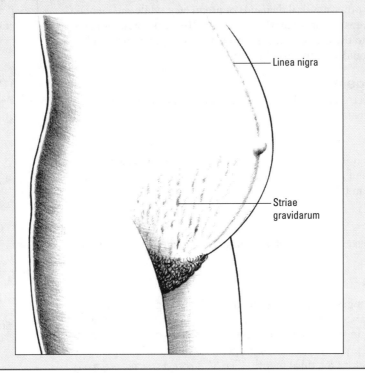

Linea nigra

Striae gravidarum

Laboratory tests

Laboratory tests for pregnancy are used to detect the presence of human chorionic gonadotropin (hCG) – a hormone created by the chorionic villi of the placenta – in the urine or blood serum of the woman. Because hCG is produced by trophoblast cells – preplacental cells that wouldn't be present in a nonpregnant woman – detection of hCG is considered a sign of pregnancy. Because laboratory tests for diagnosing pregnancy are accurate only 95–98% of the time, positive hCG results are considered probable rather than positive.

Looking for hCG in all the right places

Tests for hCG include radioimmunoassay, enzyme-linked immunosorbent assay and radioreceptor assay. For these tests, hCG is measured in milli-international units (mIU). In pregnant women, trace amounts of hCG appear in the serum as early as 24–48 hours after implantation of the fertilised ovum.

They reach a measurable level of about 50 mIU/ml between 7 and 9 days after conception. Levels peak at about 100 mIU/ml between the 60th and 80th days of gestation. After this point, the level declines. At term, hCG is barely detectable in serum or urine.

Home pregnancy tests

Home pregnancy tests, which are available over the counter, are 97% accurate when performed correctly. They're convenient and easy to use, taking only 3–5 minutes to perform.

Here's how the home pregnancy test works:
- A reagent strip is dipped into the urine stream.
- A colour change on the strip denotes pregnancy.

Most manufacturers suggest that a woman waits until the day of the missed menstrual period to test for pregnancy.

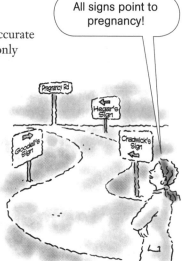

Hegar's sign

Hegar's sign is a softening of the uterine isthmus that can be felt on bimanual examination at 6–8 weeks' gestation. As pregnancy advances, the isthmus becomes part of the lower uterine segment. During labour, it expands further.

Ultrasonography

Ultrasonography, or sonographic evaluation, can detect probable and positive signs of pregnancy. At 4–6 weeks' gestation, a characteristic ring indicating the gestational sac is visible on sonographic evaluation.

Ballottement

Ballottement is passive movement of the fetus. It can be identified at 16–18 weeks' gestation.

Braxton Hicks contractions

Braxton Hicks contractions are uterine contractions that begin early in pregnancy and become more frequent after 28 weeks' gestation. Typically, they result from normal uterine enlargement that occurs to accommodate the growing fetus. Sometimes, however, they may be caused by a uterine tumour.

Positive signs of pregnancy

Positive signs of pregnancy include sonographic evidence of the fetal outline, an audible fetal heart rate and fetal movement that's felt by the examiner. These signs confirm pregnancy because they can't be attributed to other conditions.

Ultrasonography

Ultrasonography can confirm pregnancy by providing an image of the fetal outline, which can typically be seen by the 8th week. The fetal outline on the ultrasound is so clear that a crown to rump measurement can be made to establish gestational age. Fetal heart movement may be visualised as early as 7 weeks' gestation.

Audible fetal heart rate

Fetal heart rate can be confirmed by auscultation or visualisation during an ultrasound. Fetal heart sounds may be heard as early as the 10th to 12th week by Doppler ultrasonography.

Fetal movement

Even though the pregnant woman can feel fetal movement at a much earlier date (usually around 16–20 weeks), other people aren't able to feel fetal movement until the 20th to 24th week. Obese women may not feel fetal movement until later in pregnancy because of excess adipose tissue.

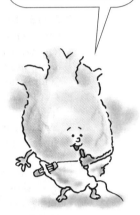

Physiological changes in body systems

As the fetus grows and hormones shift during pregnancy, physiological adaptations occur in every body system to accommodate the fetus. These changes help a pregnant woman to maintain health throughout the pregnancy and to physically prepare for childbirth. Physiological changes also create a safe and nurturing environment for the fetus. Some of these changes take place even before the woman knows that she's pregnant.

Reproductive system

In addition to the physical changes that initially indicate pregnancy, such as Hegar's sign and Goodell's sign, the reproductive system undergoes significant changes throughout pregnancy.

Out and about

External reproductive structures affected by pregnancy include the labia majora, labia minora, clitoris and vaginal introitus. These structures enlarge because of increased vascularity. Fat deposits also contribute to the enlargement of the labia majora and labia minora. These structures reduce in size after childbirth, but may not return to their pre-pregnant state because of loss of muscle tone or perineal injury (such as from a vaginal tear or an episiotomy). For example, in many women, the labia majora remain separated and gape after childbirth. In addition, varices may be caused by pressure on vessels in the perineal and perianal areas.

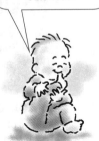

The inside story

Internal reproductive structures, including the ovaries, uterus and other structures, change dramatically to accommodate the developing fetus. These internal structures may not regain their pre-pregnant states after childbirth.

Ovaries

When fertilisation occurs, ovarian follicles cease to mature and ovulation stops. The chorionic villi, which develop from the fertilised ovum, begin to produce hCG to maintain the ovarian corpus luteum. The corpus luteum produces oestrogen and progesterone until the placenta is formed and functioning. At 8–10 weeks' gestation, the placenta assumes production of these hormones. The corpus luteum, which is no longer needed, then degrades into a corpus albicus.

Uterus

In a nonpregnant woman, the uterus is smaller than the size of a fist, measuring approximately 7.5 cm × 5 cm × 2.5 cm. It can weigh 60–70 g in a nulliparous woman (a woman who has never been pregnant) and 100 g in a parous woman (a woman who has given birth). In a nonpregnant state, a woman's uterus can hold up to 10 ml of fluid. Its walls are composed of several overlapping layers of muscle fibres that adapt to the developing fetus and help in expulsion of the fetus and placenta during labour and childbirth.

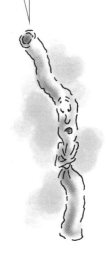

Look out! Pressure on vessels in the perineal area can cause varices.

More strength, more stretch

After conception, the uterus retains the developing fetus for approximately 280 days, or 9 calendar months. During this time, the uterus undergoes progressive changes in size, shape and position in the abdominal cavity. In the first trimester, the pear-shaped uterus lengthens and enlarges in response to elevated levels of oestrogen and progesterone. This hormonal stimulation primarily increases the size of myometrial cells (hypertrophy), although a small increase in cell number (hyperplasia) also occurs. These changes increase the amount of fibrous and elastic tissue to more than 20 times that of the nonpregnant uterus. Uterine walls become stronger and more elastic.

During the first few weeks of pregnancy, the uterine walls remain thick and the fundus rests low in the abdomen. The uterus can't be palpated through the abdominal wall. After 12 weeks of pregnancy, however, the uterus typically reaches the level of the symphysis pubis (the joint at the pubic bone) and then may be palpated through the abdominal wall.

Shape shifters

In the second trimester, the corpus and fundus become globe shaped. As pregnancy progresses, the uterus lengthens and becomes oval in shape. The uterine walls thin as the muscles stretch; the uterus rises out of the pelvis, shifts to the right and rests against the anterior abdominal wall. At 20 weeks' gestation, the uterus is palpable just below the umbilicus and reaches the umbilicus at 22 weeks' gestation.

Reach and descend

In the third trimester, the fundus reaches nearly to the xiphoid process (the lower tip of the breast bone) and the lower segment stretches. Between weeks 38 and 40, the fetus begins to descend into the pelvis (lightening), which causes fundal height to gradually drop. The uterus remains oval in shape. Its muscular walls become progressively thinner as it enlarges, finally reaching a muscle wall thickness of 5 mm or less. At term (40 weeks), the uterus typically weighs approximately 1,100 g, holds 5–10 L of fluid and has stretched to approximately 28 cm × 24 cm × 21 cm. (See *Fundal height throughout pregnancy*.) The lower uterine segment stretches too.

Endometrial development

During the menstrual cycle, progesterone stimulates increased thickening and vascularity of the endometrium, preparing the uterine lining for implantation and nourishment of a fertilised ovum. After implantation, menstruation stops.

Fundal height throughout pregnancy

This illustration shows approximate fundal heights at various times during pregnancy. The times indicated are in weeks. Note that between weeks 38 and 40, the fetus begins to descend into the pelvis.

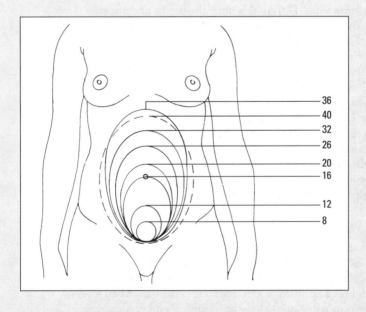

The endometrium then becomes the decidua, which is divided into three layers:

 decidua capsularis, which covers the blastocyst (fertilised ovum)

 decidua basalis, which lies directly under the blastocyst and forms part of the placenta

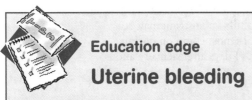 decidua vera, which lines the rest of the uterus.

Vascular growth

As the fetus grows and the placenta develops, uterine blood vessels and lymphatics increase in number and size. Vessels must enlarge to accommodate the increased blood flow to the uterus and placenta. By the end of pregnancy, an average of 500 ml of blood may flow through the maternal side of the placenta each minute. Maternal arterial pressure, uterine contractions and maternal position affect uterine blood flow throughout pregnancy.

Because one-sixth of the body's blood supply is circulating through the uterus at any given time, uterine bleeding during pregnancy is always potentially serious and can result in major blood loss. (See *Uterine bleeding*.)

Cervical changes

The cervix consists of connective tissue, elastic fibres and endocervical folds. This composition allows it to stretch during childbirth. During pregnancy, the cervix softens. It also takes on a bluish colour during the second month due to increased vascularity. It becomes oedematous and may bleed easily on examination or sexual activity.

Bacteria blocker

During pregnancy, hormonal stimulation causes the glandular cervical tissue to increase in cell number and become hyperactive, secreting thick, tenacious

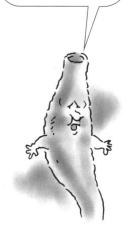

During pregnancy, it's okay for my waistline to expand a bit, too. I have to be ready to handle increased blood flow to the uterus and placenta.

Education edge

Uterine bleeding

Uterine bleeding in a pregnant woman is always potentially serious because it can result in major blood loss. She should be warned that such blood loss poses a major health risk. Advise the pregnant woman to contact her midwife, GP or obstetrician if uterine bleeding occurs.

mucus. This mucus thickens into a mucoid weblike structure, eventually forming a mucus plug that blocks the cervical canal. This creates a protective barrier against bacteria and other substances attempting to enter the uterus.

Vagina

During pregnancy, oestrogen stimulates vascularity, tissue growth and hypertrophy in the vaginal epithelial tissue. White, thick, odourless and acidic vaginal secretions increase. The acidity of these secretions helps prevent bacterial infections but, unfortunately, also fosters yeast infections, a common occurrence during pregnancy.

Other vaginal changes include:
- development of a bluish colour due to increased vascularity
- hypertrophy of the smooth muscles and relaxation of connective tissues, which allow the vagina to stretch during childbirth
- lengthening of the vaginal vault
- possible heightened sexual sensitivity.

Breasts

In addition to the presumptive signs that occur in the breasts during pregnancy (such as tenderness, tingling, darkening of the areola and appearance of Montgomery's tubercles), the nipples enlarge, become more erectile and darken in colour. The areolae widen from a diameter of less than 3 to 5 or 6 cm in the primigravid woman.

Rarely, patches of brownish discolouration appear on the skin adjacent to the areolae. These patches, known as secondary areolae, may indicate pregnancy if the woman has never breastfed an infant.

Lactation preparation

The breasts also undergo several changes in preparation for lactation. As blood vessels enlarge, veins beneath the skin of the breasts become more visible and may appear as intertwining patterns over the anterior chest wall. Breasts become fuller and heavier as lactation approaches. *They may throb uncomfortably*.

Increasing hormone levels cause the secretion of colostrum (a yellowish, viscous fluid) from the nipples. High in protein, antibodies and minerals – but low in fat and sugar relative to mature human milk – colostrum may be secreted as early as week 16 of pregnancy, but it's most common during the last trimester. It continues secreting until 2–4 days after delivery and is followed by milk production.

More change for first-timers

Breast changes are more pronounced in a primigravida woman than in a multigravida woman. In a multigravida woman, changes are even less significant if the woman has breastfed an infant within the past year because her areola are still dark and her breasts enlarged.

Endocrine system

The endocrine system undergoes many fluctuations during pregnancy. Changes in hormone levels and protein production help support fetal growth and maintain body functions.

Placenta

The most striking change in the endocrine system during pregnancy is the addition of the placenta. The placenta is an endocrine organ that produces large amounts of oestrogen, progesterone, hCG, human placental lactogen (hPL), relaxin and prostaglandins.

The oestrogen produced by the placenta causes breast and uterine enlargement as well as palmar erythema (redness in the palm of the hand). Progesterone helps maintain the endometrium by inhibiting uterine contractility. It also prepares the breasts for lactation by stimulating breast tissue development.

Relaxin is secreted primarily by the corpus luteum. It is a smooth muscle relaxant and affects the following:
- inhibits uterine activity
- helps to soften the cervix, which allows for dilation at delivery
- softens the collagen in body joints, which allows for laxness in the lower spine and helps enlarge the birth canal.

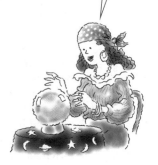

I predict palmar erythema caused by the oestrogen, produced by the placenta.

How stimulating!

Secreted by the trophoblast cells of the placenta in early pregnancy, hCG stimulates progesterone and oestrogen synthesis until the placenta assumes this role.

Alternate energy source

Also called *human chorionic somatomammotropin*, the hormone hPL is secreted by the placenta. It promotes fat breakdown (lipolysis), providing the woman with an alternate source of energy so that glucose is available for fetal growth. This hormone, however, has a complicating effect. Along with oestrogen, progesterone and cortisol, hPL inhibits the action of insulin, resulting in an increased insulin need throughout pregnancy.

Prostaglandins

Prostaglandins are found in high concentration in the female reproductive tract and the decidua during pregnancy. They affect smooth muscle contractility to such an extent that they may trigger labour at term.

Pituitary gland

The pituitary gland undergoes various changes during pregnancy. High oestrogen and progesterone levels in the placenta stop the pituitary gland from producing follicle-stimulating hormone and luteinising hormone. Increased production of growth hormone and melanocyte-stimulating hormone causes skin pigment changes.

Late-breaking developments

Late in pregnancy, the posterior pituitary gland begins to produce oxytocin, which stimulates uterine contractions during labour. Prolactin production also starts late in pregnancy as the breasts prepare for lactation after birth.

Thyroid gland

As early as the second month of pregnancy, the thyroid gland's production of thyroxine-binding protein increases, causing total thyroxine (T4) levels to rise. Because the amount of unbound T4 doesn't increase, these thyroid changes don't cause hyperthyroidism; however, they increase basal metabolic rate (BMR), cardiac output, pulse rate, vasodilation and heat intolerance. BMR increases by about 20% during the second and third trimesters as the growing fetus places additional demands for energy on the woman's system. By term, the woman's BMR may increase by 25%. It returns to the pre-pregnant level within 1 week after childbirth.

In addition to T4 level changes, increased oestrogen levels augment the circulating amounts of triiodothyronine (T3). Like the elevation of T4, the elevation of T3 levels doesn't lead to a hyperthyroid condition during pregnancy because much of this hormone is bound to proteins and, therefore, nonfunctional.

Parathyroid gland

As pregnancy progresses, fetal demands for calcium and phosphorus increase. The parathyroid gland responds by increasing hormone production during the third trimester to as much as twice the pre-pregnancy level.

Adrenal gland

Adrenal gland activity increases during pregnancy as production of corticosteroids and aldosterone escalates.

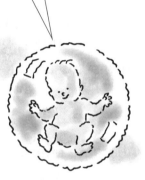

I want calcium! I want phosphorus! Hey, if you think I'm demanding now, just wait until I'm born!

Corticosteroids deployed

Some researchers believe that increased corticosteroid levels suppress inflammatory reactions and help to reduce the possibility of the woman's body rejecting the foreign protein of the fetus. Corticosteroids also help to regulate glucose metabolism in the woman.

Aldosterone zone

Increased aldosterone levels help to promote sodium reabsorption and maintain the osmolarity of retained fluid. This indirectly helps to safeguard the blood volume and provide adequate perfusion pressure across the placenta.

Pancreas

Although the pancreas itself doesn't change during pregnancy, maternal insulin, glucose and glucagon production do. In response to the additional glucocorticoids produced by the adrenal glands, the pancreas increases insulin production. Insulin is less effective than normal, however, because oestrogen, progesterone and hPL all act as antagonists to it. Despite insulin's diminished action and increased fetal demands for glucose, maternal glucose levels remain fairly stable because the mother's fat stores are used for energy.

Respiratory system

Throughout pregnancy, changes occur in the respiratory system in response to hormonal changes. These changes can be anatomical (biochemical) or functional (mechanical). As pregnancy advances, these respiratory system changes promote gas exchange, providing the woman with more oxygen.

Anatomical changes

The diaphragm rises by approximately 4 cm during pregnancy, which prevents the lungs from expanding as much as they normally do on inspiration. The diaphragm compensates for this by increasing its excursion (outward expansion) ability, allowing more normal lung expansion. In addition, the anteroposterior and transverse diameters of the rib cage increase by approximately 2 cm, and the circumference increases by 5–7 cm. This expansion is possible because increased progesterone relaxes the ligaments that join the rib cage. As the uterus enlarges, thoracic breathing replaces abdominal breathing.

All that vascularisation

Increased oestrogen production leads to increased vascularisation of the upper respiratory tract. As a result, the woman may develop respiratory congestion, voice changes and epistaxis as capillaries become engorged in the nose, pharynx, larynx, trachea, bronchi and vocal cords. Increased vascularisation may also cause the eustachian tubes to swell, leading to such problems as impaired hearing, earaches and a sense of fullness in the ears. This increased stuffiness in the nose, pharynx and larynx – combined with the pressure the enlarged uterus places on the woman's diaphragm – may make her feel as if she's short of breath.

Functional changes

Changes in pulmonary function improve gas exchange in the alveoli and facilitate oxygenation of blood flowing through the lungs. Respiratory rate typically remains unaffected in early pregnancy. By the third trimester, however, increased progesterone may increase the rate by approximately two breaths per minute.

Rising tide

Tidal volume (the amount of air inhaled and exhaled) rises throughout pregnancy as a result of increased progesterone and increased diaphragmatic excursion. In fact, a pregnant woman breathes 30–40% more air during pregnancy than she does when she isn't pregnant. Minute volume (the amount of air expired per minute) increases by approximately 50% by term.

The difference between changes in tidal volume and minute volume creates a slight hyperventilation, which decreases carbon dioxide in the alveoli. The resulting lowered partial pressure of arterial carbon dioxide in maternal blood leads to a greater partial pressure difference of carbon dioxide between fetal and maternal blood, which facilitates diffusion of carbon dioxide from the fetus.

Hyperprotective

An elevated diaphragm decreases functional residual capacity (the volume of air remaining in the lungs after exhalation), which contributes to hyperventilation. Maternal hyperventilation is considered a protective measure that prevents the fetus from being exposed to excessive levels of carbon dioxide. Vital capacity (the largest volume of air that can be expelled voluntarily after maximum inspiration) increases slightly during pregnancy. These changes, along with increased cardiac output and blood volume, provide adequate blood flow to the placenta.

Assorted aberrations

During the third month of pregnancy, increased progesterone sensitises respiratory receptors and increases ventilation, leading to a drop in carbon dioxide levels. This increases pH, which might cause mild respiratory alkalosis; however, the decreased level of bicarbonate present in a pregnant woman partially or completely compensates for this tendency.

Cardiovascular system

Pregnancy alters the cardiovascular system so profoundly that its changes would be considered pathological, and even life-threatening, outside of this situation. During pregnancy, however, these changes are vital.

Anatomical changes

The heart enlarges slightly during pregnancy, probably because of increased blood volume and cardiac output. This enlargement isn't marked and reverses after childbirth. As pregnancy advances, the uterus moves up and presses on the diaphragm, displacing the heart upward and rotating it on its long axis. The amount of displacement varies depending on the position and size of the uterus, the firmness of the abdominal muscles, the shape of the abdomen and other factors.

Auscultatory changes

Changes in blood volume, cardiac output and the size and position of the heart alter heart sounds during pregnancy.

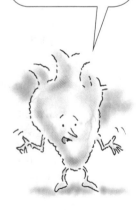

The vital changes that occur in the cardiovascular system during pregnancy would be considered life-threatening if they occurred at another time.

During pregnancy, the normal 'lub-dub' sounds may appear abnormal and murmurs or 'extra' beats may be heard on listening.

Break in rhythm

Cardiac rhythm disturbances, such as sinus arrhythmia, may occur. In the pregnant woman with no underlying heart disease, these arrhythmias don't require therapy and don't indicate the development of myocardial disease.

Haemodynamic changes

Haemodynamically, pregnancy affects heart rate and cardiac output, venous and arterial blood pressures, circulation and coagulation and blood volume.

Heart rate and cardiac output

During the second trimester, heart rate gradually increases. It may reach 10–15 beats/minute above the woman's pre-pregnancy rate. During the third trimester, heart rate may increase by 15–20 beats/minute above the woman's pre-pregnancy rate. The woman may feel palpitations occasionally throughout pregnancy; in the early months, these palpitations result from sympathetic nervous stimulation.

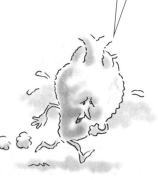

A pregnant woman's heart rate increases during the second trimester, and again during the third!

All about output

Increased tissue demands for oxygen and increased stroke volume raise cardiac output by up to 50% by the 32nd week of pregnancy. Cardiac output peaks during labour, when tissue demands are greatest.

Venous and arterial blood pressure

When the woman lies on her back, femoral venous pressure increases. This occurs because the uterus exerts pressure on the inferior vena cava and pelvic veins, slowing venous return from the legs and feet and reducing the volume of blood returning to the heart; this vaso vagal compression is sometimes known as supine or postural hypotension. The woman may feel light-headed if she rises abruptly after lying on her back. Oedema in the legs and varicosities in the legs, rectum and vulva may occur.

Progesterone to smooth muscles: Relax!

Early in pregnancy, increased progesterone levels relax smooth muscles and dilate arterioles, resulting in vasodilation. Despite the hypervolaemia that occurs during pregnancy, the woman's blood pressure doesn't normally rise because the increased action of the heart enables the body to handle the increased amount of circulating blood. In most women, blood pressure actually decreases slightly during the second trimester because of the lowered peripheral resistance to circulation that occurs as the placenta rapidly expands. Systolic and diastolic pressures may decrease by 5–10 mmHg. The pregnant woman's blood pressure is at its lowest during the second half of the second trimester; it gradually returns to first trimester levels during the third trimester. By term, arterial blood pressure approaches pre-pregnancy levels.

Position, position, position

Brachial artery pressure is lowest when the pregnant woman lies on her left side because this relieves uterine pressure on the vena cava. Brachial artery pressure is highest when the woman lies on her back (supine). The weight of the growing uterus presses the inferior vena cava against the vertebrae, obstructing blood flow from the lower extremities. This results in a decrease in blood return to the heart and, consequently, immediate decreased cardiac output and hypotension. (See *A look at supine hypotension*.)

Circulation and coagulation

Venous return decreases slightly during the eighth month of pregnancy and, at term, increases to normal levels. Blood is able to clot more easily during pregnancy and the postpartum period because of increased levels of clotting factors VII, IX and X.

Fibrin factor

Fibrinogen (a protein in blood plasma) is converted into fibrin by thrombin and is known as *coagulation factor I*. In a nonpregnant woman, levels average 250 mg/dl. In a pregnant woman, levels average 450 mg/dl, increasing as much as 50% by term. This increase

> A pregnant woman should avoid lying in a supine position. The weight of the uterus on the inferior vena cava could lead to supine hypotension.

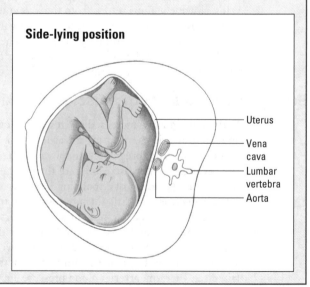

A look at supine hypotension

When a pregnant woman lies on her back, the weight of the uterus presses on the inferior vena cava and aorta, as shown below left. This obstructs blood flow to and from the legs, resulting in supine hypotension. In a side-lying position, shown below right, pressure on the vessels is relieved, allowing blood to flow freely.

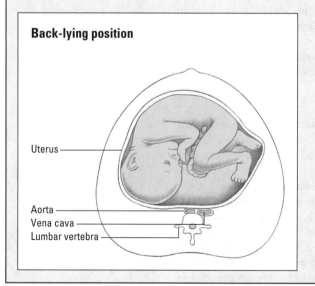

Back-lying position

Uterus

Aorta
Vena cava
Lumbar vertebra

Side-lying position

Uterus

Vena cava

Lumbar vertebra

Aorta

in the coagulation factor plays an important role in preventing maternal haemorrhage during childbirth

Blood volume

Total intravascular volume increases beginning between 10 and 12 weeks' gestation and peaks with an increase of approximately 40% between weeks 32 and 34. This increase can total 5,250 ml in a pregnant woman compared with 4,000 ml in a nonpregnant woman. Volume decreases slightly in the 40th week and returns to normal several weeks after delivery.

The ABCs of RBCs

Increased blood volume, which consists of two-thirds plasma and one-third red blood cells (RBCs), performs several functions:
- It supplies the hypertrophied vascular system of the enlarging uterus.
- It provides nutrition for fetal and maternal tissues.
- It serves as a reserve for blood loss during childbirth and puerperium.

As the plasma volume first increases, the concentration of haemoglobin and erythrocytes may decline, giving the woman physiological anaemia or pseudoanaemia. The woman's body compensates for this change by producing more RBCs. The body can create nearly normal levels of RBCs by the second trimester.

Haematological changes

Haematological changes also occur during pregnancy. Pregnancy affects iron demands and absorption as well as RBC, white blood cell (WBC) and fibrinogen levels. In addition, bone marrow becomes more active during pregnancy, producing an excess of RBCs of up to 30%.

Ironing out deficiencies

During pregnancy, the body's demand for iron increases. Not only does the developing fetus require approximately 350–400 mg of iron per day for healthy growth, but the mother's iron requirement increases as well – by 400 mg per day. This iron increase is necessary to promote RBC production and accommodate the increased blood volume that occurs during pregnancy. The total daily iron requirements of a woman and her fetus amount to roughly 800 mg. Because the average woman's store of iron is only about 500 mg, some pregnant woman may require iron supplements if they become anaemic with symptoms, e.g. fatigue, breathlessness, poor appetite and palpitations.

Iron supplements may also be necessary to accommodate for impaired iron absorption. Absorption of iron may be hindered during pregnancy as a result of decreased gastric acidity (iron is absorbed best from an acid medium). In addition, increased plasma volume (from 2,600 ml in a nonpregnant woman to 3,600 ml in a pregnant woman) is disproportionately greater than the increase in RBCs, which lowers the woman's haematocrit (the percentage of RBCs in whole blood) and may cause anaemia. Haemoglobin level also decreases. Haematocrit below 35% and haemoglobin level below 11.5 g/dl indicate pregnancy-related anaemia. Iron supplements are not prescribed in pregnancy unless clinically indicated; if the woman's haemoglobin is 11 g/dl at the first contact visit and 10.5 g/dl at 28 weeks' gestation, iron supplements may be necessary if she is symptomatic (NICE guidelines).

WBC mystery

The WBC count rises from 7,000 ml before pregnancy to 20,500 ml during pregnancy. The reason for this is unknown. The count may increase to 25,000 ml or more during labour, childbirth and the early postpartum period.

Urinary system

The kidneys, ureters and bladder undergo profound changes in structure and function during pregnancy.

Anatomical changes

Significant dilation of the renal pelves, calyces and ureters begins as early as 10 weeks' gestation, probably due to increased oestrogen and progesterone levels. As pregnancy advances and the uterus undergoes dextroversion (movement towards the right), the ureters and renal pelves become more dilated above the pelvic brim, particularly on the right side. In addition, the smooth muscle of the ureters undergoes hypertrophy and hyperplasia and muscle tone decreases, primarily because of the muscle-relaxing effects of progesterone. These changes slow the flow of urine through the ureters and result in hydronephrosis and hydroureter (distention of the renal pelves and ureters with urine), predisposing the pregnant woman to urinary tract infections (UTIs). In addition, because of the delay between urine's formation in the kidneys and its arrival in the bladder, inaccuracies may occur during clearance tests.

Maximal capacity, minimal comfort

Hormonal changes cause the bladder to relax during pregnancy, permitting it to distend to hold approximately 1,500 ml of urine. However, hormonal changes and pressure from the growing uterus cause bladder irritation, manifested as urinary frequency and urgency, even if the bladder contains little urine. Bladder vascularity increases and the mucosa bleeds easily.

When the uterus rises out of the pelvis, urinary symptoms reduce. As term approaches, however, the presenting part of the fetus engages in the pelvis, which exerts pressure on the bladder again, causing symptoms to return.

Functional changes

Pregnancy affects fluid retention; renal, ureter and bladder function; renal tubular resorption and nutrient and glucose excretion.

Fluid retention

Water is retained during pregnancy to help handle the increase in blood volume and to serve as a ready source of nutrients for the fetus. Because nutrients can only pass to the fetus when dissolved in or carried by fluid, this ready fluid supply is a fetal safeguard. This excess fluid also replenishes the mother's blood volume in case of haemorrhage.

A running theme

To provide sufficient fluid volume for effective placental exchange, a pregnant woman's total body water increases about 7.5 L from pre-pregnancy levels of 30–40 L. To maintain osmolarity, the body has to increase sodium reabsorption in the tubules. To accomplish this, the body's increased progesterone levels stimulate the angiotensin–renin system in the kidneys to increase aldosterone production. Aldosterone helps with sodium reabsorption. Potassium levels, however, remain adequate despite the increased urine output during pregnancy because progesterone is potassium sparing and doesn't allow excess potassium to be excreted in the urine.

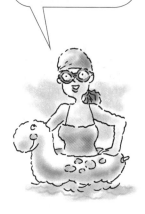

A pregnant woman's body retains water to ensure there's a medium in which nutrients can travel to get to the fetus.

Renal function

During pregnancy, the kidneys must excrete the waste products of the mother's body as well as those of the growing fetus. Also, the kidneys must be able to break down and excrete additional protein and manage the demands of increased renal blood flow. The kidneys may increase in size, which changes their structure and ultimately affects their function.

During pregnancy, urine output gradually increases to 60–80% more than pre-pregnancy output (1,500 ml/day). In addition, urine-specific gravity decreases. The glomerular filtration rate (GFR) and renal plasma flow (RPF) begin to increase in early pregnancy to meet the increased needs of the circulatory system. By the second trimester, the GFR and RPF have increased by 30–50% and remain at this level for the duration of the pregnancy. This rise is consistent with that of the circulatory system increase, peaking at about 24 weeks' gestation. This efficient GFR level leads to lowered blood urea nitrogen and lowered creatinine levels in maternal plasma.

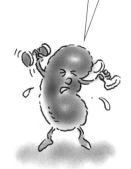

During pregnancy, I put in a double workout of excreting maternal AND fetal waste.

Glucose spill

An increased GFR leads to increased filtration of glucose into the renal tubules. Because reabsorption of glucose by the tubule cells occurs at a fixed rate, glucose sometimes is excreted, or spills, into urine during pregnancy. (See *When glucose enters urine*, page 114.) Lactose, which is being produced by the mammary glands during pregnancy but isn't being used, also spills into the urine.

Ureter and bladder function

During pregnancy, the uterus is pushed slightly towards the right side of the abdomen by the increased bulk of the sigmoid colon. The pressure on the right

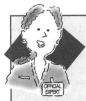

Advice from the experts

When glucose enters urine

During each antenatal visit, the woman's urine should be checked for glucose. A finding of more than a trace of glucose in a routine sample of urine from a pregnant woman is considered abnormal until proven otherwise.

Glycosuria on two consecutive occasions that isn't related to carbohydrate intake warrants further investigation. It may indicate gestational diabetes. Such a finding should be reported to the obstetrician or general practitioner. In many cases, an oral glucose screening test is ordered. A small percentage of women have glycosuria of pregnancy that isn't diabetes related but is due to a decreased kidney threshold for glucose.

Most women have a blood sample taken for glucose levels at their first booking-in visit.

ureter caused by this movement may lead to urinary stasis and pyelonephritis (inflammation of the kidney caused by bacterial infection). Pressure on the urethra may lead to poor bladder emptying and possible bladder infection, which can become more dangerous if it results in kidney infection. Infection in the kidneys, which serve as the filtering system for toxins in the blood, can be extremely dangerous to the mother. UTIs are also potentially dangerous to the fetus because they're associated with preterm labour.

Renal tubular resorption

To maintain sodium and fluid balance, renal tubular resorption increases by as much as 50% during pregnancy. The woman's sodium requirement increases because she needs more intravascular and extracellular fluid. She may accumulate 6.2–8.5 L of water to meet her needs and those of the fetus and placenta. Up to 75% of maternal weight gain is due to increased body water in the extracellular spaces. Amniotic fluid and the placenta account for about one-half of this amount; increased maternal blood volume and enlargement of the breasts and uterus account for the rest.

Posture of elimination

Late in pregnancy, changes in the woman's posture affect sodium and water excretion. For example, the woman excretes less when lying on her back because the enlarged uterus compresses the vena cava and aorta, causing decreased cardiac output. This decreased cardiac output reduces renal blood flow, which in turn decreases kidney function. The woman excretes more when lying on her left side because, in this position, the uterus doesn't compress the great vessels and cardiac output and kidney function remain unchanged.

Nutrient and glucose excretion

A pregnant woman loses increased amounts of some nutrients, such as amino acids, water-soluble vitamins, folic acid and iodine. Proteinuria (protein in the urine) can occur during pregnancy because the filtered load of amino acids may exceed the tubular reabsorptive capacity. When the renal tubules can't reabsorb the amino acids, protein may be excreted in small amounts in the woman's urine. Values of +1 protein on a urine dipstick aren't considered abnormal until the levels exceed 300 mg/24 hours. Glycosuria (glucose in the urine) may also occur as GFR increases without a corresponding increase in tubular resorptive capacity.

> Use it or lose it! My tubules can't reabsorb amino acids, so I have to excrete protein in the urine.

GI system

Changes during pregnancy affect anatomical elements in the gastrointestinal (GI) system and alter certain GI functions. These changes are associated with many of the most commonly discussed discomforts of pregnancy.

Anatomical changes

The mouth, stomach, intestines, gallbladder and liver are affected during pregnancy. (See *Crowding of abdominal contents*, page 116.)

Mouth

The salivary glands become more active in the pregnant woman, especially in the latter half of pregnancy. The gums become oedematous and bleed easily because of increased vascularity.

Stomach and intestines

As progesterone increases during pregnancy, gastric tone and motility decrease, thus slowing the stomach's emptying time and possibly causing regurgitation and reflux of stomach contents. This may cause the woman to complain of heartburn. Progesterone also makes smooth muscle – including that which appears in the intestine – less active.

Make room for the uterus

As the uterus enlarges, it tends to displace the stomach and intestines towards the back and sides of the abdomen. About halfway through the pregnancy, the pressure may be sufficient enough to slow intestinal peristalsis and the emptying time of the stomach, leading to heartburn, constipation and flatulence. Relaxin may contribute to decreased gastric motility, which may cause a decrease in blood supply to the GI tract as blood is drawn to the uterus.

The enlarged uterus also displaces the large intestine and puts increased pressure on veins below the uterus. This may predispose the woman to haemorrhoids.

Gallbladder and liver

As smooth muscles relax, the gallbladder empties sluggishly. This can lead to reabsorption of bilirubin into the maternal bloodstream, causing subclinical

> I can tell them not to push, but I know it's no use. Crowding of abdominal contents occurs late in pregnancy as a result of uterine enlargement.

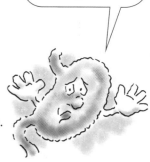

Crowding of abdominal contents

As the uterus enlarges as a result of the growing fetus, the intestinal contents are pushed upward and to the side. The uterus usually remains midline, although it may shift slightly to the right because of the increased bulk of the sigmoid colon on the left.

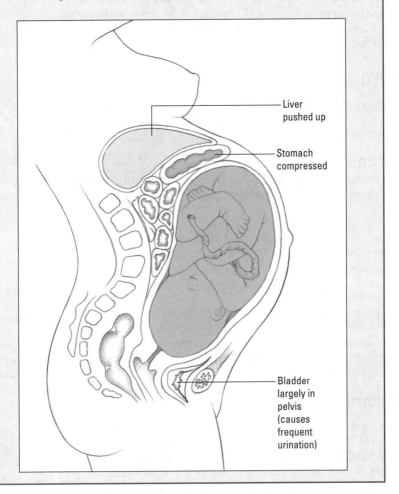

Liver pushed up

Stomach compressed

Bladder largely in pelvis (causes frequent urination)

jaundice (generalised itching). A woman who has had previous gallstone formation may have an increased tendency for stone formation during pregnancy as a result of the increased plasma cholesterol level and additional cholesterol incorporated in bile. A woman with a peptic ulcer generally finds her condition improved during pregnancy because *the acidity of the stomach decreases*.

Biliary overtime

The liver doesn't enlarge or undergo major changes during pregnancy. However, hepatic blood flow may increase slightly, causing the liver's workload to increase as BMR increases. Factors within the liver as well as increased oestrogen and progesterone decrease bile flow.

Some liver function studies show drastic changes during pregnancy, possibly caused by increased oestrogen levels. Test results may show:
• doubled alkaline phosphatase levels, caused in part by increased alkaline phosphatase isoenzymes from the placenta
• decreased serum albumin
• increased plasma globulin levels, causing decreases in albumin globulin ratios
• decreased plasma cholinesterase levels.

These changes would suggest hepatic disease in a nonpregnant woman but are considered normal in the pregnant woman.

Functional changes

Nausea and vomiting during pregnancy may affect appetite and food consumption, even when the woman's energy demand increases.

Appetite and food consumption

A pregnant woman's appetite and food consumption fluctuate. This may be due to several things. For example, she may experience nausea and vomiting that decrease her appetite and, therefore, food consumption. These symptoms are more noticeable in the morning when the woman first arises, hence the term *morning sickness*. Nausea and vomiting can also occur when the woman experiences fatigue, and may be more frequent if she smokes. Nausea and vomiting tend to be noticeable when hCG and progesterone levels begin to rise. These conditions may also be a reaction to decreased glucose levels (because glucose is being used in great quantities by the growing fetus) or increased oestrogen levels.

In addition to the reduced appetite caused by nausea and vomiting, increased hCG levels and changes in carbohydrate metabolism may also reduce the woman's appetite. When nausea and vomiting stop, her appetite and metabolic needs increase.

Carbohydrate, lipid and protein metabolism

The woman's carbohydrate needs rise to meet increasing energy demands; she needs more glucose, especially during the second half of pregnancy. Plasma lipid levels increase starting in the first trimester, rising at term to 40–50% above pre-pregnancy levels. Cholesterol, triglyceride and lipoprotein levels increase as well. The total concentration of serum proteins decreases, especially serum albumin and, perhaps, gamma globulin. The primary immunoglobulin transferred to the fetus is lowered in the woman's serum.

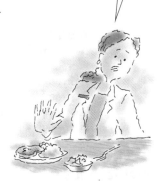

Nausea and vomiting may decrease a pregnant woman's appetite and food consumption.

Musculoskeletal system

The woman's musculoskeletal system changes in response to hormones, weight gain and the growing fetus. These changes may affect her gait, posture and comfort. In addition, increased maternal metabolism creates the need for greater calcium intake. If the woman ingests insufficient calcium, hypocalcaemia and muscle cramps may occur. Musculoskeletal changes during pregnancy include changes to the skeleton, muscles and nerves.

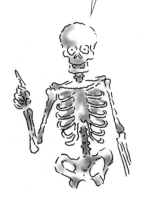

Pregnancy can make my joints relax.

Skeleton

The enlarging uterus tilts the pelvis forward, shifting the woman's centre of gravity. The lumbosacral curve increases, accompanied by a compensatory curvature in the cervicodorsal region. The lumbar and dorsal curves become even more pronounced as breasts enlarge and their weight pulls the shoulders forward, producing a stoop-shouldered stance. Increasing sex hormones (and possibly the hormone relaxin) relax the sacroiliac, sacrococcygeal and pelvic joints. These changes cause marked alterations in posture and gait. Relaxation of the pelvic joints may also cause the woman's gait to change. Shoe and ring sizes tend to increase because of weight gain, hormonal changes and dependent oedema. Although these changes may persist after childbirth, in most cases, they return to pre-pregnancy states.

Muscles

In the third trimester, the prominent rectus abdominis muscles (rectus muscles of the abdomen) separate, allowing the abdominal contents to protrude at the midline. Occasionally, the abdominal wall may not be able to stretch enough and the rectus muscles may actually separate, a condition known as *diastasis* (also called diverification of the rectus abdominus). If this happens, a bluish groove appears at the site of separation after pregnancy.

Inny to outty

The umbilicus is stretched by pregnancy to such an extent that, by the week 28 of gestation, its depression becomes obliterated and smooth because it has been pushed so far outward. In some women, it may appear as if it has turned inside out, protruding as a round bump at the centre of the abdominal wall.

Nerves

In the third trimester, carpal tunnel syndrome may occur when the median nerve of the carpal tunnel of the wrist is compressed by oedematous surrounding tissue. The woman may notice tingling and burning in the dominant hand, possibly radiating to the elbow and upper arm. Numbness or tingling in the hands also may result from pregnancy-related postural changes such as slumped shoulders that pull on the brachial plexus.

The Skin

Skin changes vary greatly among pregnant women. Of those who experience skin changes, the women with brown hair typically show more marked changes.

Because some skin changes may remain after childbirth, they aren't considered important signs of pregnancy in a woman who has given birth before. Skin changes associated with pregnancy include striae gravidarum, pigment changes, vascular markings and other changes.

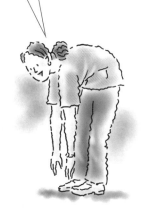

Stretch marks are most common on the skin covering the breasts, abdomen, buttocks and thighs.

Striae gravidarum

The woman's weight gain and enlarging uterus, combined with the action of adrenocorticosteroids, lead to stretching of the underlying connective tissue of the skin, creating striae gravidarum in the second and third trimesters. Better known as *stretch marks*, striae on light-skinned women appear as pink or slightly reddish streaks with slight depressions; on dark-skinned women, they appear lighter than the surrounding skin tone. They develop most commonly on the skin covering the breasts, abdomen, buttocks and thighs. After labour, they typically grow lighter until they appear silvery white on light-skinned women and light brown on dark-skinned women.

Pigment changes

Pigmentation begins to change at approximately 8 weeks' gestation, partly because of melanocyte-stimulating and adrenocorticotropic hormones and partly because of oestrogen and progesterone. These changes are more pronounced in hyperpigmented areas, such as the face, breasts (especially nipples), axillae, abdomen, anal region, inner thighs and vulva. Specific changes may include linea nigra and melasma.

Vascular markings

Tiny, bright-red angiomas may appear during pregnancy as a result of oestrogen release, which increases subcutaneous blood flow. They're called *vascular spiders* because of the branching pattern that extends from each spot. Occurring mostly on the chest, neck, arms, face and legs, they disappear after childbirth.

Pink-handed

Palmar erythemas, commonly seen along with vascular spiders, are well-delineated, pinkish areas over the palmar surface of the hands. When pregnancy ends and oestrogen levels decrease, this condition reverses.

Bubbled gums

Epulides, also known as *gingival granuloma gravidarum*, are raised, red, fleshy areas that appear on the gums as a result of increased oestrogen. They may enlarge, cause severe pain and bleed profusely. An epulis that grows rapidly may require excision.

Other skin changes

Nevi (circumscribed, benign proliferations of pigment-producing cells in the skin) may develop on the face, neck, upper chest or arms during pregnancy. Oily skin and acne from increased oestrogen may also occur. Hirsutism (excessive hair growth) may occur, but this reverses when pregnancy ends. By the sixth week of pregnancy, fingernails may soften and break easily – a problem that may be exacerbated by nail polish removers.

Immune system

Immunological competency naturally decreases during pregnancy, most likely to prevent the woman's body from rejecting the fetus. To the immune system, the fetus is a foreign object. In most cases, the immune system responds to foreign objects by sending defence cells that gang up on the foreign objects and try to destroy them. For certain types of foreign objects, such as a cold virus, this immune response is necessary to protect the body. In a situation such as organ transplantation, however, the person must be given medications to reduce the immune system response so that the body doesn't attack the transplant.

Make yourself at home

A similar process occurs naturally in a pregnant woman, whereby her immune system response decreases, allowing the fetus to remain. In particular, immunoglobulin G (IgG) production is decreased, which increases the risk of infection during pregnancy. A simultaneous increase in the WBC count may help to counteract the decrease in IgG response.

Neurological system

Changes in the neurological system during pregnancy are poorly defined and aren't completely understood. For most women, neurological changes are temporary and revert back to normal after pregnancy is over.

Nervous reactions

Functional disturbances called *entrapment neuropathies* occur in the peripheral nervous system as a result of mechanical pressure. In other words, nerves become trapped and pinched by the enlarging uterus and enlarged oedematous vessels, making them less functional. For example, the woman may experience meralgia paresthetica, a tingling and numbness in the anterolateral portion of the thigh that results when the lateral femoral cutaneous nerve becomes entrapped in the area of the inguinal ligaments. This feeling is more pronounced in late pregnancy, as the gravid uterus presses on the nerves and as vascular stasis occurs.

Psychosocial changes

Pregnancy and childbirth are events that deeply affect the lives of parents, partners and family members. The midwife faces many responsibilities and challenges regarding the expectant family's psychosocial care. Psychological, social, economic and cultural factors as well as family and individual influences towards sex-specific and family roles affect the parents' response to pregnancy and childbirth. All of these aspects of childbearing affect the health of the parents and their children.

Phases of acceptance

A woman's acceptance of the pregnancy can progress through different phases:
• During the first stage, called *full embodiment*, the woman may become dependent on her partner or significant others and may be introspective and calm. The woman, especially if she's a new mother, may initially feel some ambivalence about finding out that she's pregnant. She may spend the first few weeks imagining how the pregnancy will change her life. As the pregnancy progresses, however, the mother incorporates the fetus into her body image.
• Next comes the developmental stage of *fetal distinction*. In this stage, the woman starts to view her fetus as a separate individual. She begins to accept her new body image and may even characterise it as being 'full of life'. She may become closer or more dependent on her mother at this stage.
• The next stage is *role transition*. During this stage, the woman prepares to separate from, and give up her attachment, to the fetus. She may become anxious about labour and delivery. Discomfort and frustration over the awkwardness of her body may lead the woman to become impatient about the impending delivery. During this stage, she also begins to get ready for the baby and to mentally prepare for her role as mother.

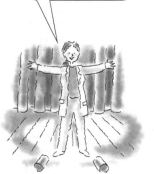

A woman's acceptance of her pregnancy can be viewed in three stages: full embodiment, fetal distinction and role transition.

Influences affecting acceptance

Such factors as cultural background, family influences and individual temperaments can affect a woman's acceptance of her pregnancy.

Cultural background
A woman's cultural background may strongly influence how she progresses through the stages of acceptance. They may also guide how actively the woman participates in her pregnancy. Certain beliefs and taboos may place restrictions on her behaviour and activities. For example, some women from ethnic minority groups may not seek antenatal care as soon as other pregnant women, because they view pregnancy as a normal condition.

Family influences
The home in which a woman was raised can also influence her beliefs about and her acceptance of pregnancy. If a woman was raised in a home in which

children were loved and viewed as pleasant additions to a happy family, she may have a more positive attitude towards pregnancy. If she was raised in a home in which children were considered intruders or were blamed for the break-up of a marriage, the woman's view of pregnancy may not be a positive one.

Like mother, like daughter

More specifically, the views of the woman's mother commonly influence her attitudes about pregnancy. If her mother hated being pregnant and always reminded her that she was a burden and that children weren't always wanted, she may view her own pregnancy in the same way. However, support and counselling may help – many women consciously choose to treat their children differently to how they were brought up.

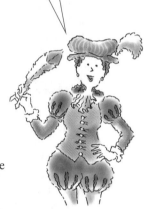

During the role transition stage, the woman begins to prepare for her new role as mother.

Individual temperament

A woman's temperament and ability to cope with or adapt to stress plays a role in how she resolves conflict and adapts to her new life after childbirth. How she accepts her pregnancy depends on her self-image and the support that's given to her. For example, a woman may view pregnancy as a situation that robs her of her career, looks and freedom; however, most women choose to be pregnant and may see it more as another facet of womanhood and an opportunity to nurture new life whilst building a family. By planning the pregnancy she will have the baby at a time in her life and her career that is suited to both her and her partner.

Make room for daddy?

A woman's relationship with the child's father also influences her acceptance of the pregnancy. If the father is there to provide emotional support, acceptance of the pregnancy is likely to be easier for the woman than if he isn't a part of the pregnancy. Whether the father of the child is able to accept the pregnancy depends on the same factors that affect the mother: cultural background, past experiences, relationship with family members and individual temperament.

Promoting acceptance of pregnancy

Pregnancy is a time of profound psychological, social and biological changes that affect the parents' responsibilities, freedoms, values, priorities, social status, relationships and self-images. The events of the childbearing year (9 antenatal and 3 postpartum months) also may be unpredictable.

Champion for change

The midwife must promote family adaptation to the new family member. To achieve these goals, the midwife should take steps to:
• Promote each family member's self-esteem.
• Elicit questions and concerns from the family and listen to them attentively.

- Discuss the roles and tasks for each family member, affirm their efforts and inquire about and show concern for each family member's health care needs. Make referrals as needed.
- Involve all family members in antenatal visits, as appropriate.
- Facilitate communication among family members and offer anticipatory guidance about family changes during pregnancy and the postpartum period.
- Help the woman maximise her family's positive contributions and minimise negative ones.

Good job!

- Praise the family's efforts.
- Offer books and other materials that address all family members.
- Promote the family's antenatal bonding (sometimes called *attachment*) with the fetus by sharing information about fetal development and helping the family identify fetal heart tones, position and movements. Reinforce bonding behaviours, such as patting the abdomen or talking to the fetus, by asking the woman or her partner to note and report fetal movements.

Conquering conflicts

- Facilitate conflict resolution related to pregnancy and childbirth. Help identify underlying conflicts through reflective communication, validation of feelings.
- Support adaptive coping patterns through realistic client and family education about pregnancy, childbirth and the postpartum period. Discuss childbirth and human responses accurately and realistically. Frankly discuss the challenges of parenting.

Proceed with care

- Deliver culturally sensitive midwifery care. Gather information about the family's customs and beliefs to add to assessment data and to individualise care.
- Identify personal attitudes and feelings about childbearing. Avoid imposing personal values, feelings and emotional reactions on others. Also avoid making assumptions about the woman and her preferences. Allow her to share her feelings freely.

First trimester

The mother copes with the common discomforts and changes of the first trimester; the father begins to accept the reality of the pregnancy.

Other psychosocial challenges that the parents face include maternal acceptance of physical changes and paternal acceptance of and preparation for fatherhood.

Parents experience mixed feelings in early pregnancy. Many women have unrealistic ideas about maternal instincts, expecting to feel only loving, happy thoughts about the fetus and motherhood. In fact, most women may feel some ambivalence about pregnancy and motherhood. Pregnancy involves stressful changes that force women to think and behave differently than they have in the past.

Sharing the joy (and the doubt)

Mixed feelings are very normal. Encourage the parents to communicate these feelings to each other. Partners who discuss these feelings usually can resolve their concerns and fears and enjoy the gratifications of expecting a child. When partners share feelings, they may find they're experiencing similar conflicts.

Dream a little dream

During this time, both partners may experience vivid dreams about the impending birth. The woman may recall her dreams with greater intensity, however, because she typically is awakened more often at night by heartburn, fetal activity and a need to urinate. Dreams tend to follow a predictable pattern during pregnancy. By exploring them, expectant parents can better understand themselves and any subconscious conflicts they may have.

Psychological responses to physical changes

In the early weeks of the first trimester, the woman watches for body changes that confirm her pregnancy. Her body image (her mental image of how her body looks, feels and moves, and how others see her) changes as her breasts enlarge, her menses cease and she begins to experience nausea, fatigue and waist thickening. Depending on her acceptance of the pregnancy, the woman may enjoy or dread these changes.

In the mood . . . or not!

A woman's response to the physical changes her body incurs during pregnancy, as well as other factors, can affect the sexual relationship between her and her partner. Women's sexual responses during pregnancy vary widely. Some women are too uncomfortable, due to the minor disorders of pregnancy (such as nausea and bladder irritability), to enjoy sexual intercourse. Others, especially those who have had a past spontaneous abortion, may fear fetal injury. Those who believe sex is only for procreation may feel guilty about sexual activity during pregnancy. Conversely, some women may feel sexually stimulated by the freedom from contraception, the joy of conception or the lack of pressure to avoid pregnancy or to have sex on a regular schedule to achieve pregnancy.

A man's sexual response also may change during his partner's pregnancy. Typically, the man worries about how the pregnancy will change his relationship with his partner. He may feel personally rejected when his partner's fatigue, nausea and other first trimester discomforts diminish her sexual interest. He may also fear causing spontaneous abortion or fetal injury during intercourse. These concerns may increase as the pregnancy advances.

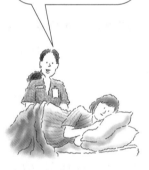

During the first trimester, it's perfectly normal for the woman to have especially vivid dreams about what's to come.

Affection prescription

Because of these fears and concerns, both partners may need extra affection from each other, especially during the first trimester. The midwife should encourage them to communicate and share their feelings and preferences about sexual activities.

Acceptance of and preparation for fatherhood

During the first trimester, the father typically finds the pregnancy unreal and untangible. The idea of the fetus may be abstract to him because he can't observe physical changes in his partner. Accepting the reality of pregnancy is the father's main psychological task in the first trimester.

You've got style

Because he isn't physically pregnant, the father can choose his degree and type of involvement in the pregnancy. There are numerous fathering styles – let's look at just a few:

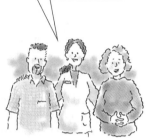

A healthy dose of affection and communication will go a long way towards helping an expectant couple to deal with their fears and concerns.

The *observer* style describes a father who's happy about the pregnancy and provides much support to his partner. However, due to personal shyness or cultural values, he doesn't participate in such activities as attending parenting education classes or helping to choose the mode of infant feeding.

The *expressive* style describes a man who shows a strong emotional response to the pregnancy and wishes to be fully involved in it. He demonstrates the same emotional ability and ambivalence as the pregnant woman and may even experience common pregnancy symptoms, such as nausea, vomiting and fatigue.

In the *instrumental* style of fathering, the man takes on the role of 'manager' of the pregnancy. He asks questions and takes pictures throughout the pregnancy, carefully plans for the birthing event, prepares to serve as labour coach and plans for the infant's arrival home. He's protective and supportive of his partner and feels responsible for the pregnancy outcome.

None of these styles is more competent or mature than another. Although each father becomes more involved as the pregnancy advances, fathering style usually remains consistent. Regardless of fathering style, the man may experience two psychosocial phenomena during the pregnancy: obsession with his role as provider and couvade symptoms (meaning, he exhibits some of the pregnancy symptoms).

Sympathy pains

Couvade syndrome describes physical symptoms – such as backache, nausea and vomiting – experienced by the man that mimic the symptoms experienced by the pregnant woman. These symptoms commonly result from stress, anxiety and empathy for the woman. Couvade symptoms aren't associated with the father's attachment to the fetus and aren't limited to first-time fathers. However, they occur most frequently in fathers who are greatly involved in the pregnancy.

Show baby the money

Because Western society values a man's provider role, the expectant father usually ponders the increased financial responsibilities a child brings. Finances remain a major focus throughout pregnancy, and the man may exert tremendous effort to attain financial security. A disproportionate emphasis on finances may reflect deep doubts about his competence as a father. The more secure he feels about his family's economic status, the more open and nurturing he may be with his partner.

Second trimester

During the second trimester, mother and father have to cope with body image and sexuality changes, and development of antenatal attachment. Parents may experience various fears. Feeling dependent and vulnerable, the woman may fear for her partner's safety. In touch with mortality, the man may consider how his death would affect his family. He may recall risks he has taken, such as driving recklessly; as a result, he may commit to being more careful to avoid the risk of abandoning his partner and fetus.

Dreams with meaning

During the second trimester, the parents' dreams may reflect concerns about the normalcy of the fetus, parental abilities, divided loyalties and related subjects. To accomplish these tasks, the couple may examine their dreams and fears.

Mother-image development

As the second trimester begins, expectant parents have completed much of the first trimester's conflicts or ambivalence. The woman has abandoned old roles and has started to determine what kind of mother she wants to be. Her mother image is a composite of mothering characteristics she has gleaned from role models, readings and her imagination.

Four aspects of the mother–daughter relationship influence the woman's mother image:

☝ her mother's availability in the past and during the pregnancy

✌ her mother's reaction to the pregnancy, her acceptance of the grandchild and her acknowledgement of her daughter as a mother

🤟 her mother's respect for the daughter's autonomy and acceptance of her as a mature adult

🖖 her mother's willingness to reminisce about her own childbearing and child-rearing experiences.

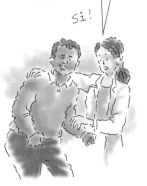

Congratulations! You're experiencing backaches and nausea and your wife is pregnant. You're the proud father of couvade symptoms.

Sí!

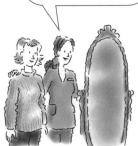

Introspection is common during the second trimester. The pregnant woman takes a good look at herself and begins to see a mother!

Expect introspection

The new mother's preoccupation with forming a mother image causes a period of introspection. As a result, she may show less affection, become more passive or withdraw from her other children, who react by becoming more demanding. Her partner also may feel neglected during this period.

Father-image development

While the woman develops her mother image, the man begins to form his father image, which is based on his relationship with his father, previous fathering experiences, the fathering styles of friends and family members and his partner's view of his role in the pregnancy.

Reach out and touch someone

As he starts to develop his father image, the man remembers his relationship with his father and sometimes increases contact with his parents. He may have difficulty viewing his father as a grandfather and coming to terms with his position as a father.

Generally, the woman's expectations about her partner's involvement and the quality of their relationship may predict the man's role in delivery and child-rearing. Some women desire privacy and modesty during childbirth and don't expect or desire to involve their partners. Others expect their partner's full involvement in tracking fetal movements, attending antenatal visits and acting as coach, advocate and primary emotional support during labour. When the woman's expectations about her partner's role don't match those of her partner, the couple may need to be referred for counselling.

Antenatal bonding

A new phase begins at approximately 17–20 weeks' gestation, when the woman feels fetal movements for the first time. Because fetal movements are a sign of good health and may dispel the fear of spontaneous abortion, the woman almost always experiences the first flutter of movement positively, even when the pregnancy is unwanted. As a result, she becomes attentive to the type and timing of movements and to fetal responses to environmental factors, such as music, abdominal strokes and meals.

Yes, sir, that's my baby

The woman may demonstrate bonding behaviours, such as stroking and patting her abdomen, talking to the fetus about eating while she eats, reprimanding the fetus for moving too much, engaging her partner in conversations with the fetus, eating a balanced diet and engaging in other health-promoting behaviours. Bonding is influenced by the woman's health, developmental stage and culture – not by obstetric complications, general anxiety or demographic variables such as socioeconomic level.

This antenatal bonding requires positive self-esteem, positive role models and acceptance of the pregnancy. Social support improves this attachment, which in turn increases the woman's feelings of maternal competence and effectiveness. In general, a woman who displays more bonding behaviours during pregnancy has more positive feelings about the neonate after delivery.

Third trimester

As the third trimester begins, the woman feels a sense of accomplishment because her fetus has reached the age of viability. She may feel sentimental about the approaching end of her pregnancy, when the mother–child relationship replaces the mother–fetus relationship. At the same time, however, she may look forward to giving birth because the last months of pregnancy involve bulkiness, insomnia, childbirth anxieties and concern about the neonate's normality.

> When parents bond with me in utero, they develop positive feelings about their roles as parents.

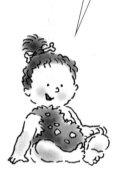

Time to address the special delivery

During the third trimester, the woman and her partner must adapt to activity changes, prepare for parenting, provide partner support, accept body image and sexuality changes, develop birth plans and prepare for labour. At this time, the woman needs to overcome any fears she may have about the unknown, labour pain, loss of self-esteem, loss of control and death.

Adaptation to activity changes

The growing fetus makes daily activities more difficult for the woman and forces her to slow down. This change can affect her emotional state and her family relationships. Decreased social support for the woman on maternity leave can add to anxiety.

> During the third trimester, it's time to prepare for the concrete realities of parenting.

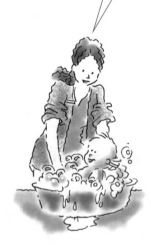

Preparation for parenting

Because the pregnant woman is more aware of what's going on in her body, she may begin to prepare for parenting before her partner. As the woman's body grows, however, typically so does the partner's acceptance of the pregnancy and anticipation of fatherhood. To prepare for parenting, the couple may now focus on concrete tasks, such as preparing the nursery, making decisions about childcare (if required) and planning postpartum events.

Partner support and nurture

The couple's ability to support each other through the childbearing cycle is paramount. In many families, men and women get their support from each other.

Easy does it

In relationships in which neither partner is dominant, there may be greater satisfaction and greater closeness during the pregnancy. Relationships that allow flexibility, growth and risk-taking ease the transition into parenthood.

Acceptance of body image and sexuality changes

A woman's body image can change as the pregnancy progresses and she gains weight. She may begin to feel less attractive. Her body image and her partner's feelings affect her sexual drive. Poor body image may cause the woman's interest in sex to drop off, or increase, depending on how she perceives herself. Some men also experience diminished sexual interest as pregnancy advances. Couples that desire sexual intimacy in the third trimester must be creative, using new positions and techniques.

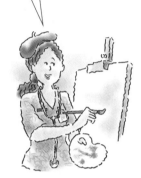

Creativity is key for the couple that wants to stay sexually intimate during the third trimester.

Preparation for labour

Childbirth education classes can prepare the woman and her partner for labour and delivery. The partner's attendance at antenatal classes and his participation in all aspects of pregnancy correlate with his degree of relationship satisfaction. Women who feel supported during the pregnancy and delivery may make the transition to motherhood more easily.

Development of birth plans

Some women, who prefer the midwife to guide them in their decision-making, may require a little more reassurance and advice to enable them to make informed decisions. A more independent woman may seek health care that's comfortable to her (and her partner) and that fits with her beliefs and knowledge, thus ensuring that her wishes are honoured during labour. It is the midwife's role to give appropriate information and guidance but ultimately the mother should be able to make informed decisions as to what she wants in labour and also for her delivery and be supported in these.

The woman ideally shapes her childbirth experience and develops realistic expectations of the event more easily when she has been given all facts. Many community midwives should discuss the woman's birth plan at 36 weeks – this can be done in the woman's home or at the antenatal clinic.

Quick quiz

1. Nausea and vomiting are common during pregnancy because of:
    A. increased progesterone levels.
    B. decreased progesterone levels.
    C. increased hCG and oestrogen levels.
    D. decreased oestrogen levels.

Answer: C. Nausea and vomiting may occur as a systemic reaction to increased hCG and oestrogen levels.

2. Which change in respiratory function during pregnancy is considered normal?

    A. Increased tidal volume
    B. Increased expiratory volume
    C. Decreased inspiratory capacity
    D. Decreased oxygen consumption

Answer: A. A pregnant woman breathes more deeply, which increases the tidal volume of gas moving in and out of the respiratory tract with each breath.

3. Decreased gastric motility may occur around mid-pregnancy because of:

    A. oestrogen.
    B. progesterone.
    C. relaxin.
    D. folic acid.

Answer: C. Relaxin (a hormone produced by the ovaries) can contribute to decreased gastric motility, which may cause a decrease in blood supply to the GI tract as blood is drawn into the uterus.

4. Which condition is common in the second trimester of pregnancy?

    A. Mastitis
    B. Metabolic acidosis
    C. Physiological anaemia
    D. Respiratory acidosis

Answer: C. Haemoglobin and haematocrit values decrease during pregnancy and the increase in plasma volume exceeds the increase in red blood cell production.

5. Which cardiac condition is normal during pregnancy?

    A. Cardiac tamponade
    B. Heart failure
    C. Endocarditis
    D. Systolic murmur

Answer: D. Systolic murmurs are heard in up to 90% of pregnant women, and the murmur disappears soon after birth.

Scoring

✩✩✩ If you answered all five questions correctly, bravo! You're a pregnancy adaptations star!

✩✩ If you answered three or four questions correctly, take a bow! Your brain has adapted to all of your new knowledge!

✩ If you answered fewer than three questions correctly, the show must go on! Do a quick review, then get ready for the next act!

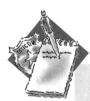

5 Antenatal care

Just the facts

In this chapter, you'll learn:

♦ components of an antenatal maternal history and physical assessment

♦ different types of antenatal testing

♦ nutritional needs of the pregnant woman

♦ common discomforts of pregnancy and ways to minimise them.

A look at antenatal care

Antenatal care is essential to the overall health of the infant and the mother. Traditional elements of antenatal care include assessing the woman, performing antenatal screening, providing nutritional care and minimising the discomforts of pregnancy. However, that isn't where antenatal care ends – or, should we say, where it begins.

Pre-pregnancy

Believe it or not, antenatal care begins long before pregnancy, when the expectant mother herself is still a child! Ideally, to reduce the risk of complications during pregnancy, a woman needs to maintain good health and nutrition throughout her life. For example, adequate calcium and vitamin D intake during the woman's infancy and childhood helps to prevent rickets, which can distort pelvic size, resulting in difficulties during birth. Maintaining immunisations protects her from viral diseases such as rubella. In addition, such healthy lifestyle practices as eating a nutritious diet, having positive attitudes about sexuality, practising safer sex and receiving prompt treatment for sexually transmitted infections (STIs) also contribute to the woman's health status throughout pregnancy.

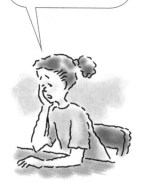

Clean your room! Do your homework! Prevent rickets? A kid's work is never done!

After the fact

Antenatal care after the woman has conceived consists of a thorough assessment, including a health history and physical examination, antenatal testing, nutritional care and reduction of discomfort. Each of these factors should be addressed at the first antenatal visit.

Occasion for education

The first antenatal visit is also the time when the pregnant woman and her family can receive information on and counselling about what to expect during pregnancy, including necessary care. This promotes the development of healthy behaviours and helps to prevent complications. Keep in mind that the client education you provide during pregnancy should vary depending on the age and parity of the woman as well as her cultural background. Warn the woman ahead of time that her first visit may be a long one.

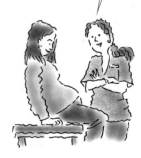

Developing and maintaining healthy behaviours during pregnancy helps prevent complications.

Assessment

The first antenatal visit is the best time to establish baseline data. A thorough assessment of the reproductive system should be included. As with other body systems, this assessment depends on an accurate history (see *Tips for a successful interview*, page 133) and a thorough physical examination.

Share and share alike

Remember to keep the woman informed about assessment findings. Sharing this information with her may help her to comply with health care recommendations and encourage her to seek additional information about any problems or questions that she has later in the pregnancy.

Health history

Information obtained from the woman's health history helps establish baseline data, which can be used to plan health-promotion strategies for every subsequent visit and identify potential complications. (See *Formidable findings*, page 134.)

The health history you conduct should be extensive. Be sure to include biographic data, information on the client's nutritional status, a medical history, a family history, a gynaecologic history and an obstetric history.

Biographic data

When obtaining biographic data, assure the woman that the information will remain confidential. Topics to discuss include age; cultural considerations, such as ethnicity and religion; marital status; occupation and education.

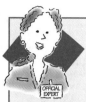

Advice from the experts

Tips for a successful interview

Here are some tips that can help you obtain an accurate and thorough client history.

Location

Pregnancy is too private to be discussed in public areas. Make every effort to interview your client in a private, quiet setting. Trying to talk to a pregnant woman in a crowded area, such as a busy waiting room in a clinic, is rarely effective. Remember client confidentiality and respect her privacy, especially when discussing intimate topics.

Checklist

To ensure that your history is complete, be sure to ask about:

- overall patterns of health and illness
- medical and surgical history
- history of pregnancy or abortion
- the date of the woman's last menses and whether her menses are regular or irregular
- sexual history, including number of partners, frequency, current method of birth control and satisfaction with chosen method of birth control
- family history
- any allergies the woman has
- health-related habits, such as smoking and alcohol use.

Age

The woman's age is an important factor because reproductive risks increase among adolescents younger than age 15 and women older than age 35. For example, pregnant adolescents are more likely to have pre-eclampsia, whereas expectant mothers older than age 35 are at risk for other problematic conditions, including placenta praevia; hydatidiform mole and vascular, neoplastic and degenerative diseases. (See Chapter 6, *High-risk pregnancy*.)

Ethnicity and religion

The woman's ethnicity and religion, as well as other cultural considerations, may also impact on the pregnancy. Obtaining information from your client about these topics can help you plan care. (See *Cultural considerations for assessment*, page 135.) It also gives you greater insight into the woman's behaviour, potential problems in health promotion and maintenance and ways of coping with illness.

It's important to learn about the cultural communities in which you work, and become familiar with the cultural practices of those communities.

Formidable findings

When performing your health history and assessment, look for the following findings to determine if a pregnant woman is at risk for complications.

Obstetric history

- History of infertility
- Grandmultiparity
- Incompetent cervix
- Uterine or cervical anomaly
- Previous preterm labour or preterm birth
- Previous caesarean birth
- Previous infant with macrosomia
- Two or more spontaneous or elective abortions
- Previous hydatidiform mole or choriocarcinoma
- Previous ectopic pregnancy
- Previous stillborn neonate or neonatal death
- Previous multiple gestation
- Previous prolonged labour
- Previous low-birthweight infant
- Previous midforceps delivery
- Diethylstilbestrol exposure in utero
- Previous infant with neurological deficit, birth injury or congenital anomaly
- Less than 1 year since last pregnancy

Medical history

- Cardiac disease
- Metabolic disease
- Renal disease
- Recent urinary tract infection or bacteriuria
- GI disorders
- Seizure disorders
- Family history of severe inherited disorders
- Surgery during current pregnancy

- Emotional disorders or learning disability
- Previous surgeries, particularly those involving the reproductive organs
- Pulmonary disease
- Endocrine disorders
- Haemoglobinopathies
- Sexually transmitted infections (STIs)
- Chronic hypertension
- History of abnormal cervical smear
- Malignancy
- Reproductive tract anomalies

Current obstetric status

- Inadequate antenatal care
- Intrauterine growth-restricted fetus
- Large-for-gestational-age fetus
- Pregnancy-induced hypertension
- Pre-eclampsia
- Abnormal test results: CTG, Cord Doppler, Liquor volume ↓
- Polyhydramnious
- Placenta praevia
- Abnormal presentation
- Maternal anaemia
- Overweight or underweight status: BMI >30 or <18
- Fetal or placental malformation
- Rh sensitisation
- Preterm labour
- Multiple gestation
- Premature rupture of membranes
- Abruptio placentae
- Postmature pregnancy
- Fibroid tumours
- Fetal manipulation

- Cervical cerclage (purse string suture placed around incompetent cervix to prevent premature opening and subsequent spontaneous abortion)
- STI
- Maternal infection
- Poor immunisation status

Psychosocial factors

- Inadequate finances
- Social problems
- Adolescent
- Poor nutrition
- More than two children at home with no additional support
- Lack of acceptance of pregnancy
- Attempt at or ideation of suicide
- Poor housing
- Lack of involvement of father of baby
- Minority status
- Antenatal occupation
- Inadequate support systems
- Dysfunctional grieving
- Psychiatric history
- Maternal age younger than 16 or older than 35

Lifestyle

- Smoking (more than ten cigarettes per day)
- Substance abuse
- Long commute to work
- Alcohol consumption
- Heavy lifting or long periods of standing
- Unusual stress
- Lack of smoke detectors in the home

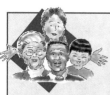

Bridging the gap

Cultural considerations for assessment

Encourage the woman to discuss her cultural beliefs regarding health, illness and health care. Be considerate of the woman's cultural background. Also, be aware that members of many cultures are reluctant to talk about sexual matters and, in some cultures, sexual matters aren't discussed freely with members of the opposite sex. It is vital that the midwife seeks the help of an interpreter when taking a history from the woman – it is not ideal to use a family member as her interpreter, as this may lead to inaccurate interpretations of the woman's true wishes when formulating her care plan.

A race to detect disease

Because some diseases are more common among certain ethnic groups, asking the client about this can be an important part of your assessment. It may help guide your antenatal screening. For example, a pregnant black woman should be screened for sickle cell trait because this trait primarily occurs in people of African or Mediterranean descent. A Jewish woman of Eastern European ancestry should be screened for Tay-Sachs disease.

Believe it or not

Religious beliefs and practices can also affect the client's health during pregnancy and can predispose her to complications. For example, women of the Seventh-Day Adventists faith traditionally exclude dairy products from their diets, and women who are of Jehovah's Witnesses faith refuse blood transfusions as well as blood products such as Anti-D. Because these practices could impact antenatal care and the client's risk of complications, you should ask about them when you take her history.

> Asking about a client's occupation will help to identify potential risks during pregnancy.

Marital status

Knowing the client's marital status may help you determine whether family support systems are available. Marital status can also provide information on the size of the woman's home, financial status and possible stress factors.

All midwives are now required to talk with the mother in private so that they have the opportunity to ask about domestic violence. It is vital the woman doesn't feel threatened or afraid to talk openly with the midwife about potential threats to her safety. The midwife has to build a relationship with the mother in a short period of time – enough to gain the mother's trust and allow her to confide in the midwife. If the mother cannot speak English it is important that an interpreter is involved – family members cannot speak for the woman in cases where violence is likely.

The mother should always be given a contact card which she can use to access a helpline in emergencies, and the issue of domestic violence should be revisited throughout her pregnancy.

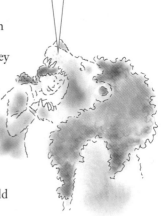

Occupation

Ask about the client's occupation and work environment to assess possible risk factors. If the woman works in a high-risk environment that exposes her to such hazards as chemicals, inhalants or radiation, inform her of the dangers of these substances as well as the possible effects on her pregnancy. Knowing the client's occupation can also help you to identify such risks as working long hours, lifting heavy objects and standing for prolonged periods.

Education

The woman's formal education and her life experiences may influence several aspects of the pregnancy, including:

- her attitude towards the pregnancy
- her willingness to seek antenatal care
- the adequacy of her at-home antenatal care and nutritional status
- her knowledge of infant care
- her emotional response to childbirth and the responsibilities of parenting.

  Obtaining information about the client's education can help you to plan appropriate teaching.

Nutritional status

Adequate nutrition is especially vital during pregnancy so it is useful to enquire as to the kind of diet the woman takes on a daily basis. For more information, see 'Nutritional care', page 161.

Medical history

When taking a medical history, find out whether the woman is taking any prescription or over-the-counter (OTC) drugs, including vitamins and herbal remedies. Also ask about her smoking practices, alcohol use and use of illegal drugs. Many drugs – except those with very large molecules, such as insulin and heparin – are able to cross the placenta and affect the fetus. All of the medications the client is currently taking (including vitamins and herbal remedies) should be carefully evaluated, and the benefits of each medication should be weighed against the risk to the fetus.

Brushing up on current events

Ask the client about previous and current medical problems that may jeopardise the pregnancy. For example:

- Diabetes can become unstable during pregnancy and harm the mother and fetus. Even a woman who has been successfully managing her diabetes may find it challenging during pregnancy because the glucose-insulin regulatory system changes during pregnancy. Every woman appears to develop insulin resistance during pregnancy. In addition, the fetus uses maternal glucose, which may lead to hypoglycaemia in the mother. When glucose regulation is poor, the mother is at risk of pregnancy-induced hypertension and infection, especially monilial infection. The fetus is at risk of abnormality, preterm delivery, asphyxia and stillbirth. Macrosomia (an abnormally large body) may also occur, resulting in an increased risk of birth complications.

- Maternal hypertension, which is more common in women with essential hypertension, renal disease or diabetes, increases the risk of abruptio placentae.
- Rubella infection during the first trimester can cause malformation in the developing fetus.
- Genital herpes can be transmitted to the neonate during birth. A woman with a history of this disease should have cultures done throughout her pregnancy and may need to deliver by caesarean birth to reduce the risk of transmission, e.g. active herpes.

Obstacle course

Specific problems that you should ask the pregnant woman about include cardiac disorders, respiratory disorders such as tuberculosis; reproductive disorders, such as STIs and endometriosis; phlebitis; epilepsy and gallbladder disorders. Also, ask the woman if she has a history of urinary tract infections (UTIs), cancer, alcoholism, smoking, drug addiction or psychiatric problems.

Consider the woman's education level when using medical or scientific terms. For example, she may answer 'No' when asked if she has hypertension, but 'Yes' when asked if she has high blood pressure.

Family history

Knowing the medical histories of the woman's family members can help you plan care and guide your assessment by identifying complications for which she may be at greater risk. For example, if the woman has a family history of varicose veins, she may inherit a weakness in blood vessel walls that becomes evident when she develops varicosities during pregnancy. Pregnancy-induced hypertension (PIH) has also been shown to have a familial tendency, so a family history of PIH means that the woman is at greater risk for this complication. Be sure to ask whether there's a family history of multiple births, abnormalities or learning disability.

Don't dismiss Dad!

When possible, obtain a medical history from the child's father as well. Note that some fetal congenital anomalies may be traced to the father's exposure to environmental hazards.

Gynaecological history

The gynaecological portion of your assessment should include a menstrual history and contraceptive history.

Menstrual history

When obtaining a menstrual history, be sure to ask the client:
- When did your last menstrual period begin?
- How many days are there between the start of one of your periods and the start of the next?
- Was your last period normal? Was the one before that normal?
- How many days does your flow usually last, and is it light, moderate or heavy?
- Have you had bleeding or spotting since your last normal menstrual period?

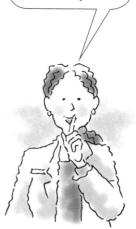

No need to whisper; menstrual and contraceptive information are important parts of a pregnant woman's history.

Contraceptive history

To obtain a contraceptive history, ask the client:
• What form of contraception did you use before your pregnancy?
• How long did you use it?
• Were you satisfied with the method?
• Did you experience any complications while on this type of birth control?

Clients who took hormonal contraceptives before becoming pregnant should be asked how long it took to become pregnant once the contraceptives were stopped.

Contraceptive catastrophes

A woman whose pregnancy results from contraceptive failure needs special attention to ensure her medical and emotional well-being. Because the pregnancy wasn't planned, the woman may have emotional and financial issues. Offering support and referring her to counsellors may help her work through these issues and resolve any ambivalence.

If the client has an intrauterine contraceptive device (IUCD) in place when she becomes pregnant, it will need to be removed immediately because of the risk of spontaneous abortion or preterm labour and delivery.

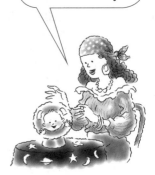

A crystal ball is fun, but *Nägele's rule* is much more reliable for calculating a client's estimated date of delivery.

Calculating estimated date of delivery

Based on information obtained in the client's menstrual history, you can calculate the estimated date of delivery (EDD) using *Nägele's rule:* first day of last normal menses, minus 3 months, plus 7 days. Because *Nägele's rule* is based on a 28-day cycle, you may need to vary the calculation for a woman whose menstrual cycle is irregular, prolonged or shortened.

Obstetric history

Obtaining an obstetric history is another important part of your assessment. The obstetric history provides important information about the client's past pregnancies. No matter what age she is, don't assume that this is her first pregnancy.

Getting the details

The obstetric history should include specific details about past pregnancies, including whether the woman had difficult or long labours and whether she experienced complications. Be sure to document each child's sex and the location and date of birth.

Do it in order

Always record the client's obstetric history chronologically. For a list of the types of information you should include in a complete obstetric history, see *Taking an obstetric history*, page 139.

Taking an obstetric history

When taking the pregnant woman's obstetric history, be sure to ask her about:

- genital tract anomalies
- medications used during this pregnancy
- history of hepatitis, pelvic inflammatory disease, acquired immunodeficiency syndrome, blood transfusions and herpes or other sexually transmitted infections (STIs)
- partner's history of STIs
- previous abortions
- history of infertility.

Pregnancy particulars

Also ask the client about past pregnancies. Be sure to note the number of past full-term and preterm pregnancies and obtain the following information about each of the past pregnancies, if applicable:

- Was the pregnancy planned?
- Did any complications – such as spotting, swelling of the hands and feet, surgery or falls – occur?
- Did the woman receive antenatal care? If so, when did she start?
- Did she take any medications? If so, what were they? How long did she take them? Why?
- What was the duration of the pregnancy?

- How was the pregnancy overall for the woman?

Birth and baby specifics

Also obtain the following information about the birth and postpartum condition of all previous pregnancies:

- What was the duration of labour?
- What type of birth was it?
- What type of anaesthesia, if any, did the woman have?
- Did the woman experience any complications during pregnancy or labour?
- Confirm the birthplace, condition, sex, weight and Rh factor of the neonate.
- Was the labour as she had expected it? Better? Worse?
- Did she have sutures after birth?
- What was the condition of the infant after birth?
- What was the infant's Apgar score?
- Was special care needed for the infant? If so, what?
- Did the neonate experience any problems during the first several days after birth?
- What's the child's present state of health?
- Was the infant discharged from the maternity unit with the mother?
- Did the woman experience any postpartum problems?

Pregnancy classification system

When referring to the obstetric and pregnancy history of a client, keep these terms in mind:

- A *primigravida* is a woman who's pregnant for the first time.
- A *primipara* is a woman who has delivered one child past the age of viability.
- A *multigravida* is a woman who has been pregnant before but may not necessarily have carried to term.
- A *multipara* is a woman who has carried two or more pregnancies to viability.
- A *nulligravida* is a woman who has never been and isn't currently pregnant.

What's your type?

In addition to asking about pregnancy history, ask the woman if she knows her blood type. If the woman's blood type is Rh-negative, ask if she received Anti-D after miscarriages, abortions or previous births so that you'll know whether Rh sensitisation occurred. If she didn't receive Anti-D after any of these situations, her present pregnancy may be at risk for Rh sensitisation again. Also ask if she's ever had a blood transfusion to establish possible risk of hepatitis B and human immunodeficiency virus (HIV) exposure.

Gravida and para

Two important components of a woman's obstetric history are her gravida and para status. *Gravida* represents the number of times the woman has been pregnant. *Para* refers to the number of children above the age of viability the woman has delivered. The age of viability is the earliest time at which a fetus can survive outside the womb, generally at age 24 weeks, at a weight of more than 400 g (14.1 oz) or showing signs of life. This information is important but provides only the most rudimentary information about the woman's obstetric history.

Preventing history from repeating itself

If the woman is a multigravida, you'll want to know about any complications that affected her previous pregnancies. A woman who has delivered one or more large neonates (more than 4.1 kg) or who has a history of recurrent Candida infections or unexplained unsuccessful pregnancies should be asked about a family history of diabetes. A history of recurrent second-trimester abortions may indicate an incompetent cervix.

Physical assessment

Physical assessment should occur throughout pregnancy, starting with the mother's first antenatal visit and continuing throughout labour, delivery and the postnatal period. Physical assessment includes evaluation of maternal and fetal well-being. At each assessment stage, keep in mind the interdependence of the mother and fetus. Changes in the mother's health may affect fetal health, and changes in fetal health may affect the mother's physical and emotional health.

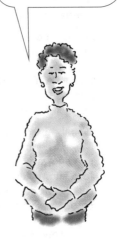

We're in this together! Changes in my health affect my baby and changes in my baby's health affect me.

Rounding the baselines

At the first antenatal visit, measurements of height and weight establish baselines for the woman and allow comparison with expected values throughout the pregnancy. (Fewer maternity units actually do this now.) Vital signs, including blood pressure and pulse rate, are also measured for baseline assessment. (See *Monitoring vital signs*, page 141.)

Scheduled surveillance

Antenatal care visits are scheduled according to the woman's parity, according to her health needs and depending on who is providing her care, e.g. midwife, obstetrician or general practitioner (GP). Women who have known risk factors for complications and those who develop complications during the pregnancy require more frequent visits and their care will be shared between the obstetrician and the physician or specialist.

Advice from the experts

Monitoring vital signs

Monitoring the woman's vital signs, especially blood pressure, during each antenatal visit is an important part of ongoing assessment. A sudden increase in blood pressure is a danger sign of gestational hypertension. Likewise, a sudden increase in pulse or respiratory rate may suggest bleeding, such as in an early placenta praevia or an abruption.

Be sure to report any of these signs or alterations in the woman's vital signs to the midwife or obstetrician, for further assessment and evaluation.

And now back to our regularly scheduled visit

Regular antenatal visits usually consist of vital sign checks, palpation of the abdomen, fundal height checks and urinalysis. You should also assess the mother for preterm labour symptoms, fetal heart rate and oedema. Also, be sure to ask her if she has felt her baby move. (See *Assessing pregnancy by weeks*, pages 142 and 143.)

Getting started

At the start of an antenatal visit, the woman should empty her bladder. Emptying the bladder makes the abdominal palpation more comfortable for her, allows for easier identification of pelvic organs and provides a urine specimen for laboratory testing.

General appearance

Inspect the woman's general appearance. This helps form an impression of the woman's overall health and well-being. The manner in which a woman dresses and speaks, in addition to her body posture, can reveal how she feels about herself. It might be useful to pick up on pallor, signs of tiredness, facial expression, e.g. anxiety. Be sure to document your findings.

Mouth

Examine the inside and outside of the mouth. Cracked corners may reveal a vitamin A deficiency. Pinpoint lesions with an erythematous base on the lips suggest herpes infection. Gingival (gum) hypertrophy may result from oestrogen stimulation during pregnancy; the gums may be slightly swollen and tender to the touch. (See *Taking care of the teeth*, page 143.)

Neck

Slight thyroid hypertrophy may occur during pregnancy because overall metabolic rate is increased. Lymph nodes normally aren't palpable and, if enlarged, may indicate an infection.

Assessing pregnancy by weeks

Here are some assessment findings you can expect as pregnancy progresses.

Weeks 1–4

- Amenorrhoea occurs.
- Breasts begin to change.
- Immunological pregnancy tests become positive: radioimmunoassay test results are positive a few days after implantation; urine human chorionic gonadotropin test results are positive 10–14 days after amenorrhoea occurs.
- Nausea and vomiting may begin between the 4th and 6th weeks.

Weeks 5–8

- Goodell's sign occurs (softening of cervix and vagina).
- Ladin's sign occurs (softening of uterine isthmus).
- Hegar's sign occurs (softening of lower uterine segment).
- Chadwick's sign appears (purple-blue colouration of the vagina, cervix and vulva).
- McDonald's sign appears (easy flexion of the fundus towards the cervix).
- Braun von Fernwald's sign occurs (irregular softening and enlargement of the uterine fundus at the site of implantation).
- Piskacek's sign may occur (asymmetrical softening and enlargement of the uterus).
- The cervical mucus plug forms.
- Uterus changes from pear shape to globular.
- Urinary frequency and urgency occur.

Weeks 9–12

- Fetal heartbeat is detected using an ultrasonic stethoscope.
- Nausea, vomiting and urinary frequency and urgency lessen.
- By the 12th week, the uterus is palpable just above the symphysis pubis.

Weeks 13–17

- Mother gains 4.5–5.5 kg during the second trimester.
- Uterine soufflé (sound made by the blood within the arteries of a gravid uterus) is heard on auscultation.

- Mother's heartbeat increases by about 10 beats/minute between 14 and 30 weeks' gestation. The rate is maintained until 40 weeks' gestation.
- By the 16th week, the mother's thyroid gland enlarges by about 25%, and the uterine fundus is palpable halfway between the symphysis pubis and the umbilicus.
- Maternal recognition of fetal movements, or quickening, occurs between 16 and 20 weeks' gestation.

Weeks 18–22

- The uterine fundus is palpable just below the umbilicus.
- Fetal heartbeats are heard with a fetoscope at 20 weeks' gestation.
- Fetal rebound or ballottement is possible.

Weeks 23–27

- The umbilicus appears to be level with abdominal skin.
- Striae gravidarum are usually apparent.
- The uterine fundus is palpable at the umbilicus.
- The shape of the uterus changes from globular to ovoid.
- Braxton Hicks contractions start.

Weeks 28–31

- The mother gains 3.5–4.5 kg in the third trimester.
- The uterine wall feels soft and yielding.
- The uterine fundus is halfway between the umbilicus and xiphoid process.
- Fetal outline is palpable.
- The fetus is mobile and may be found in any position.

Weeks 32–35

- The mother may experience heartburn.
- Striae gravidarum become more evident.
- The uterine fundus is palpable just below the xiphoid process.

Assessing pregnancy by weeks (continued)

- Braxton Hicks contractions increase in frequency and intensity.
- The mother may experience shortness of breath.

Weeks 36–40

- The umbilicus protrudes.
- Varicosities, if present, become very pronounced.

- Ankle oedema is evident.
- Urinary frequency recurs.
- Engagement, or lightening, occurs.
- The mucus plug is expelled.
- Cervical effacement and dilation begin.

Education edge

Taking care of the teeth

Advise the woman that dental hygiene and taking care of dental caries are important during pregnancy and she gets her treatment free! Dental x-rays can be taken during pregnancy as long as the woman reminds her dentist that she's pregnant and wears a lead apron. Extensive dental work requiring anaesthesia shouldn't be done during pregnancy without approval from the woman's doctor.

Breasts

During pregnancy, the areola may darken, breast size increases and breasts become firmer. Blue streaking of veins may occur on the breasts. Colostrum may leak as early as 16 weeks' gestation. Montgomery's tubercles may become more prominent.

Although the woman will not have her breasts examined at the initial visit, it is good to enquire about her choices for infant feeding and also whether she actually checks her breasts on a regular basis. If she wishes, the midwife can instruct her on how to perform a breast self-examination (BSE). Also educate her on the ongoing changes she'll experience during pregnancy, as appropriate. Some mothers will ask for advice on care of their breasts and appropriate underwear for pregnancy.

Heart

Heart rate should range from around 70 to 80 beats/minute. If the woman is considered high risk for cardiac disease then she may have her chest sounds auscultated by the doctor. Occasionally a benign functional heart murmur that's caused by increased vascular volume may be auscultated. If this occurs, the woman needs further evaluation to ensure that the condition is only a physiological change related to the pregnancy and not a previously undetected heart condition. In this instance her care will be shared between the obstetrician and the cardiologist.

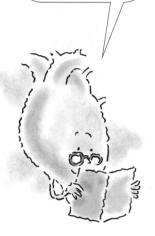

A pregnant woman's heart rate should range from around 70 to 80 beats per minute. I can handle that!

Advice from the experts

Measuring fundal height

Measuring the height of the uterus above the symphysis pubis reflects the progress of fetal growth, provides a gross estimate of the duration of pregnancy and may indicate intrauterine growth retardation (IUGR). Excessive increase in fundal height could mean a large fetus, multiple pregnancy or hydramnios (an excess of amniotic fluid), but you also need to look at the stature of the woman. How much space has she between her xiphisternum and her pelvis – how much room does the fetus have to stretch out?

A reduced increase in fundal height could mean a small fetus (SGA) due to IUGR, oligohydramnios or perhaps a transverse lie?

To measure fundal height, use a pliable (not stretchable) tape measure to measure from the notch of the symphysis pubis to the top of the fundus, without tipping back the corpus. The centimetres measured equal the number of weeks gestation, e.g. 37 cm = 37 weeks' gestation.

The uterus can be palpated at various places at differing gestations.

12 weeks – at the symphysis pubis

16 weeks – halfway between the symphysis pubis and the umbilicus

24 weeks – at the umbilicus

32 weeks – halfway between the umbilicus and the xiphisternum

36 weeks – at the xiphisternum

40 weeks – halfway between the xiphisternum and umbilicus (on the way down again!)

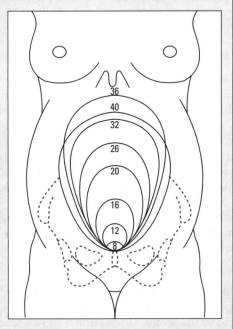

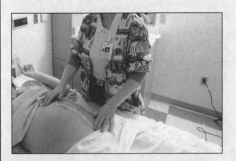

Midwives tend to use 'landmarks' on the woman's abdomen when assessing fundal height.

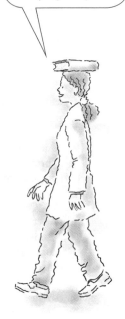

Even a 'charm-school' dropout should be taught that proper posture and walking prevent musculoskeletal and gait problems later in pregnancy.

Pelvic shape and potential problems

The shape of a woman's pelvis can affect the delivery of her fetus. Her pelvis may be one of four types.

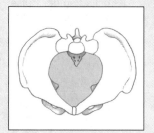 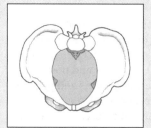 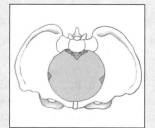 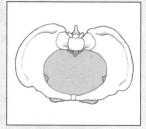

Android pelvis

In an *android* pelvis, the pelvic arch forms an acute triangle, making the lower dimensions of the pelvis extremely narrow. A pelvis of this shape is typically associated with males, but can also occur in women. A pregnant woman with this pelvic shape may experience difficulty delivering the fetus because the narrow shape makes it difficult for the fetus to exit.

Anthropoid pelvis

In an *anthropoid* pelvis, also known as an *ape-like pelvis*, the transverse diameter is narrow and the anteroposterior diameter of the inlet is larger than normal. This pelvic shape doesn't accommodate a fetal head as well as a gynecoid pelvis because the transverse diameter is narrow.

Gynecoid pelvis

In a *gynecoid* pelvis, the inlets are well rounded in both the forward and backward diameters and the pubic arch is wide. The sacrum is concave allowing good rotation inside the cavity. This type of pelvis is ideal for childbirth.

Platypelloid pelvis

In a *platypelloid*, or flattened, pelvis, the inlet is oval and smoothly curved but the anteroposterior diameter is shallow. Problems may occur during childbirth for a woman with this pelvic shape if the fetal head is unable to rotate to match the curves of the spine because the anteroposterior diameter is shallow and the pelvis is flat.

Antenatal testing

The fetus is assessed by using direct and indirect monitoring techniques. Common tests include fetal heart rate (FHR) monitoring, ultrasonography, fetal activity determination, maternal urinalysis and serum assays, amniocentesis, chorionic villi sampling (CVS), percutaneous umbilical blood sampling (PUBS), fetoscopy and blood studies.

Fetal heart rate

You can obtain an FHR by placing a Pinard's stethoscope or Doppler ultrasound stethoscope on the mother's abdomen and counting fetal heartbeats. Simultaneously palpating the mother's pulse helps you to avoid confusion between maternal and fetal heartbeats.

Heart to heart

A Pinard's stethoscope can detect fetal heartbeats as early as 20 weeks' gestation. The Doppler ultrasound stethoscope, a more sensitive instrument, can detect fetal heartbeats as early as 10 weeks' gestation and remains a useful tool throughout labour.

To determine the FHR at fewer than 20 weeks' gestation, place the head of the Doppler stethoscope at the midline of the woman's abdomen above the pubic hairline. After 20 weeks' gestation, when fetal position can be determined, palpate for the back of the fetal thorax and position the instrument directly over it. Locate the loudest heartbeats and palpate the maternal pulse. Count fetal heartbeats for at least 60 seconds while monitoring maternal pulse. Abdominal palpation can be used to determine fetal position, presentation and attitude.

Because FHR usually ranges from 120 to 160 beats/minute, auscultation yields only an average rate at best. It can detect gross (but commonly late) signs of fetal distress, such as tachycardia and bradycardia, and is thus recommended only for a woman with an uncomplicated pregnancy. For a woman with a high-risk pregnancy, indirect or direct electronic fetal monitoring provides more accurate information on fetal status. (See *Abdominal palpation*, pages 147 and 148.)

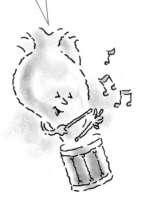

Whose beat is whose? My mum's may be louder, so avoid confusion by palpating her pulse while you listen for my FHR.

Ultrasonography

Through the use of sound waves bouncing off internal structures, ultrasonography allows visualisation of the fetus without the hazards of x-rays. Ultrasonography allows the parents to see their baby and even produces an image.

How ultra-useful!

Ultrasonography is used to:
- verify the due date and correlate it with fetus size
- evaluate the condition of the fetus through observation of fetal activity, breathing movements and amniotic fluid volume
- determine the condition of the fetus when there's a greater than average risk of an abnormality or a greater than average concern
- rule out pregnancy by week 7 if there has been a suspected false-positive pregnancy test
- determine the cause of bleeding or spotting in early pregnancy
- locate an IUCD that was in place at the time of conception
- locate the fetus before amniocentesis and during CVS
- determine the condition of the fetus if no heartbeat has been detected by week 14 with a Doppler device or if no fetal movement has occurred by week 22
- diagnose multiple pregnancy, especially if the woman has taken fertility drugs or the uterus is larger than it should be for the expected due date

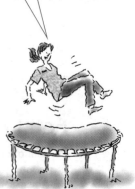

In ultrasonography, sound waves bounce off internal structures to let you see the fetus.

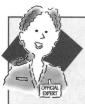

Advice from the experts

Abdominal palpation

You can determine fetal position, presentation and attitude by performing an abdominal palpation. Gain consent, ask the woman to empty her bladder, assist her to a supine position and expose her abdomen. Then perform the palpation in the following order:

1. **Assessing fundal height.** Face the woman and warm your hands. Placing your hands on the woman's abdomen to determine fundal height. Using a tape measure, measure the fundal height – from the upper border of the symphysis pubis to the top of the fundus – in centimetres. This is equivalent to the number of weeks' gestation, e.g. 32 cm = 32 weeks' gestation. Or alternatively, place your hand gently on the fundus and use the nearest landmark to assess the number of weeks gestation.

woman's feet. Place your hands gently on the woman's abdomen – with your thumbs just below her umbilicus. Place your index and middle fingers above her symphysis pubis and press downwards and inwards simultaneously – this will enable you to feel the presenting part – hopefully either a head or a breech. If the fetus is in the vertex (cephalic) position and hasn't descended, you'll feel the head. If the fetus is in the vertex position and has descended, you'll feel a less distinct mass. If the fetus is in the breech position, you'll also feel a less distinct mass, which could be the bottom, the feet or knees. There is no need to palpate too deeply before 36 weeks as there is little likelihood of any part of the fetus being engaged.

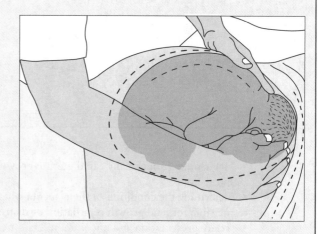

2. **Deep pelvic palpation.** This should only be done after 36 weeks' gestation. The aim is to ascertain which part of the fetus is presenting. Face the

3. **Lateral palpation.** Turn around to face the woman again. Place one hand on the side of her abdomen and use the other to move up the opposite side of the abdomen, applying gentle pressure. If the fetus

(continued)

Abdominal palpation *(continued)*

is in the vertex position, you'll feel a smooth, hard surface on one side – the fetal back. Palpate the other side – on the opposite side, you'll feel lumps and knobs – the knees, hands, feet and elbows. If the fetus is in the breech position, you may not feel the back at all.

Once you have attempted to feel which side the back is on – try carrying out a procedure called 'walking the abdomen'. This entails you gently 'tiptoeing' with your fingers, from one side across the abdomen to the other side – so instead of moving up and down the abdomen, you are moving across it. The aim here is to see which side you feel a solid mass on and which side feels more 'empty' – the side with the solid mass is more likely to be the back.

4. **Fundal palpation.** You go back to the fundal area again to confirm the opposite pole of what you felt in the deep pelvic palpation, i.e. if you felt the fetus was cephalic presentation then you should feel a breech in the fundus.

5. **Auscultation.** You listen to the fetal heart on the side where you palpated a back – you should listen with a Pinard's stethoscope and count the fetal heart for a full minute while checking the maternal pulse rate. If you have difficulty locating the heart – use a sonicaid to avoid distressing the mother. But do try to get used to 'listening in' with a Pinard's stethoscope – it is a skill which takes much practice to perfect!

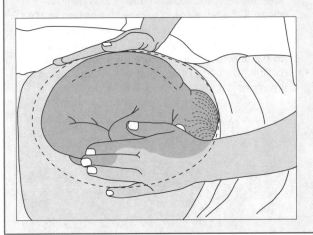

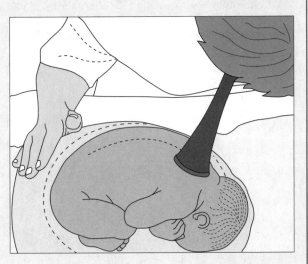

• determine if abnormally rapid uterine growth is being caused by excessive amniotic fluid

• determine the condition of the placenta when deterioration might be responsible for fetal growth retardation or distress

• verify presentation and uncommon fetal or cord position before delivery.

Screen debut

Here's how it's usually done. An ultrasonic transducer that's placed on the mother's abdomen transmits high-frequency sound waves through the abdominal wall. These sound waves deflect off the fetus, bounce back to the transducer and are transformed into a visual image on a monitoring screen.

A fluid fill-up

To prepare a mother for an abdominal ultrasound, have her drink approximately 1 L of fluid 1–2 hours before the test. Instruct her not to void before the test because a full bladder serves as a landmark to define other pelvic organs.

A bladder-friendly version

Transvaginal ultrasonography is another type of imaging. It's well tolerated because it eliminates the need for a full bladder and is usually used during the first trimester of pregnancy. It also lets you – and the parents – see the developing fetus at a much earlier gestation. This method can be particularly useful in very early pregnancy when abdominal scans do not produce a good quality image.

Fetal activity determination

The activity of the fetus (kick counts) determines its condition in utero. Daily evaluation of movement provides an inexpensive, noninvasive way of assessing fetal well-being. Decreased activity in a previously active fetus may reflect a disturbance in placental function.

As early as 7 weeks' gestation, the embryo can produce spontaneous movements; however, these movements don't become apparent to the mother until sometime between weeks 14 and 26 (but generally between weeks 18 and 22). The first noticeable movement of the fetus by the mother is called *quickening*. The acknowledgement of fetal movements may be delayed if the due date is miscalculated or if the mother doesn't recognise the sensation. A woman who has had a baby before is likely to recognise movement earlier. If the mother hasn't felt any movements by week 22 and the Doppler fails to detect a fetal heart, an ultrasound may be ordered to assess the condition of the fetus.

Looking for some fetal action

Fetal movements may be elicited by having the woman lie down for about an hour after having a glass of milk or another snack. The jolt of energy produced by a light snack commonly produces fetal movement. If the woman isn't feeling fetal movement as often as she should, she may be asked to record fetal movements in a 12-hour period, so if, from 8 a.m. to 8 p.m. she had not felt 8–10 movements, she should be seen by a professional.

Maternal urinalysis

During pregnancy, the woman is monitored routinely for potential problems. Some problems may be detected by a simple urine test. The urine specimen should be obtained from the woman during her regularly scheduled visit using a clean-catch technique. The specimen is examined for bacteriuria as well as

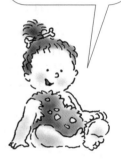

As you can imagine, I've had lots of practice posing. My first 'photo opportunity' was courtesy of an ultrasonic scan.

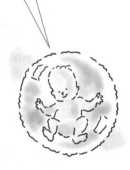

I'm kicking up a storm in here! It's just my way of letting mum know I'm doing great – and the placenta is working just fine, thank you!

protein, glucose and ketones. Urinalysis can detect such problems as infection and diabetes before the woman shows any signs.

Maternal serum assays

Serum assays – including those for oestrogens, human placental lactogen (hPL) and human chorionic gonadotropin (hCG) – are used in addition to urinalysis to monitor the pregnant woman for problems.

Oestrogens

Three major oestrogens exist: oestrone, oestradiol and oestriol. Production of oestrogens, particularly oestriol, increases during pregnancy. During pregnancy, levels of oestrone and oestradiol increase to about 100 times their nonpregnancy levels, whereas oestriol levels increase 1,000 times. Oestrogen production depends on the interaction of the maternal fetal–placental unit. Oestriol is secreted by the placenta into the maternal circulation and is eventually excreted in maternal urine.

The old oestriol test just ain't what it used to be

In the past, a mother's urinary oestriol levels were measured regularly to assess fetal and placental well-being. Today, however, oestriol levels are measured only as part of the triple screen test. (For more information, see 'Triple screen', page 160.)

Serial evaluation

A radioimmunoassay measures plasma hPL levels. The test may be required in high-risk pregnancies, such as those involving diabetes mellitus, hypertension or suspected placental tissue dysfunction. Because values vary widely during the latter half of pregnancy, serial determinations over several days provide the most reliable test results.

For pregnant women, normal hPL levels slowly increase throughout pregnancy, reaching 7 mg/ml at term. Low hPL concentrations are also characteristically associated with postmaturity syndrome, intrauterine growth retardation, pre-eclampsia and eclampsia. However, low hPL concentrations don't confirm fetal distress. Conversely, concentrations over 4 mg/ml after 30 weeks' gestation don't guarantee fetal well-being because elevated levels have been reported after fetal death. An hPL value above 6 mg/ml after 30 weeks' gestation may suggest an unusually large placenta, common in women with diabetes mellitus, multiple pregnancy and Rh isoimmunisation.

Human chorionic gonadotropin

Although the precise function of hCG (a glycoprotein hormone produced in the placenta) is still unclear, it appears that hCG and progesterone maintain the corpus luteum during early pregnancy. Production of hCG increases steadily during the first trimester, peaking around 10 weeks' gestation. Levels then fall to less than 10% of first-trimester peak levels during the remainder

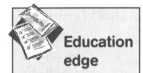

Education edge

Monitoring for fetal distress

If the woman is recording the episodes of fetal activity, make sure that she rests during the counting period. If she's walking around or otherwise physically moving, she may not feel the movements as much as if she were at rest. If 12 hours go by without 6–8 movements, she should promptly contact her midwife. Absence of fetal activity doesn't necessarily mean there's a problem but, in some cases, it indicates fetal distress. Immediate action may be needed.

of the pregnancy. About 2 weeks after delivery, the hormone may no longer be detectable.

The serum test for hCG, which is more sensitive and costly than the routine pregnancy test using a urine sample, provides a quantitative analysis. It's used to:

- detect pregnancy
- determine adequacy of hormonal production in high-risk pregnancies
- aid diagnosis of trophoblastic tumours, such as hydatidiform moles and choriocarcinoma
- detect tumours that ectopically secrete hCG
- monitor treatment for induction of ovulation and conception.

Levelling with you

Normal hCG levels are less than 4 IU/l. During pregnancy, hCG levels vary widely, depending partly on the number of days after the last normal menses. Elevated hCG levels indicate pregnancy; significantly higher concentrations are present in a multiple pregnancy. Low hCG levels can occur in ectopic pregnancy or pregnancy of less than 9 days. Unfortunately, hCG levels can't differentiate between pregnancy and tumour recurrence because levels are high in both conditions.

Down and out

In addition, researchers have found that a high level of hCG in a pregnant woman's blood means she's at greater risk for having a baby with Down syndrome. If conception occurs, a specific assay for hCG, commonly called the *beta-subunit assay*, may detect this hormone in the blood as soon as 9 days after ovulation. This interval coincides with the implantation of the fertilised ovum into the uterine wall. If hCG levels are indicative of Down syndrome, amniocentesis is used to confirm.

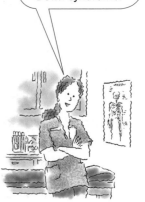

A high level of hCG in a pregnant woman's blood means she's at greater risk for having a baby with Down syndrome.

Amniocentesis

Amniocentesis is the sterile needle aspiration of fluid from the amniotic sac for analysis. This procedure is recommended when:

- the mother is older than age 40
- the couple has already had a child with a chromosomal abnormality (such as Down syndrome) or a metabolic disorder (such as Hunter's syndrome)
- the mother is a carrier of an X-linked genetic disorder, such as haemophilia, which she has a 50% chance of passing on to a son
- a parent is known to have a condition, such as Huntington's chorea, that's passed on by autosomal dominant inheritance, giving the baby a one in two chance of inheriting the disease
- both parents are carriers of an autosomal recessive inherited disorder, such as Tay-Sachs disease or sickle cell anaemia, and thus have a one in four chance of bearing an affected child

- results of triple screening tests and ultrasonography are abnormal and amniotic fluid evaluation is necessary to determine whether there's a fetal abnormality.

Oh, the uses you'll find

Amniocentesis is valuable because it can be used to:
- detect fetal abnormalities, particularly chromosomal and neural tube defects
- detect haemolytic disease of the fetus
- diagnose metabolic disorders, amino acid disorders and mucopolysaccharidosis
- assess fetal lung maturity (the lungs are the last organs ready to function on their own)
- determine fetal age and maturity, especially
- detect the presence of meconium or blood
- measure amniotic levels of oestriol and fetal thyroid hormone
- identify fetal gender.

Diagnostic second-trimester amniocentesis is usually performed between weeks 16 and 18 of pregnancy, although it may be done as early as week 14 or as late as week 20. Most tests require cells to be cultured in the laboratory and take from 24 to 35 days to complete. A few tests – such as those used to detect Tay-Sachs disease, Hunter's syndrome and neural tube defects – can be performed immediately.

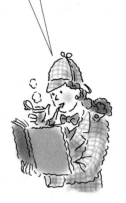

Very interesting, my dear midwives. Apparently, amniocentesis is a great detective in its own right – of fetal abnormalities, haemolytic disease, metabolic disorders and more!

Aspiring towards aspirate

To begin, ask the woman to empty her bladder. Then explain that she'll be positioned on the examining table on her back and her body will be draped so that only her abdomen is exposed. During the test, FHR, maternal vital signs and ultrasonography are monitored. The doctor:
- prepares the skin with antiseptic and alcohol
- injects the skin with lidocaine to numb the area
- inserts a 20 G spinal needle with a stylet into the amniotic cavity
- aspirates amniotic fluid and places it in an amber or foil-covered test tube.

Generally speaking, not for general use

Complications of amniocentesis include spontaneous abortion, trauma to the fetus or placenta, bleeding, premature labour, infection and Rh sensitisation from fetal bleeding into the maternal circulation. Because of the potential severity of possible complications, amniocentesis is contraindicated as a general screening test.

Meaning in amnio

Abnormal test results or failure of the tissue cultures to grow may necessitate repetition of the test. (See *Amniotic fluid analysis findings*, page 153.)

Amniotic fluid analysis findings

Amniotic fluid analysis can provide important information about the condition of the mother, fetus and placenta. This table shows normal findings as well as abnormal findings and their implications.

Test component	Normal findings	Abnormal findings and fetal implications
Colour	Clear, with white flecks of vernix caseosa in a mature fetus	Blood of maternal origin is usually harmless. 'Port wine' fluid may indicate abruptio placentae. Fetal blood may indicate damage to the fetal, placental or umbilical cord vessels.
Bilirubin	Absent at term	High levels indicate haemolytic disease of the neonate in isoimmunised pregnancy.
Meconium	Absent (except in breech presentation)	Presence indicates fetal hypotension or distress.
Creatinine	More than 2 mg/dl in a mature fetus	Decrease may indicate immature fetus (less than 37 weeks).
Lecithin-sphingomyelin ratio	More than 2 generally indicates fetal pulmonary maturity	A ratio of less than 2 indicates pulmonary immaturity and subsequent respiratory distress syndrome.
Phosphatidylglycerol	Present	Absence indicates pulmonary immaturity.
Glucose	Less than 45 mg/dl	Excessive increases at term or near term indicate hypertrophied fetal pancreas and subsequent neonatal hypoglycaemia.
Alpha-fetoprotein	Variable, depending on gestation age and laboratory technique; highest concentration (about 18.5 µg/ml) occurs at 13–14 weeks	Inappropriate increases indicate neural tube defects, such as spina bifida or anencephaly, impending fetal death, congenital nephrosis or contamination of fetal blood.
Bacteria	Absent	Presence indicates chorioamnionitis.
Chromosome	Normal karyotype	Abnormal karyotype may indicate fetal sex and chromosome disorders.
Acetylcholinesterase	Absent	Presence may indicate neural tube defects, exomphalos or other serious malformations.

Chorionic villi sampling

Performed between 8 and 10 weeks' gestation, CVS involves aspirating chorionic villi from the placenta for antenatal diagnosis of genetic disorders. Chorionic villi are fingerlike projections that surround the embryonic membrane and eventually give rise to the placenta. Cells obtained from the sample are of fetal – rather than maternal – origin and thus can be analysed for fetal abnormalities. Experts believe that villi in the chorion frondosum reflect fetal chromosome, enzyme and deoxyribonucleic acid (DNA) content. (See *A look at CVS*, page 154.)

Trans times two

Either a transcervical or transabdominal approach can be used to obtain a CVS specimen. In transcervical sampling, a sterile catheter is introduced into

A look at CVS

Chorionic villi sampling (CVS) is an antenatal test for quick detection of fetal chromosomal and biochemical disorders that's performed during the first trimester of pregnancy. Preliminary results may be available within 1 hour; complete results, within a few days.

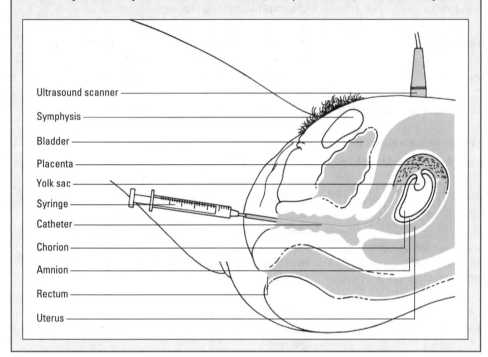

Labels (top to bottom): Ultrasound scanner, Symphysis, Bladder, Placenta, Yolk sac, Syringe, Catheter, Chorion, Amnion, Rectum, Uterus

the cervix using direct visualisation with real-time ultrasonography. A small portion of chorionic villi is aspirated through the catheter into a syringe. In transabdominal sampling, the maternal abdomen is cleaned and an 18–20 G needle is inserted into the chorion frondosum under ultrasound guidance. The specimen is then aspirated into a syringe. Aspirated villi are placed into a sterile medium for cytogenic analysis.

Painting a picture of the fetus

The cells from the villi normally have the same genetic and biochemical make-up as the embryo. Therefore, examining villi cells provides a complete picture of the genetic make-up of the developing fetus. CVS can detect fetal karyotype, haemoglobinopathies (such as sickle cell anaemia, alpha-thalassaemias and some beta-thalassaemias), phenylketonuria, alpha-1 antitrypsin deficiency, Down syndrome, Duchenne's muscular dystrophy and factor IX deficiency. The test also identifies sex, allowing early detection of X-linked conditions in male fetuses.

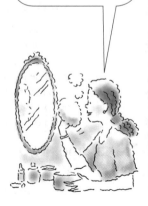

Chorionic villi sampling can provide a complete picture of the genetic 'make-up' of the fetus.

Complicated matters

Test complications include failure to obtain tissue, ruptured membranes or leakage of amniotic fluid, bleeding, intrauterine infection, spontaneous abortion, contamination of the specimen and possible Rh isoimmunisation. If the woman is Rh-negative, administer Anti-D, as ordered, to cover the risk of Rh sensitisation from the procedure. Also, recent research indicates an incidence of limb malformations in neonates whose mothers have undergone CVS. However, this incidence appears to be low when CVS is performed after 10 weeks' gestation.

Many women feel physically and emotionally drained after undergoing this procedure. Advise the woman to have someone drive her home. Tell her not to make other plans for the rest of the day. Instruct her to call her midwife, GP or obstetrician with any concerns or symptoms of complications, such as fever, vaginal discharge, vaginal bleeding or cramping.

Percutaneous umbilical blood sampling

PUBS, which is used to obtain blood samples directly from the fetal circulation, is indicated for antenatal diagnosis of inherited blood disorders, detection of fetal infection and assessment of the acid–base status of a fetus with intrauterine growth retardation. PUBS can also be used to administer blood products or drugs directly to the fetus. Allowing for treatment of the fetus in utero, PUBS reduces the risk of prematurity and mortality for a neonate with erythroblastosis fetalis (haemolytic disease of the newborn due to Rh incompatibility).

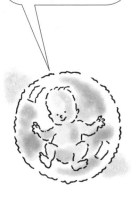

PUBS? I'm not even born yet and already I'm getting my first blood test! Let me know when it's over!

Point of origin

In PUBS, a fine needle is passed through the mother's abdomen and uterine wall into a vessel in the umbilical cord. Ultrasonography is used for guidance. The mobility of the cord complicates the procedure. Although the cord is more stable close to the placenta – allowing for a more accurate puncture – maternal intervillous blood lakes occupy this site, creating a risk of contamination with maternal blood. The Betke–Kleihauer procedure, which is used to detect fetal cells in maternal blood, is immediately performed on the blood sample obtained to ensure that it's fetal in origin.

Direct access

Performed anytime after 16 weeks' gestation, PUBS can help diagnose fetal coagulopathies, haemoglobinopathies, haemophilias and congenital infections. It also provides for rapid fetal karyotyping. Rather than analysing amniotic fluid to detect abnormalities, PUBS directly assesses fetal blood. This is especially helpful in a woman who may have an isoimmunised pregnancy from Rh disease or another antibody sensitisation.

Fetoscopy

Fetoscopy is a procedure in which a fetoscope – a telescope-like instrument with lights and lenses – is inserted into the amniotic sac, where it can view and photograph the fetus. This procedure makes it possible to diagnose, through blood and tissue sampling, several blood and skin diseases that amniocentesis can't detect. Fetoscopy is a relatively risky procedure and, because other safer techniques are becoming available to detect the same disorders, it isn't widely used.

Internal observation

Fetoscopy is typically performed at or after 16 weeks' gestation. The woman's abdomen is swabbed with antiseptic solution and numbed with a local anaesthetic. Tiny incisions are made in the abdomen and uterus. Using ultrasonography to guide the instrument, a fibre-optic endoscope is passed through the incisions and into the uterus. The fetus, placenta and amniotic fluid are observed and blood samples are taken from the junction of the umbilical cord and the placenta. A small piece of fetal or placental tissue may also be removed for examination.

The procedure carries with it a 3–5% chance of fetal loss. Though this risk is greater than that of other diagnostic tests, it's outweighed for some women by the benefit of discovering – and possibly treating or correcting – a defect in the fetus.

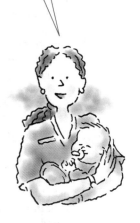

Long before this little one was born, a biophysical profile allowed assessment of his well-being as a fetus.

Biophysical profile

A biophysical profile assesses fetal well-being in the later stages of pregnancy and is used to aid in detecting central nervous system depression in the fetus. It utilises five variables: amniotic fluid volume, fetal body movements, fetal breathing movements, FHR reactivity and fetal muscle tone. Each variable can score a maximum of 2 points. The total score is then calculated. A score of 8–10 indicates a potentially healthy fetus; a score of 6 is suspicious and a score of 4 indicates that the fetus may be in jeopardy. (See *Scoring the biophysical profile*, page 157.)

Blood studies

During pregnancy, blood studies are ordered to assess the mother's health, screen for maternal conditions that may endanger the fetus, detect genetic defects and monitor fetal well-being. Initial studies include blood typing, a complete blood count (CBC) with differential, antibody screening tests, and a serologic test for syphilis and gonorrhoea. Other tests may be performed to assess alpha-fetoprotein (AFP) levels, blood glucose and other chemicals, if indicated.

Scoring the biophysical profile

Parameter	Diagnostic tool	Factor for a score of 2
Amniotic fluid volume	Ultrasound	Presence of a pocket of amniotic fluid measuring more than 1 cm in vertical diameter
Fetal breathing movements	Ultrasound	At least one episode of 30 seconds of sustained fetal breathing movements within 30 minutes of observation
Fetal heart rate reactivity	Nonstress test	Two or more fetal heart rate accelerations of at least 15 beats/minute above baseline and 15 seconds' duration occurring with fetal movement over a 20-minute period
Fetal body movements	Ultrasound	At least three separate episodes of fetal limb or trunk movement within a 30-minute observation
Fetal muscle tone	Ultrasound	Extension and then flexing of the spine or extremities at least once in 30 minutes

Blood typing

Blood typing, including Rh factor, is performed to determine the woman's blood type and detect possible blood type incompatibilities. The woman's Rh status is also tested to determine if she's Rh-negative or Rh-positive.

Complete blood count

A CBC includes haemoglobin level, haematocrit, red blood cell (RBC) index, and platelet and white blood cell (WBC) counts. Haemoglobin level and haematocrit help to determine the presence of anaemia. The RBC index helps to classify anaemia, if present. Platelet count estimates clotting ability. An elevated WBC count may indicate an infection.

Antibody screening tests

The blood studies performed during pregnancy also include antibody screening tests for Rh compatibility (indirect Coombs' test), rubella and hepatitis B. Antibodies for varicella (chickenpox) may also be assessed.

Indirect Coombs' test

The indirect Coombs' test screens maternal blood for RBC antibodies.

A sensitive situation

This test should be performed on a woman who's Rh-negative; if her fetus is Rh-positive and its blood mixes with the maternal blood during pregnancy or delivery, the woman's immune system produces antibodies against the fetus's RBCs. This antibody response is called *Rh sensitisation*. Rh sensitisation usually isn't a problem with the first Rh-positive fetus. However, future Rh-positive fetuses are in danger of having their RBCs destroyed by the mother's immune system. After sensitisation has occurred, the fetus can develop mild to severe problems, such as Rh disease or haemolytic disease of the newborn.

All women are given Anti-D prophylactically at 28 weeks' and 34 weeks' gestation and any time when a placental incident occurs. The Coomb's test is carried out again after the birth of the baby.

Rubella titre

A rubella (German measles) titre detects antibodies in maternal blood for the virus that causes rubella. If antibodies are found, the woman is immune to rubella. Most women have either had the virus as a child or have received a vaccination for rubella and, therefore, have antibodies in the blood.

Rubella exposure during pregnancy can lead to blindness, deafness and heart defects in the fetus. If tests reveal that the woman isn't immune, she should avoid anyone who has the infection. She can't receive the vaccination while she's pregnant, but she should get the vaccine after she gives birth to provide protection during future pregnancies.

Hepatitis B

Another antibody screening test, called the *hepatic antibody surface antigen* (HbsAg) test, is used to determine if a woman has hepatitis B. In many cases, the HbsAg test is the only way to tell if she has hepatitis B because many people who carry the virus have no symptoms. If the woman is a carrier, she could pass this to her baby during labour or delivery.

If the woman tests positive for hepatitis B, the neonate must receive injections of hepatitis B immunoglobulin and hepatitis B vaccine immediately after birth to prevent liver damage. The neonate then receives additional doses of the vaccine at 2–4 months and again at 6–18 months.

> All pregnant women should be tested for HIV, even if they don't think they're at risk.

HIV testing

HIV screening is offered to all women booking into the Antenatal clinic. This test uses an enzyme-linked immunosorbent assay on a blood sample to determine the presence of HIV antibodies. If the HIV screening test is positive, findings are confirmed by a second test – the Western blot test. However, in some cases, a pregnant woman won't pursue HIV testing because she doesn't want to know if she's infected. Screening for all pregnant women is recommended, but it is especially important for women who:

• have a history of I.V. drug use
• have unprotected sex
• have multiple sex partners
• have had a sexual partner who was infected with HIV or was at risk for contracting it (because he was bisexual, an I.V. drug user or a haemophiliac)
• received a blood transfusion between 1977 and 1985.

Damage control

A woman who's antibody-positive for HIV may begin therapy with zidovudine (AZT) to decrease the risk of transmitting the disease to her fetus. Alternatively, she may choose to terminate the pregnancy to avoid giving birth to a baby who has a high risk of developing the disease. When discussing test results with the woman, keep in mind that a positive test result or an antibody-positive result indicates that she has been exposed to the disease – she doesn't necessarily have the disease.

Support

Positive HIV screening results should be presented with tact and compassion. Results are confidential; the information should be reported only to the woman. Extra support and counselling needs to be given to the woman who tests positive because although life expectancy is longer than it was a few years ago, there's no known cure for the infection.

Serologic tests

The Venereal Disease Research Laboratories (VDRL) test and rapid plasma reagin (RPR) test are serologic tests for syphilis. Syphilis needs to be treated early in pregnancy, before fetal damage occurs.

Pregnant women who test positive for syphilis must receive treatment before 16 weeks' gestation. Untreated syphilis infection during pregnancy can cause miscarriage, premature birth, stillbirth or birth defects.

Alpha-fetoprotein testing

AFP testing – sometimes called the *MSAFP* test or *maternal serum AFP* test – is usually used to detect neural tube defects. AFP is a protein that's secreted by the fetal liver and excreted in the mother's blood. When testing by immunoassay, AFP values are less than 15 ng/ml in nonpregnant women.

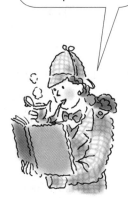

Even the best detective can use some help! AFP levels can be used to detect neural tube defects, abdominal wall defects, low birthweight and other complications.

'MOM' levels

The test is considered positive for an increased risk of neural tube defect when the AFP level is greater than 2.5 times the median (midpoint of levels of a group of clients at the same gestational age), or 2.5 MOM (multiples of median).

AFP testing can also indicate:
• abdominal wall defects
• oesophageal and duodenal atresia
• renal and urinary tract anomalies
• Turner's syndrome
• low birthweight
• placental complications.

Congenital anomalies, such as Down syndrome, may be associated with low maternal serum AFP concentrations. Elevated maternal serum AFP levels may suggest neural tube defects or other anomalies. Maternal AFP levels rise sharply in the blood of about 90% of women carrying a fetus with anencephaly and in about 50% of those carrying a fetus with spina bifida. Definitive diagnosis requires ultrasonography and amniocentesis. High AFP levels can also indicate intrauterine death or other anomalies, such as duodenal atresia, omphalocele, Fallot's tetralogy and Turner's syndrome.

Glucose-tolerance testing

If the woman has a history of previously unexplained fetal loss, has a family history of diabetes, has previously delivered a large-for-gestational age baby (over 4.1 kg), is obese or has glycosuria, a 75 mg oral 2-hour glucose-loading or glucose-tolerance test should be scheduled towards the end of the first trimester. This test is performed to rule out or confirm gestational diabetes. It's done between 16 and 18 weeks' gestation to evaluate insulin-antagonistic effects of placental hormones but, in high-risk pregnancies, testing should be performed earlier. Fasting plasma glucose levels shouldn't be above 140 mg/dl.

Triple screen

The triple screen is a blood test routinely offered between weeks 15 and 20. It measures three chemicals: AFP, unconjugated oestriol and hCG.

The triple screen uses chemical patterns to predict any increased risk of a chromosomal abnormality in the fetus.

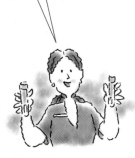

Picking up on patterns

By detecting chemical patterns, the test predicts if there's an increased risk of bearing a child with a chromosomal abnormality or open-tube defect, including:
• Down syndrome – extra chromosome 21 that results in mental retardation
• trisomy 18 – extra chromosome 18 that results in mental retardation that's much more serious than Down syndrome; the baby usually dies within hours of birth but may live for months or, in rare cases, years
• spina bifida – fetal spine doesn't close properly; size and location of opening determine severity; surgery is required at birth; it may cause paralysis
• anencephaly – the most severe type of neural tube defect in which the brain and skull don't form properly; babies are stillborn or die within a few weeks
• omphalocele and gastroschisis – improper closure of the abdominal wall; severity depends on size and location of opening; surgery may correct problem; prognosis depends upon severity.

Suggestive, not definitive

Triple screening doesn't definitively answer whether a fetus has a birth defect. It only suggests that there's a possibility for birth defects. In some cases, results appear to be abnormal because the fetus is younger or older than initially estimated. Suspicions can be confirmed by amniocentesis.

Nutritional care

Nutritional needs must also be addressed as a part of antenatal care. A pregnant woman's nutritional intake – including calories, protein, fat, vitamins, minerals and fluid – needs to be increased to provide sufficient nutrients for her growing fetus. In most cases, the woman doesn't have to increase the quantity of food she eats; she simply needs to increase the quality of the food she eats.

Let the pyramid be your guide

A pregnant woman's food choices should be based on the diet in pregnancy. When discussing nutrition with the woman, refer to servings of food rather than milligrams or percentages. (See *Diet in pregnancy*.)

Diet in pregnancy

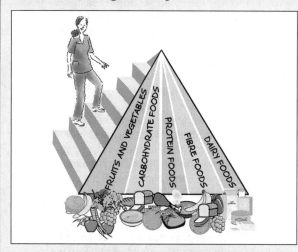

It's important to try to eat a variety of foods including:

- Fruits and vegetables (fresh, frozen, tinned, dried or a glass of juice). Aim for at least five portions of a variety each day.
- Carbohydrate foods such as bread, pasta, rice and potatoes.
- Protein foods such as wholegrains, lean meat and chicken, fish (aim for at least two servings of fish a week, including one of oily fish), eggs and pulses (such as beans and lentils).
- Fibre foods such as wholegrain bread, pasta, rice, pulses and fruit and vegetables. This helps prevent constipation.

- Dairy foods such as milk, cheese and yoghurt, which contain calcium.

Eating for two?

It's also a good idea to cut down on foods such as cakes and biscuits, because these are high in fat and sugar. This can also help you to avoid putting on too much weight during pregnancy.

Healthy snacks to have instead include malt loaf; currant buns without icing; sandwiches or pitta bread filled with cottage cheese, chicken or lean ham; low-fat yoghurts; vegetable and bean soups and fruit including fresh, tinned in juice or dried fruit such as raisins or apricots.

Folic acid

You should take a daily 400 μg folic acid supplement from the time you stop using contraception until the 12th week of pregnancy.

You should also eat foods containing folate – the natural form of folic acid – such as green vegetables and brown rice, fortified bread and breakfast cereals.

Folic acid has been shown to reduce the risk of neural tube defects such as spina bifida. If you would like to take your folic acid in a supplement that contains other vitamins, make sure it contains 400 μg folic acid and doesn't contain vitamin A.

If you have already had a pregnancy affected by a neural tube defect, ask your GP for advice.

(continued)

Diet in pregnancy *(continued)*

Iron

Pregnant women can become deficient in iron, so make sure you have plenty of iron-rich foods such as red meat, pulses, green leafy vegetables and cereals. Try to have some food or drink containing vitamin C, such as fruit or vegetables or a glass of fruit juice, with any iron-rich meals to help your body absorb iron. Avoid drinking tea or coffee with, or after, your main meals as this reduces absorption of iron.

If the iron level in your blood becomes low, your GP or midwife will advise you to take iron supplements.

Vitamin D

Vitamin D intake is vital for calcium synthesis and development of fetal bones and teeth as well as making sure mum does not become deficient during the pregnancy.

What to avoid

There are certain foods that you should avoid when you're pregnant, because they might make you ill or harm your baby.

- *Some types of cheese.* Avoid cheeses such as Camembert, Brie or chevre (goats' cheese) or others that have a similar rind. You should also avoid blue cheeses. These cheeses are made with mould and they can contain listeria, a type of bacteria that could harm your unborn baby.
- *Pâté.* Avoid all types of pâté, including vegetable. This is because pâté can contain listeria.
- *Raw or partially cooked eggs.* Avoid eating raw eggs and food containing raw or partially cooked eggs. Only eat eggs cooked enough for both the white and yolk to be solid. This is to avoid the risk of salmonella, which causes a type of food poisoning.
- *Raw or undercooked meat.* Make sure you only eat meat that has been well cooked. This is especially important with poultry and products made from minced meat, such as sausages and burgers. Make sure these are cooked until they are piping hot all the way through and no pink meat is left.

Always wash your hands after handling raw meat, and keep it separate from foods that are ready to eat. This is because raw meat contains bacteria that can cause food poisoning.

- *Liver products and supplements containing vitamin A.* Make sure you don't have too much vitamin A. This means you should avoid eating liver and liver products such as pâté and avoid taking supplements containing vitamin A or fish liver oils (which contain high levels of vitamin A). You need some vitamin A, but having too much means that levels could build up and may harm your unborn baby. Ask your GP or midwife if you want more information.
- *Some types of fish.* You can eat most types of fish when you're pregnant, but there are a few types you should avoid and some others where you should limit the amount you eat. Limit the amount of tuna you eat to no more than two tuna steaks a week. This is because of the levels of mercury in these fish. At high levels, mercury can harm a baby's developing nervous system.

Have no more than two portions of oily fish a week. Oily fish includes fresh tuna (not canned tuna, which is not considered an oily fish), mackerel, sardines and trout.

- *Undercooked ready meals.* Avoid eating ready meals that are undercooked. Make sure you heat them until they are piping hot all the way through.
- *Alcohol and caffeine.* When you're pregnant, it's best to stop drinking alcohol altogether. But if you do drink, have no more than 1 or 2 units of alcohol, once a week (A unit is half a pint of standard strength beer, lager or cider, or a pub measure of spirit. A glass of wine is about 2 units and alcopops are about 1.5 units.)

You should limit the amount of caffeine you have each day, but you don't need to cut it out completely. Caffeine occurs naturally in a range of foods, such as coffee, tea and chocolate, and it's also added to some soft drinks and 'energy' drinks.

It's important not to have more than 300 mg a day. This is because high levels of caffeine can result in babies having a low birthweight, or even miscarriage.

Remember that caffeine is also found in certain cold and flu remedies, so always check with your GP or another health professional before taking any of these.

More information is available about diet in pregnancy on www.food.gov.uk

Education edge

Foods to avoid during pregnancy

Although several nutritional needs increase during pregnancy, other food restrictions become necessary. Tell the client to avoid the following food products.

Artificial sweeteners and additives

Artificial sweeteners, such as saccharin and aspartame, aren't recommended during pregnancy. According to the results of some animal studies, a large intake of saccharin may be carcinogenic. Some studies also suggest that saccharin may cross the placental barrier. Although no definitive study has been performed that indicates that aspartame crosses the placental barrier, a woman should still be advised to avoid ingesting food products with this substance during pregnancy.

A pregnant woman should also avoid foods that contain additives because the effects of many of these additives are unknown.

Cholesterol

A pregnant woman should limit her cholesterol intake. Encourage her to eat lean meats, to cook with olive oil instead of lard or butter and to remove the skin from poultry. Even though such foods as eggs are good sources of protein, a woman who has a family history of high cholesterol shouldn't consume more than one egg per week.

Infliction of restriction

Although certain nutritional requirements increase during pregnancy, certain restrictions also become necessary to protect the health of the baby. (See *Foods to avoid during pregnancy*.)

Calories

During the first trimester, the energy needs of a pregnant woman are essentially the same as those of a nonpregnant woman. In the second and third trimesters, however, the increased need for energy ranges from 300 to 400 calories per day. Because nutrient needs increase more than calorie needs, a pregnant woman's food choices need to be nutrient-dense. More calories (2,700–3,000 per day) may be needed for active, large or nutritionally deficient women. Inadequate calorie intake can lead to protein breakdown for energy, depriving the fetus of essential protein and, possibly, resulting in ketoacidosis and neurological defects.

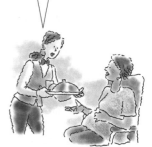

We're only going to increase your calorie intake by 300 calories. That should provide the extra energy that you need.

Meal plan

To help a woman plan for increased calorie intake, consider her lifestyle. Many women skip meals, have erratic eating patterns, and rely on fast or convenience foods. Help her plan on adding calories by eating foods rich in protein, iron and other essential nutrients rather than eating empty-calorie foods, such as cakes and doughnuts. Suggest such snacks as carrot sticks or cheese and crackers. Encourage the woman to have these snacks on hand ahead of time to provide needed nutrients.

Protein

Recommended protein intake during pregnancy increases only 10–15 g/day to 60 g/day total. Many pregnant women consume more than this already and don't need to increase protein intake.

You complete me

Good animal sources of protein include meat, poultry, fish, cheese, yogurt, eggs and milk. Because the protein in these forms contains all nine essential amino acids, it's considered *complete protein*. However, cooked meats such as bologna and salami shouldn't be consumed regularly because they're high in fat and aren't typically good sources of protein.

Full of complements

The protein found in nonanimal sources doesn't contain all nine essential amino acids. Vitamin B12 is found exclusively in animal proteins. Therefore, a pregnant woman who excludes animal proteins from her diet may have a vitamin B_{12} deficiency. Complete protein can be obtained through nonanimal sources by cooking different protein sources together. For example, eating complementary proteins, such as beans and rice, legumes and rice, or beans and wheat together, can provide the woman with all nine essential amino acids.

Got milk?

Milk products are also rich in protein and may be consumed in various forms – buttermilk, yogurt, cheese, custards and cream soups – to meet daily protein requirements. If the woman is lactose intolerant, lactose supplements may be purchased over the counter. These supplements predigest milk and make it palatable for her.

Fats

Linoleic acid is an essential fatty acid that's necessary for new cell growth. It isn't manufactured in the body but can be found in such vegetable oils as safflower, corn, olive, peanut and cottonseed. In addition, these vegetable oils are low in cholesterol compared with animal oils such as lard. They're also recommended for all adults to prevent hypercholesterolaemia and atherosclerosis.

Vitamins

Requirements of fat-soluble and water-soluble vitamins increase during pregnancy to support the growth of new fetal cells. A healthy, varied diet with plenty of fruits and vegetables usually allows the pregnant woman to

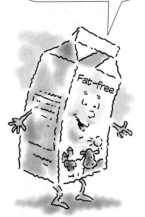

Milk products are great sources of protein, calcium and vitamin D – which are all necessary nutrients.

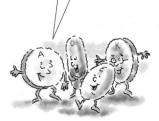

Warn your client to take us fat-soluble vitamins only as prescribed. Too much of us can be toxic!

meet these requirements. A specially designed multivitamin supplement can be prescribed if she is unable to eat the correct nutrients in pregnancy. The woman should be advised to take these vitamins as directed and the recommended dose shouldn't be exceeded because fat-soluble vitamins can be toxic.

Restock the stores

A woman who was taking hormonal contraceptives before she became pregnant also needs to include good sources of vitamin A, vitamin B_6 and folic acid in her diet in early pregnancy because hormonal contraceptives may deplete her stores of these vitamins. Vitamin A can be found in milk, eggs, yellow fruits and vegetables, dark green fruits and vegetables; vitamin B_6, in whole grains, organ meats, brewer's yeast, blackstrap molasses and wheat germ; folic acid, in citrus fruits, tomatoes and other vegetables, grain products and most ready-to-eat cereals (fortified with folic acid).

Too little . . .

Vitamin deficiencies can cause many problems. For example:
• Vitamin D deficiency may result in the breakdown of fetal and maternal mineral bone density (vitamin D is necessary for calcium and phosphorus absorption).

. . . too much

Likewise, an overdose of vitamins can also cause problems:
• Vitamin A excess can result in fetal malformation and congenital anomalies. Such an excess can occur through the body's absorption of isotretinoin (Accutane), a medication for acne.
• Megadoses of vitamin C may cause withdrawal scurvy in the infant at birth.

Folic acid

Folic acid (folacin) is a water-soluble B_9 vitamin that's necessary for RBC formation. A folic acid deficiency may result in megaloblastic anaemia (development of large but ineffective RBCs). If evidence of folic acid deficiency is present at the time of birth, the newborn infant may be affected as well. Low levels of folic acid in pregnant women have been associated with premature separation of the placenta, spontaneous abortions and neural tube defects. Good sources of folic acid include fruits and vegetables. Folic acid supplements are essential – they can be bought from the chemist and should be taken pre-conceptually and for the first 12 weeks of pregnancy to prevent neural tube defects.

Minerals

Minerals are needed for fetal cell development. They're found in many foods, so most mineral deficiencies in pregnant women are rare. For women whose intake of minerals is below daily requirements, supplements may be necessary.

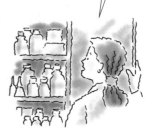

Remind the woman that all vitamins should be kept out of reach of small children because the folic acid and iron in these pills may be poisonous.

Calcium and phosphorus

Calcium and phosphorus are vital to the structure of bones and teeth. Between 1,200 and 1,500 mg of calcium and 1,200 mg of phosphorus are recommended per day during pregnancy. In the last trimester of pregnancy, fetal skeletal growth is greatest and the fetus draws calcium directly from the mother's stores. In addition, clinical trials have shown that adequate calcium intake during pregnancy lowers blood pressure and may reduce the incidence of premature births.

Because calcium and phosphorus help with tooth and bone formation in the fetus, a maternal diet high in calcium and vitamin D (a vitamin needed for calcium to enter bones) is necessary. If a woman can't drink milk or eat milk products, a daily calcium supplement may be prescribed. Inadequate calcium intake can result in diminished maternal bone density. The woman should eat foods that are high in protein to ensure adequate phosphorus intake because most foods that are high in protein are also high in phosphorus.

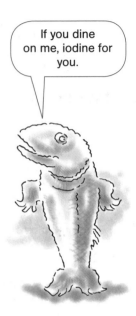

If you dine on me, iodine for you.

Iodine

The recommended daily requirement of iodine during pregnancy is 175 mg. Iodine is essential for the formation of thyroxine and proper functioning of the thyroid gland. The best sources of this mineral are ocean fish, including cod, haddock, sole and ocean perch.

If iodine deficiency occurs, it may result in thyroid enlargement (goitre) in the woman or fetus and, in extreme cases, can cause hypothyroidism in the fetus. Thyroid enlargement in the fetus at birth is serious because the increased pressure the enlarged gland places on the airway can result in early respiratory distress. If not discovered at birth, hypothyroidism may lead to cognitive impairment. In areas where water and soil are known to be iodine deficient, women should use iodised salt and include a serving of seafood in their diet at least once per week.

Iron

The recommended daily allowance (RDA) of iron for pregnant women is 30 mg. In most cases, about one-half of this intake comes from supplements because dietary intake alone can't provide sufficient iron. Remember to tell the woman to take iron supplements with orange juice to enhance absorption. Inform her that they may cause her stools to be black and that constipation may develop if she doesn't include enough fluids and fibre in her diet.

Pumping iron

Iron is necessary to build high levels of haemoglobin, which is needed for fetal oxygenation during pregnancy and after the baby is born. After the 20th week of pregnancy, the fetus begins to store iron in the liver. These stores need to be adequate to last through the first 3 months of life, when intake consists mainly of milk (which is typically low in iron). The pregnant woman also needs iron to increase her RBC volume and to replace iron lost in blood at delivery.

Because the richest sources of iron are also the most expensive – organ meats, eggs, green leafy vegetables, whole grain, enriched breads, dried fruits – a woman with a low income may have trouble taking in adequate amounts of iron in her diet. Today, many cereals are iron fortified, but even these foods may not supply the amount of iron that the woman needs.

Fluoride

Fluoride helps to form sound teeth. If the pregnant woman doesn't drink fluoridated water, supplemental fluoride may be recommended. Because large amounts of fluoride stain teeth brown, a woman shouldn't take a supplement if her water contains fluoride and she shouldn't take supplements more often than prescribed.

Sodium

Sodium is a major electrolyte that regulates fluids in the body. It helps with retention of fluid in the maternal circulation to ensure a pressure gradient for optimal exchange across the placenta. It also plays a role in maintaining the acid–base balance of blood and helps nutrients cross cell membranes.

During pregnancy and lactation, a woman's sodium metabolism (utilisation) is altered by hormone activity. As a result, sodium needs are slightly higher during these times. However, there's rarely a need for additional sodium intake because a typical diet usually provides adequate amounts. Unless the woman is hypertensive or has heart disease, seasoning foods as usual is recommended during pregnancy. However, extremely salty foods, such as cooked meats and crisps, should be avoided. Additives, such as monosodium glutamate, should also be avoided. Excessive salt intake could result in fluid retention, which strains the heart.

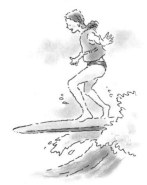

Excessive salt intake leads to fluid retention, which strains the heart.

Zinc

Zinc is necessary for synthesis of DNA and ribonucleic acid as well as cell division and growth. Zinc deficiency has been associated with preterm birth. The RDA of zinc during pregnancy is 15 mg daily. Meat, liver, eggs, seafood and antenatal vitamins are good sources of zinc.

Fluid

Because a pregnant woman is excreting not only her own waste products but also those of her fetus, her body requires extra water to promote kidney function. In addition, fluids:
- keep skin soft
- lessen the likelihood of constipation
- rid the body of toxins and waste products
- reduce excessive swelling.

Recommended fluid intake is 8 cups daily. Fluid sources include juices, milk, soups and other beverages. The woman should avoid excess intake of caffeinated and carbonated beverages.

Minimising discomforts of pregnancy

Being aware of maternal discomforts during pregnancy allows you to provide information on how to alleviate them. In addition, early monitoring of certain conditions can help to reduce their occurrence.

Have them share so you can provide care

A pregnant woman may not mention her concerns or discomforts unless she's specifically asked because she isn't aware of the significance of her problems or she's reluctant to take up a lot of time during a antenatal visit. Encourage the woman to discuss whatever concerns she has at her visits. Although some issues may represent minor common discomforts associated with normal pregnancy, others may be early indicators of potential problems. For example, a problem such as constipation, which the woman may consider a minor discomfort, may result in haemorrhoids, which can become a long-term problem if left to progress throughout the pregnancy.

On the other hand, a woman may see the discomforts of pregnancy as deterrents to good health. The minor discomforts of pregnancy may not seem minor to the woman, especially if they occur daily and make her wonder if she'll ever feel like herself again. You need to provide empathetic and sound advice for relieving discomforts and helping promote the overall health and well-being of a pregnant woman. (See *Dealing with pregnancy discomforts*, page 169.)

A pregnant woman should be encouraged to discuss the discomforts she's experiencing. Some can be easily allayed but others may be problematic.

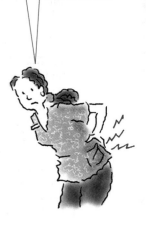

First trimester

Although a pregnant woman may be excited about pregnancy and childbirth, the many discomforts that occur during the first trimester can take away from the joyful feelings of motherhood. Such discomforts are usually accepted as an expected part of pregnancy. However, there are ways to ease discomforts and prevent further complications. You should pass this information along to her as necessary.

Nausea and vomiting

Nausea and vomiting are the most common discomforts during the first trimester. Although these symptoms are commonly referred to as *morning sickness*, they can last all day for some women. Nausea and vomiting rarely interfere with proper nutrition enough to harm the developing fetus.

Many women experience nausea normally during pregnancy. Medications are rarely prescribed to relieve nausea because they may adversely affect the fetus.

At least half of pregnant women experience the joys of nausea!

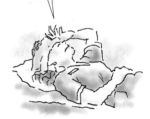

Queasiness cause

Although a specific cause of nausea during pregnancy hasn't been determined, it has been suggested that nausea is the body's reaction to the high levels

Education edge

Dealing with pregnancy discomforts

This table lists common discomforts associated with pregnancy and suggestions that you can give to the woman on how to prevent and manage them.

Discomfort	Client teaching	Discomfort	Client teaching
Urinary frequency	• Void as necessary. • Avoid caffeine. • Perform Kegel exercises.	Nasal stuffiness	• Use a cool-mist vaporiser. • Use saline nose drops. • Avoid medicated nasal sprays because of rebound stuffiness with repeated use.
Fatigue	• Try to get a full night's sleep. • Schedule a daily rest time. • Maintain good nutrition.	Haemorrhoids	• Avoid constipation. • Set a regular time for bowel movements. • Use the bidet with warm water, as often as needed to relieve discomfort. • Apply ice packs (for short periods) for reduction of swelling, if preferred over heat.
Breast tenderness	• Wear a supportive bra. • Wear a bra at night if breast discomfort interferes with sleep.		
Vaginal discharge	• Wear cotton underwear. • Avoid tight-fitting tights. • Bathe daily.	Varicosities	• Exercise regularly. • Rest with the legs elevated daily. • Avoid standing or sitting for long periods. • Avoid crossing the legs. • Avoid wearing constrictive knee-high stockings, wear support stockings instead. • Keep within the recommended weight range during pregnancy.
Backache	• Avoid standing for long periods. • Keep within the recommended weight range during pregnancy. • Avoid high-heeled shoes. • Bend at the knees, not the waist.		
Round ligament pain	• Slowly rise from a sitting position. • Bend forward to relieve pain. • Avoid twisting motions. • Lie on the side opposite the discomfort.	Ankle oedema	• Avoid standing or sitting for long periods. • Rest with the feet elevated. • Avoid wearing garments that constrict the lower extremities.
Constipation	• Increase fibre intake in the diet. • Set a regular time for bowel movements. • Drink more fluids, including water and fruit juices (unless contraindicated). Avoid caffeinated drinks.	Leg cramps	• Straighten the leg and dorsiflex the ankle. • Avoid pointing the toes. • Rest frequently with legs elevated.

of hCG that occur during the first trimester. Other possible contributors to nausea include the rapid stretching of the woman's uterine muscles, the relative relaxation of the muscle tissue in the digestive tract (making digestion less efficient), excess acid in the stomach and the woman's enhanced sense of smell. (See *Reducing nausea*, page 170.)

Nausea and vomiting are considered abnormal if:

• the woman is losing weight instead of gaining it
• lost meals are unable to be made up for during some time of the day

Education edge

Reducing nausea

To help the woman relieve nausea during pregnancy, give her these tips:

- Before getting out of bed in the morning, eat a high-carbohydrate food, such as saltines, melba toast or other crackers.
- Eat small, frequent meals rather than large, infrequent ones.
- Avoid greasy and highly seasoned foods.
- Delay breakfast (or dinner, if experiencing evening nausea) until nausea passes. Make up for missed meals at another time to maintain nutrition.
- Avoid sudden movements and fatigue, which are known to increase nausea.
- If breakfast is usually eaten late in the morning, eat a snack before bedtime to help avoid long periods between meals.
- Buy a wrist acupressure band (available at travel stores), which may help to reduce motion sickness.
- Sip carbonated beverages, water or herbal decaffeinated tea.
- Take a walk outside or take deep breaths through an open window to inhale fresh air.

- signs of dehydration, such as little urine output, are present
- nausea lasts past the 12th week of pregnancy
- the woman vomits more than once daily.

To prevent potential complications, such as hyperemesis gravidarum (severe nausea and vomiting during pregnancy that result in dehydration and loss of at least 4.5 kg), inform the obstetrician/midwife if these signs and symptoms occur. (For more information on hyperemesis gravidarum, see Chapter 6, *High-risk pregnancy*.)

Nasal stuffiness

Nasal stuffiness is common during pregnancy and may persist during all three trimesters. Oestrogen contributes to vasocongestion and makes the nasal mucosa more friable, possibly leading to epistaxis.

Urinary frequency

Urinary frequency occurs in the first trimester because of increasing blood volume and an increased glomerular filtration rate (GFR). It may last for about 3 months and disappears in mid-trimester, when the uterus rises above the bladder. It commonly returns again in late pregnancy as the fetal head presses against the bladder.

If a woman reports urinary frequency, ask her if she has experienced burning or pain on urination or if she has noticed blood in her urine – both signs of a UTI. After infection is ruled out, focus on teaching her ways to alleviate discomfort. Suggest to the woman that she reduce the amount of caffeine she drinks, if applicable. She can also perform Kegel exercises to help strengthen the pelvic muscles so that the feeling of urgency is less noticeable later in pregnancy. Kegel exercises also help with urinary control.

Breast tenderness

Breast tenderness is commonly noticed early in pregnancy and may be most noticeable when the woman is exposed to cold air. For most women, tenderness is minimal and transient. Many are aware of it but aren't distressed by it.

If breast tenderness causes the woman discomfort, recommend that she wear a bra with wide shoulder straps for support and dress warmly to avoid cold drafts (if cold increases symptoms). Wearing a bra at night may help if breast discomfort is preventing her from getting a good night's sleep. If actual pain exists, suspect the presence of an underlying condition, such as nipple fissures or mastitis.

Fatigue

Fatigue is common early in pregnancy and may be caused by the body's increased metabolic requirements. Fatigue can also intensify morning sickness; for example, if the woman becomes too tired, she may not eat properly. If she remains on her feet without at least one break during the day, the risk of varicosities and thromboembolitic complications increases.

Putting fatigue to rest

Increasing the amount of rest and sleep may relieve the woman's fatigue. During antenatal visits, ask her whether she manages to take at least one short rest period every day. Modifying her routine to allow rest periods is advised. If the woman has a sedentary job inside or outside of the home, she needs to increase her activity, such as by walking or using a treadmill. By balancing rest and exercise, she can reduce her fatigue.

A modified Sims' position with the top leg forward is a good resting position. This puts the weight of the fetus on the bed, not on the woman and allows good circulation to the lower extremities.

Increased vaginal discharge

Leucorrhoea is another discomfort of pregnancy. It's a whitish, viscous vaginal discharge or an increase in the amount of normal vaginal secretions. It's caused by the high oestrogen levels and increased blood supply to the vaginal epithelium and cervix that occur during pregnancy. A woman who's uncomfortable about discussing this part of her body or who associates vaginal infections with poor hygiene or STIs may be reluctant to mention an irritating vaginal discharge. Be sure to ask every woman at antenatal visits whether she is experiencing this problem.

Deterring discharge

Tell the woman that a daily bath or shower can help wash away accumulated secretions and prevent vulvar excoriation. Warn her not to douche; this is contraindicated throughout pregnancy. She can also use perineal pads to

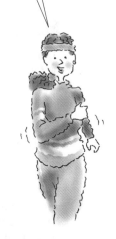

Balancing sedentary activities with physical activities can help reduce fatigue during pregnancy.

control discharge; she shouldn't use tampons, however, because they promote stasis of secretions, which can lead to infection. Wearing cotton underwear and sleeping without underwear are helpful in reducing moisture and possible excoriation. Tell the woman that she should avoid tight-fitting underwear and tights to prevent yeast infections.

Advise her to contact the midwife/obstetrician if there's a change in the colour, odour or character of the discharge as this could indicate infection. Vulvar pruritus (itching of the vulva) also needs evaluation because this sign also strongly indicates infection.

Second and third trimesters

Although the woman may be focused on bonding with the fetus, she must be reminded to report any discomforts to ensure that nothing serious is occurring. In addition, at the midpoint of pregnancy, review with the woman precautionary measures that help prevent constipation, varicosities and haemorrhoids and discuss with her the new symptoms that may occur.

Indigestion

Indigestion may be caused by large amounts of progesterone and oestrogen, which tend to relax smooth muscle tissue throughout the body – including the GI tract. This causes food to move through the system more slowly and may result in bloating and indigestion. This slowdown is beneficial because it allows for better absorption of nutrients into the bloodstream and subsequently into the fetus's system.

Feeling the burn

Heartburn results when the cardiac sphincter relaxes, allowing food and digestive juices to back up from the stomach into the oesophagus. This irritates the lining, causing a burning sensation. This problem may increase later in pregnancy because of the pressure of the fetus on the mother's internal organs. (See *Relieving heartburn and indigestion*, page 173.)

If measures fail to relieve symptoms, a low-sodium antacid or other medication that's safe to use during pregnancy may be prescribed by the doctor. Sodium or sodium bicarbonate solutions should be avoided because they can exacerbate heartburn.

Ankle oedema

Most women experience some swelling of the ankles and feet during late pregnancy, most noticeably at the end of the day. It may result from reduced blood circulation in the lower extremities caused by uterine pressure and general fluid retention. The woman may become aware of it if she takes off her shoes and then can't get them back on again comfortably. As long as proteinuria and hypertension aren't present, ankle oedema is a normal occurrence.

To help relieve oedema, tell the woman to rest in a left side-lying position; this increases the GFR. Sitting for half an hour in the afternoon and again in

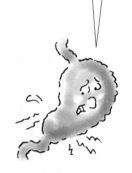

Indigestion and heartburn may result when the relaxation of smooth muscle tissue and the cardiac sphincter cause food processing to slow down.

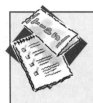

Education edge

Relieving heartburn and indigestion

To decrease the incidence of heartburn and indigestion in the pregnant woman, advise her to:

- avoid gaining too much weight (this puts excess pressure on the stomach)
- avoid wearing clothing that's tight around the abdomen and waist
- eat frequent, small meals instead of three large ones
- eat slowly and chew thoroughly
- avoid highly seasoned foods, fried and fatty foods, processed meats, chocolate, coffee, alcohol, carbonated beverages and spearmint or peppermint
- chew raw ginger/try ginger sweets or biscuits
- avoid smoking
- avoid bending at the waist
- sleep with her head elevated about 15 cm.

the evening with the legs elevated should also help. Tell the woman to avoid constricting panty girdles or knee-high stockings because these garments impede lower-extremity circulation and venous return.

Don't discount a report of lower-extremity oedema until you're certain the woman doesn't exhibit signs of proteinuria, oedema of other nondependent parts, or sudden weight increase that's indicative of gestational hypertension.

Varicose veins

Varicose veins are tortuous veins that commonly appear during pregnancy. They develop because the weight of the distended uterus puts pressure on the veins returning blood from the lower extremities. This causes blood to pool in the vessels, and the veins become engorged, inflamed and painful. Varicose veins are common in women with a family history and in women who have a large fetus or multiple pregnancies. Sitting for prolonged periods with the legs dependent also promotes venous stasis.

Simple Sims'

Resting in Sims' position for 15–20 minutes twice daily is a good preventive measure against varicose veins. Advise the woman to avoid sitting with her legs crossed or her knees bent and to avoid wearing constrictive knee-high socks. Elastic medical support stockings, such as TEDS, should be used to relieve varicose veins and should be applied before the woman arises in the morning to be most effective. Alternating exercise with rest periods is also effective in alleviating varicose veins. The woman should be advised to break up periods of sitting or standing with a walk at least twice daily. Vitamin C may also be helpful in reducing the size of varicose veins because it's involved in forming collagen and endothelium for blood vessels. Ask at antenatal visits whether fresh fruit is included in the woman's diet.

Surgical removal of varicose veins isn't recommended during pregnancy. In most cases, they improve on their own after delivery, usually by the time pre-pregnancy weight is reached.

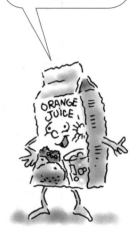

Vitamin C may help reduce the size of varicose veins.

Haemorrhoids

Haemorrhoids are varicosities of the rectal veins. They occur commonly in pregnancy because the bulk of the growing uterus puts pressure on the veins. Measures taken early in pregnancy to prevent their occurrence are key to reducing their incidence as well as severity.

Resting in a modified Sims' position daily helps to reduce the discomfort of haemorrhoids. Tell the woman to assume a knee-chest position at the end of the day to reduce pressure on rectal veins. Because this position can result in light-headedness, advise her to start by doing this for only a few minutes and gradually increasing to 10–15 minutes. Stool softeners may be recommended as well as application of witch hazel or cold compresses to help relieve pain.

Constipation

As pregnancy progresses, the growing uterus presses against the bowel and slows peristalsis, resulting in constipation and sometimes flatulence. Prescribed oral iron supplements also contribute to constipation. Reinforce the need for the supplements to build fetal iron stores but also help the woman to find a method to relieve or prevent constipation.

Advise the woman not to use home remedies, such as mineral oil and enemas. Mineral oil interferes with the absorption of fat-soluble vitamins (A, D, E and K), which are necessary for fetal growth. Enemas might initiate labour through their action. Over-the-counter laxatives and all drugs are contraindicated during pregnancy unless specifically prescribed or authorised by the woman's doctor. (See *Preventing constipation*, page 175.)

If the woman experiences excessive flatulence, recommend that she avoid gas-forming foods, such as cabbage and beans. In addition, if dietary measures and regular bowel evacuation fail, a stool softener (such as lactulose) and evacuation suppositories (such as glycerine) may be prescribed.

Backache

As pregnancy advances, a lumbar lordosis occurs and postural changes necessary to maintain balance may lead to backache. Backache can also be an initial sign of bladder or kidney infection. To determine the cause of the woman's backache, assess the manner in which she walks, determine what type of shoes she wears and obtain a detailed account of her symptoms.

Education edge

Preventing constipation

When teaching the pregnant woman about preventing constipation, include these tips:

- Encourage her to evacuate her bowels regularly.
- Advise her to increase the amount of roughage in her diet by eating raw fruits, bran and vegetables.
- Instruct her to drink extra amounts of water daily.
- Drink some fruit juice daily – take it with the iron tablets – helps absorption!

To help alleviate pain, instruct her to wear shoes with low-to-moderate height heels. Such shoes reduce the amount of spinal curvature necessary to maintain an upright posture. Advise the woman to walk with her pelvis tilted forward. This helps to alleviate back pain by putting pelvic support under the weight of the uterus. Local heat and a firmer mattress (or a board placed under the mattress) can help to relieve discomfort. Pelvic rocking or tilting can also be beneficial. To avoid back strain, advise the woman to squat – not bend over – to lift objects and to hold objects close to the body when lifting.

Tell the woman not to take muscle relaxants or analgesics (as well as other medications) for back pain without first consulting her practitioner. Generally, paracetamol or co-codamol is considered safe and effective for relieving this type of pain during pregnancy. (Check that the woman is not asthmatic or allergic to either of these medications.)

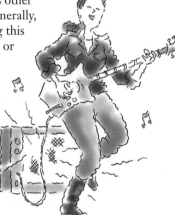

Rock on! Pelvic rocking can help alleviate back pain.

Leg cramps

Decreased serum calcium, increased serum phosphorus and interference with circulation commonly cause muscle cramps of the lower extremities during pregnancy. The pain may be extreme and the intensity of the contraction frightening. Make sure to ask the woman at antenatal visits if she's having leg cramps. If leg cramps are a problem, provide her with information on techniques for relieving discomfort.

Extend and elevate

The best way to relieve symptoms is to have the woman lie on her back momentarily and extend the involved leg while keeping her knee straight and dorsiflexing the foot until the pain is gone. Elevating the lower extremities frequently during the day to improve circulation and avoiding full leg extension, such as stretching with the toes pointed, may also be beneficial.

If the woman is having frequent leg cramps, her doctor may prescribe aluminium hydroxide gel (Amphojel) to bind phosphorus in the intestinal tract, lowering it in the circulation. Lowering milk intake to only a pint daily and supplementing this with calcium lactate may also help to reduce her phosphorus level.

Light-headedness

Light-headedness in the first trimester may be caused by a blood supply that inadequately fills the rapidly expanding circulatory system. During the second trimester, the pressure of the expanding uterus on maternal blood vessels may cause it. Faintness can occur anytime the woman rises from a sitting or prone position (postural hypotension) because the blood suddenly shifts away from the brain when blood pressure drops rapidly. Advise her to get up slowly in these situations.

Light-headedness may also be the result of low glucose levels caused by skipping meals. Carrying fruit or crackers to snack on is helpful to quickly increase glucose levels.

If the woman feels faint, advise her to lie down with her legs elevated or sit down and place her head between her knees until faintness subsides. She should also report to her midwife or doctor any light-headedness because it can be a sign of severe anaemia or another illness and should be evaluated.

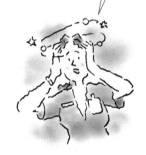

Lying down and elevating the legs helps to relieve light-headedness.

Shortness of breath

As the expanding uterus puts pressure on the diaphragm, the lungs may compress, causing dyspnoea (shortness of breath). This may be more noticeable to the woman on exertion or during the night, when her body is flat.

Sitting upright and allowing the weight of the uterus to fall away from the diaphragm can help relieve the problem. As pregnancy progresses, the woman may require two or more pillows to sleep on at night to avoid dyspnoea.

Always question the woman about shortness of breath at antenatal visits to be certain the sensation isn't continuous. Constant shortness of breath may indicate cardiac problems or a respiratory tract infection.

Insomnia

Insomnia is common during pregnancy. It's difficult for a pregnant women to rest physically because her large abdomen makes it difficult to get comfortable, and mentally because she has a lot on her mind. In cases of insomnia, it's helpful to review stress-reduction and relaxation techniques to help her get in the frame of mind for a good night's sleep. In addition, a comfortable bed and pillows to support the head, back and abdomen are helpful. Eating a light snack before bedtime and avoiding caffeine after lunchtime is also beneficial. If the woman naps during the day, suggest shortening the nap and trying to stay up to promote better sleep at night. If measures fail, suggest that she get out of bed and read, knit or do a favourite activity until she's drowsy and able to fall asleep.

Abdominal discomfort and Braxton Hicks contractions

A woman may experience uncomfortable feelings of abdominal pressure early in pregnancy. A woman with a multiple pregnancy may notice this throughout pregnancy. She can relieve this pressure by putting gentle pressure on the uterine fundus or by standing with her arms crossed in front.

Pain around the round ligaments

When a woman stands up quickly, she may experience a pulling pain in the right or left lower abdomen from tension on the round ligaments. It can be very sharp and frightening and may be prevented by always rising slowly from a lying to a sitting position or from a sitting to a standing position. Keep in mind that round ligament pain may simulate the abrupt pain that occurs with ruptured ectopic pregnancy. The woman's description of the pain needs to be evaluated carefully.

As early as the 12th week of pregnancy, the uterus periodically contracts and relaxes again. These contractions, termed *Braxton Hicks contractions*, usually aren't noticeable early in pregnancy. In the mid-trimester and late pregnancy, the contractions become stronger, causing the woman to tense and possibly feel minimal pain, similar to a hard menstrual cramp. These feelings are normal and aren't a sign of beginning labour.

Be certain the woman understands that a rhythmic pattern of contractions, characteristic of labour, shouldn't be mistaken for Braxton Hicks contractions.

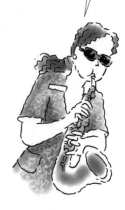

I've got rhythm, but a rhythmic pattern of contractions is characteristic of labour.

Quick quiz

1. A pregnant woman who's older than age 35 is at greater risk for having:
   A. a low-birthweight infant.
   B. a preterm infant.
   C. gestational hypertension.
   D. placenta praevia.

Answer: D. Expectant mothers who are older than age 35 are at risk for placenta praevia, hydatidiform mole, and vascular, neoplastic and degenerative diseases. They're also at risk for having fraternal twins or infants with genetic abnormalities, especially Down syndrome.

2. Which familial factor is most likely to cause discomfort during pregnancy?
   A. Anaemia
   B. Varicose veins
   C. Cancer
   D. Colitis

Answer: B. Varicose veins are an inherited weakness in blood vessel walls that become evident during pregnancy and can cause the woman discomfort.

3. A woman reports that the first day of her last normal menses was January 7. The calculated EDD is:
   A. October 14.
   B. April 14.
   C. September 31.
   D. April 7.

Answer: A. Based on information obtained in the woman's menstrual history, you can calculate the woman's EDD using *Nägele's rule:* take the first day of the last normal menses, subtract 3 months, and then add 7 days.

4. Normal FHR is:
   A. 110–150 beats/minute.
   B. 120–160 beats/minute.
   C. 130–170 beats/minute.
   D. 140–180 beats/minute.

Answer: B. Normal FHR usually ranges from 120 to 160 beats/minute.

5. Triple screening combines data from which antenatal tests?
   A. Ultrasound, amniocentesis and serum oestriol
   B. Serum hPL, serum oestriol and urinalysis
   C. Serum hCG, serum oestriol and urinalysis
   D. MSAFP, serum hCG and unconjugated oestriol

Answer: D. Triple screening combines data from MSAFP, hCG and unconjugated oestriol.

6. A pregnant woman who's fatigued is likely to be more comfortable in which position?
   A. Modified Sims'
   B. Supine with legs elevated
   C. Supine with head elevated
   D. Sitting upright with legs elevated

Answer: A. A good resting position is a modified Sims' position with the top leg forward. This puts the weight of the fetus on the bed, not on the woman, and allows good circulation in the lower extremities.

Scoring

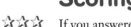 If you answered all six questions correctly, wow! You've sailed through antenatal care!

If you answered four or five questions correctly, great job! You have smooth seas ahead!

If you answered fewer than four questions correctly, don't go overboard! Forge ahead after a quick review!

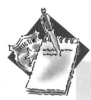

6 High-risk pregnancy

Just the facts

In this chapter, you'll learn:

♦ factors that contribute to high-risk pregnancy
♦ ways to identify high-risk situations based on key assessment findings
♦ appropriate treatments for high-risk pregnancies
♦ relevant midwifery/obstetric interventions for high-risk pregnancies.

A look at high-risk pregnancy

Most women progress through pregnancy without serious problems. They enter pregnancy in good health and give birth to healthy neonates. However, problems sometimes develop that put a woman and her fetus in jeopardy. These problems may result from a chronic illness in the mother, a complication that develops during the pregnancy or an external factor that impacts the health and well-being of the mother or the fetus.

Mother + fetus = one

Keep in mind that the health of a woman and her fetus are interdependent. Changes in the woman's health may affect fetal health, and changes in fetal health may affect the mother's physical and emotional health.

Group effort

Rarely is just one risk factor responsible for a high-risk pregnancy. Several factors can work together to contribute to a high-risk situation. For example, a pregnant adolescent is considered at higher risk; however, it isn't simply her age that places her in this category. Rather, her age is an indication of other factors that contribute to increased risk. First, as a pregnant adolescent, she faces a personal developmental crisis. In addition, adolescents, if unsupported, often lack proper nutrition, or adequate finances

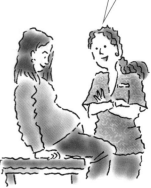

You can depend on it! The health of a woman and her fetus are interdependent.

to live in a warm, hygienic environment. These factors, together with the fact that she may have little knowledge of pregnancy and it's effects, are all contributors of increased risk. She may not feel she can attend hospital for care, as she feels isolated and afraid of the pregnancy and how her family and friends will react to it.

Maternal age

Reproductive risks increase among adolescents younger than age 15 and women older than age 35. The adolescent woman faces serious risks, including increased incidence of low birthweight (<2.5 kg) and preterm neonates, anaemia, labour dysfunction and cephalopelvic disproportion. Conditions such as iron deficiency anaemia, gestational hypertension and preterm labour occur more commonly in adolescents than in older women.

Expectant mothers older than age 35 are at risk for placenta praevia, hydatidiform mole and vascular, neoplastic and degenerative diseases. They're also at risk for having twins or infants with genetic and chromosomal abnormalities, e.g. Down's Syndrome.

Maternal parity

Maternal parity may place a pregnant woman at high risk. For example, a multigravida who has had five or more pregnancies lasting at least 20 weeks is considered high risk. In addition, if the current pregnancy occurs within 3 months of the last delivery, the pregnancy is considered high risk.

Maternal obstetric and gynaecologic history

Many factors in the mother's obstetric and gynaecologic history can place a pregnancy at high risk. These factors may include:
• two or more premature deliveries or spontaneous abortions
• one or more stillbirths at term
• one or more babies born with gross anomalies
• pelvic inadequacy or abnormal shaping
• cervical incompetency
• uterine incompetency, position or structural anomalies
• history of multiple pregnancy, placental anomalies, amniotic fluid abnormalities or poor weight gain
• history of gestational diabetes, gestational hypertension or infection
• history of delivering a postterm neonate
• history of dystocia, precipitous delivery, cervical or vaginal lacerations caused by labour and delivery, cephalopelvic disproportion, haemorrhage during labour and delivery or retained placenta
• lack of previous antenatal care.

In addition, a pregnancy that occurs within 3 years of menarche indicates an increased risk of maternal mortality and morbidity. Such a pregnancy also places the woman at risk for delivering a baby who's small for gestational age. (Birthweight falls below the 10th centile for that gestational age.)

Maternal medical history

Medical problems can cause complications during pregnancy. For example, abdominal trauma may lead to premature rupture of membranes (PROM) or abruptio placentae. Severe cardiac disease can adversely affect placental perfusion, thus jeopardising fetal nutrition. As a result, the baby may be born with a low birthweight. Gestational hypertension, which commonly develops in women with essential hypertension, renal disease or diabetes, increases the risk of placental abruption.

Insulin influx

Diabetes can worsen during pregnancy and harm the mother and fetus. Because pregnant women typically develop insulin resistance, women with diabetes need increased amounts of insulin during pregnancy. The fetus of a woman with diabetes tends to be large because the increased insulin production needed to counteract the overload of glucose from the mother stimulates fetal growth. This, in turn, can lead to problems of cephalopelvic disproportion and shoulder dystocia for the mother at delivery.

Gravida aggravations

Stomach displacement by the gravid uterus, along with cardiac sphincter relaxation and decreased gastrointestinal (GI) motility caused by increased progesterone, may aggravate symptoms of peptic ulcer disease such as gastric reflux. Also, the increase in blood volume and cardiac output associated with pregnancy can exhaust a woman with underlying cardiac disease.

Maternal lifestyle

Lifestyle and occupation can adversely affect a pregnancy. Make the woman aware that what she consumes and what she's exposed to can seriously affect her pregnancy. For example, taking over the counter and prescription drugs can be detrimental to the fetus. In addition, cigarette smoking is associated with intrauterine growth retardation and low birthweight babies. Exposure to toxic substances, such as lead, organic solvents, radiation and carbon monoxide, can also lead to fetal malformations.

Substance sabotage

Substance use or abuse of drugs or alcohol is another cause of fetal anomalies. After birth, the neonate may experience withdrawal. Substance abuse may also interfere with the pregnant woman's ability to obtain adequate nutrition,

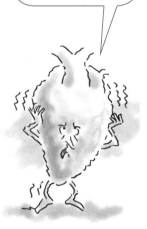

The increase in blood volume and cardiac output associated with pregnancy can be quite taxing on me!

which can adversely affect fetal growth. Additionally, if the substance abuse involves injection, the pregnant woman is at risk for infection with hepatitis B and human immunodeficiency virus (HIV).

Nourish to flourish

Adequate nutrition is especially vital during pregnancy. Inadequate nutrition can lead to a deficiency of iron, folic acid or protein. Iron deficiency anaemia during pregnancy is associated with low fetal birthweight and preterm birth. Folic acid deficiency is associated with neural tube defects. Protein deficiency can lead to poor development of the fetus and growth restriction.

Cultural and ethnic background

Several genetic disorders are associated with specific ethnic groups. For example, sickle cell anaemia occurs primarily in persons of African and Mediterranean descent. Tay-Sachs disease is about 100 times more common in people of Eastern European Jewish (Ashkenazi) ancestry than in the general population.

Family history

Certain conditions and disorders that contribute to high-risk pregnancy are familial. For example, a family history of multiple births, congenital diseases or deformities, or mental disability may place a pregnancy at higher risk.

Don't forget dad

Some fetal congenital anomalies may be traced to the father's exposure to environmental hazards. The father's blood type and Rh status are also important because isoimmunisation in the fetus may occur if the father is Rh-positive, the mother is Rh-negative and the fetus is Rh-positive.

On the home front

The family environment is also important in determining whether a pregnancy is high risk. A history of domestic abuse, a lack of support persons, inadequate housing or lack of adequate finances can increase risk during pregnancy.

Cardiac disease

The pregnant woman with preexisting cardiac disease is considered high risk. Despite improvements in early identification and management of cardiac problems, these disorders contribute to complications in approximately 1% of pregnancies.

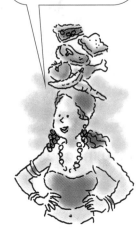

Food, glorious food! Adequate nutrition is especially vital during pregnancy.

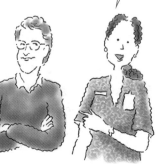

It isn't just mum. Dad also plays a role in fetal congenital anomalies, specifically related to his exposure to environmental hazards and his blood type and Rh status.

Cardiac disease classification

Here are the New York Heart Association's guidelines for classifying the degree of compromise in a pregnant woman with cardiac disease. Typically, a woman with Class I or II cardiac disease can complete a pregnancy and delivery without major complications. A woman with Class III cardiac disease usually must maintain complete bed rest during the pregnancy. A woman with Class IV cardiac disease is a poor candidate for pregnancy and should be strongly urged to avoid becoming pregnant.

Class	Description
I	*Uncompromised* – The woman has unrestricted physical activity. Ordinary physical activity causes no discomfort, cardiac insufficiency or anginal pain.
II	*Slightly compromised* – The woman has a slight limitation on physical activity. Ordinary activity causes excess fatigue, palpitations, dyspnoea or anginal pain.
III	*Markedly compromised* – The woman has a moderate or marked limitation on physical activity. With less than ordinary activity, she experiences excessive fatigue, palpitations, dyspnoea or anginal pain.
IV	*Severely compromised* – The woman can't engage in any physical activity without experiencing discomfort. Cardiac insufficiency or anginal pain occurs even at rest.

Adapted with permission from Criteria Committee of the New York Heart Association. *Nomenclature and Criteria for Diagnosis of Diseases of the Heart and Great Vessels*, 9th edn. Boston: Little, Brown, & Co., 1994: 253–256.

Rating the risk

The type and extent of the woman's cardiac disease determine whether she can successfully complete a pregnancy. Guidelines developed by the New York Heart Association could be used to predict a pregnancy's outcome. These guidelines categorise pregnancy based on the degree of compromise. (See *Cardiac disease classification*.)

What causes it

The most common underlying cause of cardiac disease in pregnancy involves congenital anomalies, such as atrial septal defect and coarctation of the aorta that hasn't been corrected. Valvular disease caused by rheumatic fever or Kawasaki disease may also be an underlying problem. Moreover, with an increase in the number of women becoming pregnant at an older age, the incidences of ischaemic cardiac disease and myocardial infarction are increasing.

On rare occasion

Peripartal cardiomyopathy (cardiac disease that manifests primarily with pregnancy) is rare. Although the exact cause is unknown, it's believed to result from the effects of pregnancy on the circulatory system. In many cases, previously undiagnosed cardiac disease is the cause.

The weaker weeks

The most dangerous time for a pregnant woman with cardiac disease and her fetus is between weeks 28 and 32 of gestation. During this time, blood volume peaks and the woman's heart may be unable to compensate adequately for the increase. As a result, cardiac decompensation can occur, causing the woman's cardiac output to drop, possibly to such an extent that perfusion to vital organs, including the placenta, is significantly affected. Consequently, oxygen and nutrients aren't delivered in adequate amounts to the cells, including those of the fetus.

What to look for

Signs and symptoms of cardiac disease in a pregnant woman depend on the type and severity of the underlying disease. Primarily, these signs and symptoms are those associated with heart failure. (See *The weaker weeks*.) Fetal signs of maternal cardiac disease are nonspecific – such as abnormally low fetal heart rate (FHR) and fetal growth retardation – so diagnosis depends mainly on maternal signs and symptoms.

Failure to the left

Left-sided heart failure occurs with such conditions as mitral valve disorder and congenital coarctation of the aorta. Common signs and symptoms are those associated with pulmonary hypertension and pulmonary oedema and may include:
- decreased systemic blood pressure
- productive cough with blood-streaked sputum
- tachypnoea
- dyspnoea on exertion, progressing to dyspnoea at rest
- tachycardia
- orthopnoea
- paroxysmal nocturnal dyspnoea
- oedema.

Failure to the right

Right-sided heart failure can occur in a woman with a congenital heart defect, such as atrial and ventricular septal defect and pulmonary valve stenosis. Signs and symptoms may include:
- hypotension
- jugular vein distention
- liver and spleen enlargement
- ascites
- dyspnoea and pain.

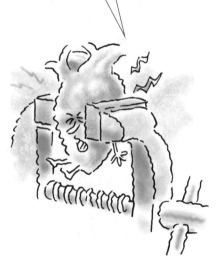

I've got coarctation to the left of me, defects to the right. Here I am, stuck in the middle.

Myocardial failure

For the woman with peripartal cardiac disease, signs and symptoms typically reflect myocardial failure. Shortness of breath, chest pain and oedema are common. Cardiomegaly also may occur.

What tests tell you

An electrocardiogram (ECG) may show cardiac changes in the mother but may be less accurate later in pregnancy as the enlarged uterus pushes the diaphragm upward and displaces the heart. Echocardiography shows cardiomegaly. If the mother's cardiac decompensation has reached the point of placental insufficiency and incompetency, late decelerations during fetal monitoring may indicate fetal distress. Ultrasonography may show growth retardation.

How it's treated

Treatment focuses on ensuring the health and safety of the mother and fetus. Commonly, more frequent antenatal visits are scheduled, such as every 2 weeks and then every week during the last month, to achieve this goal. The mother may need to spend some time in hospital prior to delivery.

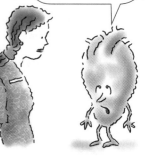

ECG may be less accurate later in pregnancy because the enlarged uterus displaces the heart.

No wonder! I thought it was getting crowded around here!

Minor adjustments

If the woman was taking cardiac medications before becoming pregnant, the medications are typically continued during pregnancy. However, maintenance doses may need to be increased to aid in compensating for the increased blood volume associated with pregnancy.

The deal with other drugs

If the woman required digoxin (Lanoxin) before her pregnancy, she can continue use during pregnancy without risk. Even if she wasn't taking digoxin before her pregnancy, she may require it to help increase or strengthen her cardiac output as her pregnancy advances. The effects on pregnancy of propranolol (Inderal), a beta-adrenergic blocker commonly used for cardiac arrhythmias, aren't known; however, the drug doesn't appear to cause fetal abnormalities. The effects of nitroglycerin, a compound commonly prescribed for angina, are also unknown; however, the drug appears to be safe. A woman who's taking heparin for venous thromboembolitic disease shouldn't take any after labour begins. If the woman has had a valve replacement and is receiving warfarin therapy, warfarin – which is associated with an increase in fetal anomalies – is discontinued and heparin is used instead.

Prophylactic tactics

For women with valvular or congenital cardiac disease, some practitioners may begin prophylactic antibiotic therapy near to the mother's expected due date to prevent the development of possible subacute bacterial endocarditis, secondary to bacterial invasion from the placental site into the bloodstream. If the woman was taking prophylactic antibiotics to prevent a recurrence of rheumatic fever before becoming pregnant, they're continued during pregnancy.

Rest for the weary

Another key area of treatment is rest. A pregnant woman with cardiac disease requires more rest than the average pregnant woman. In addition, practitioners commonly recommend complete bed rest for the woman after gestational week 30 to ensure the fetus is carried to term or at least to week 36.

A weighty subject

Maintaining good nutrition is an important component of ensuring a healthy mother and fetus. For the woman with cardiac disease, it's especially important that weight gain be balanced to ensure that the nutritional needs of the mother and fetus are met, while also ensuring that the mother's heart isn't overburdened. As a general practice, salt intake may be limited; however, it shouldn't be severely restricted because sodium is needed for fluid volume. Antenatal vitamins are essential to help ensure adequate iron intake and avoid anaemia, which reduces the blood's capacity to carry oxygen. The pregnant woman with cardiac disease and her fetus need as much oxygen as possible, so anaemia must be avoided.

> The prescription for some pregnant women with cardiac disease is complete bed rest after week 30. Unfortunately, there's no such prescription for midwives!

What to do

Assess maternal vital signs and cardiopulmonary status closely for changes; question the mother about increased shortness of breath, palpitations or oedema; monitor FHR for changes.

- Monitor weight gain throughout pregnancy. Assess for oedema and note any pitting.
- Explain signs and symptoms of worsening disease and tell the mother to report them immediately.
- Reinforce use of prescribed medications to control cardiac disease. Explain possible adverse reactions to these medications and instruct the mother to report these reactions immediately.
- Anticipate the need for increased doses of maintenance medications; explain to the mother the rationale for this increase.
- Assess the woman's nutritional pattern. Work with her to develop a feasible meal plan. Stress the need for antenatal vitamins.
- Assess FHR and ultrasound results to monitor fetal growth.
- Encourage frequent rest periods throughout the day. Discuss measures for pacing activities and conserving energy.
- Advise the woman to immediately report signs and symptoms of infection, such as upper respiratory or urinary tract infection (UTI), to prevent overtaxing the heart.

> Weight gain should meet the nutritional needs of the mother and fetus but shouldn't overburden mum's heart.

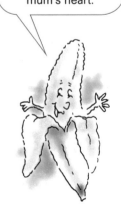

- Advise the woman to rest in the left lateral recumbent position to prevent supine hypotension and provide the best possible oxygen exchange to the fetus; if necessary, use semi-Fowler's position to relieve dyspnoea.
- Prepare the woman for labour, anticipating the use of epidural anaesthesia to avoid overtaxing the mother's heart.
- Monitor FHR, uterine contractions and maternal vital signs closely for changes during labour.
- Assess vital signs closely after delivery. Anticipate anticoagulant and cardiac glycoside therapy immediately after delivery for the woman with severe heart failure.
- Encourage ambulation, as ordered, as soon as possible after delivery.
- Anticipate administration of prophylactic antibiotics, if not already ordered, after delivery to prevent subacute bacterial endocarditis.

Diabetes mellitus

Diabetes mellitus is a metabolic disorder characterised by hyperglycaemia (elevated serum glucose level) resulting from lack of insulin, lack of insulin effect or both. It's a disorder of carbohydrate, protein and fat metabolism.
    Two general classifications are recognised.

1. *Insulin-dependent diabetes* (absolute insulin insufficiency) usually occurs before age 30, although it may occur at any age. The woman is typically thin and requires exogenous insulin and dietary management to achieve control.
2. *Gestational diabetes* (diabetes that emerges during pregnancy) typically develops during the middle of the pregnancy when insulin resistance is most apparent.

Losing balance

Diabetes affects approximately 3–12% of all pregnancies. The overall challenge associated with diabetes and pregnancy is controlling the balance between glucose levels and insulin requirements. Poor glucose control can adversely affect the mother, the fetus or both. The risk of pregnancy-induced hypertension (PIH) and infection (most commonly candidal infections) is higher in pregnant women with diabetes. Moreover, continued fetal consumption of glucose may lead to maternal hypoglycaemia, especially between meals and during the night. Additionally, polyhydramnios (increased amount of amniotic fluid) may occur because of increased fetal urine production caused by fetal hyperglycaemia.
    Babies who are born to mothers with diabetes typically are large, possibly more than 4.5 kg (10 lb). This large size may complicate labour and delivery (poor progress in 1st stage and 2nd stage, shoulder dystocia) necessitating a caesarean birth. The risks of congenital anomalies, birth traumas, spontaneous abortions and stillbirths also increase in women with diabetes.

Don't wait! A pregnant woman with cardiac disease should immediately report signs of upper respiratory tract infection . . .

. . . and other kinds of infection too.

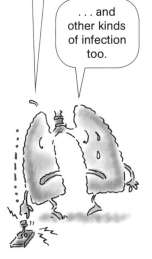

What causes it

Evidence indicates that diabetes has various causes, including:
- heredity
- environment (infection, diet, exposure to toxins and stress)
- lifestyle in genetically susceptible persons.

Insulin-dependent diabetes (IDD)

Although the cause of IDD isn't known, scientists believe that the tendency to develop diabetes may be inherited and related to viruses. In persons with a supposed genetic predisposition to IDD, a triggering event (possibly infection with a virus) spurs the production of autoantibodies that destroy the pancreas's beta cells. The destruction of beta cells causes insulin secretion to decrease or ultimately stop. When more than 90% of the beta cells have been destroyed, the subsequent insulin deficiency leads to hyperglycaemia, enhanced lipolysis (decomposition of fat) and protein catabolism.

Gestational diabetes

Gestational diabetes occurs when a woman who hasn't been previously diagnosed with diabetes shows glucose intolerance during pregnancy. Of those women who don't have diabetes when they become pregnant, approximately 3% develop gestational diabetes. It isn't known whether gestational diabetes results from inadequate insulin response to carbohydrates, excessive insulin resistance or both. Identifiable risk factors include:
- obesity
- history of delivering large neonates (usually more than 4.5 kg), unexplained fetal or perinatal loss, or evidence of congenital anomalies in previous pregnancies
- age older than 25
- family history of diabetes.

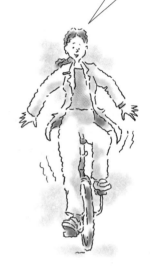

Mum and fetus can be adversely affected by poor glucose control. The key is to maintain balance between glucose levels and insulin.

What to look for

The signs and symptoms noted in the pregnant woman with diabetes are the same as those for any person with diabetes. Common signs and symptoms include hyperglycaemia, glycosuria and polyuria. Dizziness and confusion may be related to hyperglycaemia. In addition, the woman may experience an increased incidence of monilial infections. Hydramnios may be present along with poor FHR and variability arising from inadequate tissue (placental) perfusion.

The woman with type 1 or 2 diabetes may also exhibit signs and symptoms related to microvascular and macrovascular changes, such as peripheral vascular disease, retinopathy, nephropathy and neuropathy.

What tests tell you

Women who are perceived as high risk are screened for gestational diabetes during pregnancy; this screening includes:
• testing of urine for glycosuria and if present, subsequent random plasma glucose (RPG) testing
• routine RPG's during pregnancy – usually around 24 weeks' gestation
• if the RPG level is raised then further screening is required in the form of a glucose tolerance test (GTT) – this is recognised as the 'gold standard' in screening for diabetes.

Glucose tolerance test

The mother has a sample of blood for fasting blood glucose levels, then she has a glucose loaded drink (75 g). Another sample of blood is taken 1–2 hours later for glucose levels. The results of this test will determine whether the mother is a gestational diabetic.

The World Health Organisation (WHO) definition of gestational diabetes is a mother whose fasting blood glucose is ≥7.0 mmol/L or 2 hours result of ≥11.1 mmol/L.

Internationally, these levels may differ and professionals should realise that there are independent risk factors for gestational diabetes which need to be considered, such as:
• body mass index (BMI) $\geq$30 Kg/m^2
• previous macrosomic babies
• previous gestational diabetes in another pregnancy
• family history of diabetes (1st degree relative)
• ethnic origin
Refer to the National Institute of Clinical Excellence (NICE) guidelines for antenatal care, available on http://www.nice.org.uk/guidance/

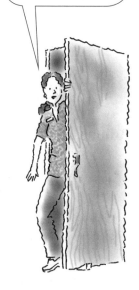

Come one, come all! During pregnancy, all women are screened for gestational diabetes.

How it's treated

Any woman with diabetes, whether preexisting or gestational, requires more frequent antenatal visits to ensure optimal control of glucose levels, minimising the risks to the woman and her fetus. Additionally, treatment focuses on balancing rest with exercise and maintaining adequate nutrition for fetal growth and control of blood glucose levels.

Ideally, the woman with preexisting diabetes should consult with her general practioner or physician before becoming pregnant to ensure the best possible health for herself and her fetus. At that time, blood glucose levels can be assessed closely and medication adjustments can be made to ensure optimal regulation before she becomes pregnant.

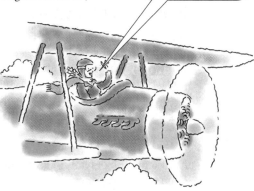

Pregnant women with diabetes will rack up lots of frequent-flier miles! Frequent antenatal visits are needed to keep glucose under control.

Crucial calories

Nutritional therapy is crucial in the treatment of women with diabetes. Typically, 1,800–2,200-calorie diet is prescribed for the pregnant woman with diabetes. Alternatively, caloric requirements may be calculated at 35 kcal/kg of ideal body weight. The caloric requirement is usually divided among three meals and three snacks, allowing the calories to be distributed throughout the day in an attempt to maintain constant glucose levels.

Additional dietary recommendations include reduced saturated fat and cholesterol and increased dietary fibre. Carbohydrates should make up more than half of daily caloric intake, with protein and fat supplying the remainder. The goal is to allow a weight gain of approximately 11.3–13.6 kg so that the neonate doesn't grow too large and vaginal delivery remains a possibility.

Nutrition is the star of the show when it comes to ensuring a healthy pregnancy for a woman with diabetes.

Adjust, reduce, increase

For the woman with preexisting diabetes, insulin adjustments are necessary. Early in pregnancy, insulin may be reduced because of the increased utilisation of glucose by the fetus for growth. However, later in pregnancy, an increase in insulin typically occurs because of an increase in the woman's metabolism. Insulin therapy dosages and types are highly individualised. A continuous subcutaneous insulin infusion via a pump may be ordered to maintain constant blood glucose levels. The woman with gestational diabetes may require insulin if diet therapy doesn't adequately control blood glucose levels.

Check 1: Glucose levels

To assist with blood glucose control, fingerstick blood glucose monitoring is important. For the woman with preexisting diabetes, typically this monitoring is performed as often as four times per day. For women with gestational diabetes, however, blood glucose monitoring may be performed on a daily or weekly basis, depending on how stable her blood glucose results are. Regardless of monitoring frequency, the goal is to obtain fasting blood glucose levels below 5.9 mmol/L and 1-hour postprandial values below 7.8 mmol/L.

Check 2: Eyes and urinary tract

Throughout the pregnancy, follow-up monitoring is performed. A urine culture may be done each trimester to detect UTIs that produce no symptoms. Ophthalmic examination may be done at each trimester for the woman with preexisting diabetes and at least once during the pregnancy for the woman with gestational diabetes. Retinal changes may develop or progress during pregnancy.

Check 3: The fetus

Because the risk of fetal complications is high, fetal monitoring is crucial. A serum alpha-fetoprotein (AFP) level may be offered at 15–17 weeks' gestation to assess for neural tube defects. Ultrasonography will be done at 18–20 weeks to detect gross abnormalities, and then serial growth scans are done at intervals to determine fetal growth, amniotic fluid volume, placental location and biparietal diameter. Mothers may be scanned more frequently during their pregnancy depending on their condition.

Preferred delivery route

The mode of delivery is discussed with the woman, taking all factors into consideration before a decision is made. During labour, uterine contractions and FHR are monitored continuously. The mother's glucose level is regulated with I.V. infusions of regular insulin based on blood glucose levels that are obtained hourly.

What to do

- Carefully monitor the woman's weight gain, blood glucose levels and nutritional intake as well as fetal growth parameters throughout pregnancy.
- Review results of fingerstick blood glucose monitoring; assess for signs and symptoms of hypoglycaemia and hyperglycaemia.
- Assist with scheduling of follow-up laboratory studies, including glycosylated haemoglobin levels and urine studies as necessary.
- Encourage the woman to maintain a consistent exercise programme and explain the benefits of eating certain snacks before exercise. (See *Preventing hypoglycaemia during exercise.*)

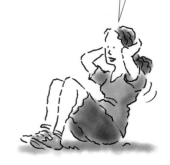

Encourage the pregnant woman with diabetes to maintain a consistent exercise programme.

Education edge

Preventing hypoglycaemia during exercise

Hypoglycaemia during exercise is a common problem for women with diabetes, but there's an easy solution for the sensible woman.

The problem

During exercise, the muscles increase their uptake of glucose, causing blood glucose levels to decrease. This effect can last up to 12 hours after exercise. In addition, if the woman injects insulin into the extremity involved in exercise, the insulin is released more quickly. As a result, blood glucose levels decrease even more dramatically, causing hypoglycaemia.

The solution

To prevent hypoglycaemia, encourage the woman with diabetes to eat a snack consisting of a protein or a complex carbohydrate before she exercises, and to maintain a consistent exercise pattern each day.

Education edge

Teaching topics for pregnant women with diabetes

Be sure to cover these topics when teaching a pregnant woman with diabetes.

- Insulin type and dosage
- Insulin syringe preparation and injection technique or insulin pump use and care
- Sites to use (Most women prefer not to use the abdomen as an injection site.)
- Site rotation (Insulin is absorbed more slowly from the thigh than from the upper arm.)
- Blood glucose monitoring technique, including frequency of monitoring and desired glucose levels

- Nutritional plan, including suggestions for appropriate foods to include and avoid
- Consistent exercise regimen
- Signs and symptoms of urinary tract and monilial infections, including the need to report one immediately
- Signs and symptoms of hypoglycaemia and hyperglycaemia
- Measures to prevent and manage hypoglycaemia and hyperglycaemia
- Preparations for labour and delivery
- Care after delivery

- Instruct the woman in all aspects of managing diabetes, including insulin administration techniques, self-monitoring, nutrition and danger signs and symptoms. (See *Teaching topics for pregnant women with diabetes*.)
- Arrange for a consultation with a dietitian.
- Assist with preparations for labour, including explanations about possible labour induction and required monitoring.
- Closely assess the woman in the postpartum period for changes in blood glucose levels and insulin requirements. Typically, the woman with preexisting diabetes will require no insulin in the immediate postpartum period (because insulin resistance is gone), and won't return to her pre-pregnancy insulin requirements for several days. The woman with gestational diabetes usually exhibits normal blood glucose levels within 24 hours after delivery, requiring no further insulin or diet therapy.
- Encourage the woman with gestational diabetes to keep all follow-up appointments so that glucose testing can be performed to detect possible type 2 diabetes.

Ectopic pregnancy

Ectopic pregnancy is the implantation of a fertilised ovum outside the uterine cavity. It most commonly occurs in the fallopian tube but may occur in other sites as well. (See *Sites of ectopic pregnancy*, page 193.)

The prognosis for the woman is good with prompt diagnosis, appropriate surgical intervention and control of bleeding. It would be very rare, in cases of abdominal implantation, for the fetus to survive to term. Rupture of the tube causes life-threatening complications, including haemorrhage, shock and peritonitis. The woman may need to have the affected tube removed.

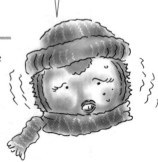

Brrr! What am I doing outside the uterine cavity? It must be ectopic pregnancy.

Sites of ectopic pregnancy

In most women with ectopic pregnancy, the ovum implants in the fallopian tube, either in the imbria, ampulla or isthmus. Other possible sites of implantation include the interstitium, tubo-ovarian ligament, ovary, abdominal viscera and internal cervical os.

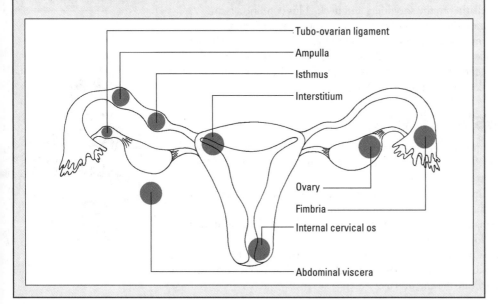

Tubo-ovarian ligament
Ampulla
Isthmus
Interstitium
Ovary
Fimbria
Internal cervical os
Abdominal viscera

What causes it

Conditions that prevent or slow the fertilised ovum's passage through the fallopian tube into the uterine cavity include:
• Pelvic inflammatory disease (PID), an inflammatory reaction that causes folds of the tubal mucosa to agglutinate, narrowing the tube
• diverticula (blind pouches that cause tubal abnormalities)
• tumours pressing against the tube
• previous surgery, such as tubal ligation or resection, or adhesions from previous abdominal or pelvic surgery
• transmigration of the ovum from one ovary to the opposite tube resulting in delayed implantation.

Ectopic pregnancy may also result from congenital defects in the reproductive tract or ectopic endometrial implants in the tubal mucosa. Additional factors include sexually transmitted tubal infections as well as intrauterine and assisted fertility, e.g. In Vitro Fertilisation (IVF).

What to look for

Symptoms of ectopic pregnancy are sometimes similar to those of a normal pregnancy, making diagnosis difficult. Mild abdominal pain may occur, especially in cases of abdominal pregnancy. Typically, the woman reports amenorrhoea or abnormal menses (in cases of fallopian tube implantation), followed by slight vaginal bleeding and unilateral pelvic pain over the mass. During a vaginal examination, the woman may report extreme pain when the cervix is moved (cervical excitation) and the adnexa is palpated. The uterus feels boggy and is tender. If the tube ruptures, the woman may complain of sharp lower abdominal pain, possibly radiating to the shoulders and neck. This condition is an emergency situation that requires immediate transport to a hospital.

The woman may complain of lower abdominal pain precipitated by activities that increase abdominal pressure, such as a bowel movement. She may also experience shoulder tip pain caused by blood irritating the diaphragm or rectal pain caused by blood in the pouch of Douglas.

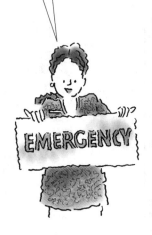

Complaints of sharp lower abdominal pain indicate tube rupture – a medical emergency

What tests tell you

Differential diagnosis is necessary to rule out intrauterine pregnancy, ovarian cyst or tumour, PID, appendicitis and spontaneous abortion. The following tests confirm ectopic pregnancy:
• Real-time ultrasonography performed after a positive serum pregnancy test detects intrauterine pregnancy or ovarian cyst.
• Serum pregnancy test results show an abnormally low level of human chorionic gonadotropin (hCG)
• Laparoscopy, performed if culdocentesis (the extraction of fluid from the rectouterine pouch posterior to the vagina through a needle) is positive, may reveal pregnancy outside the uterus.

How it's treated

Treatment is surgical, medical or conservative

Surgical treatment
Laparoscopic treatment is preferable – in most cases, a laparoscopic salpingectomy (removal of tube) is performed provided the other tube is healthy. If the woman is in a collapsed state or unwell, she may require a laparotomy and salpingectomy. Abdominal pregnancy requires a laparotomy to remove the fetus, except in rare cases, when the fetus survives to term or calcifies undetected in the abdominal cavity.

Medical treatment
This involves oral administration of methotrexate, a chemotherapeutic drug and folic acid inhibitor that stops cell production. The drug destroys remaining trophoblastic tissue, thus avoiding the need for laparotomy.

Conservative treatment
Conservative treatment is recommended as long as the hCG levels are dropping and the woman's condition remains stable. Treatment includes whole blood or packed red blood cells (RBCs) to replace excessive blood loss,

broad-spectrum I.V. antibiotics for sepsis, supplemental iron (either oral or I.M.) and a high-protein diet.

Grief counselling for the loss of the pregnancy is also recommended.

What to do

• Ask the woman the date of her last period, and obtain serum hCG levels as ordered.
• Assess vital signs, and monitor vaginal bleeding for extent of fluid loss.
• Check the amount, colour and odour of vaginal bleeding; monitor perineal pad count.
• Withhold food and fluid orally in anticipation of possible surgery; prepare the woman for surgery as indicated.
• Assess for signs and symptoms of hypovolaemic shock secondary to blood loss from tubal rupture. Monitor closely for decreased urine output, which suggests fluid volume deficit.
• Document all observations, treatment and drugs given.
• Administer blood transfusions, as ordered, and provide emotional support.
• Record the location and character of the pain, and administer analgesics as ordered.
• Determine if the woman is Rh-negative. If she is, administer anti-D, as ordered after treatment or surgery.
• Provide a quiet, peaceful environment and encourage the woman and her partner to express their feelings of fear, loss and grief. Help them to develop effective coping strategies.
• To prevent recurrent ectopic pregnancy from diseases of the fallopian tube, urge the woman to get prompt treatment of pelvic infections.
• Inform women who have undergone surgery involving the fallopian tubes or those with confirmed PID that they're at increased risk for another ectopic pregnancy.
• Refer the woman to a grief counsellor or support group.

> There's plenty of folic acid in a well-balanced diet, but this important B vitamin is easily destroyed by cooking, and 20% is excreted unabsorbed.

Folic acid deficiency anaemia

Folic acid deficiency anaemia is a common, slowly progressive, megaloblastic (involving enlarged RBCs) form of anaemia. Folic acid, or folacin, is a B vitamin needed for RBC formation and deoxyribonucleic acid (DNA) synthesis. It's also thought to play a role in preventing neural tube defects in the developing fetus.

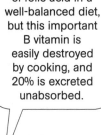

Folic acid deficiency anaemia is a risk factor in approximately 1–5% of pregnancies, becoming most apparent during the second trimester. It's believed to be a risk factor contributing to early spontaneous abortion and abruptio placentae.

Folic folly

Folic acid is found in most body tissues. It acts as a co-enzyme in metabolic processes. Although its body stores are relatively small, folic acid can be found in most well-balanced diets. Even so, folic acid is water-soluble and is affected by heat, so it's easily destroyed by cooking. Moreover, about 20% of folic acid intake is excreted unabsorbed. Insufficient intake – typically less than 50 mcg/day – usually results in folic acid deficiency anaemia within 4 months.

What causes it

Alcohol abuse, which suppresses the metabolic effects of folic acid, is probably the most common cause of folic acid deficiency anaemia. During pregnancy, folic acid deficiency anaemia occurs most commonly in women with multiple pregnancy, probably because of the increased fetal demand for folic acid. Folic acid deficiency anaemia is also seen in women who have underlying haemolytic illness that results in rapid destruction and production of RBCs. In addition, certain drugs – such as phenytoin, an anticonvulsant agent that interferes with folate absorption, and hormonal contraceptives – have a role in folic acid deficiency anaemia.

What to look for

The main symptom of folic acid deficiency anaemia is a history of severe, progressive fatigue. Associated findings include shortness of breath, palpitations, diarrhoea, nausea, anorexia, headaches, forgetfulness and irritability. The impaired oxygen-carrying capacity of the blood from lowered haemoglobin levels may produce complaints of weakness and light-headedness.

Assessment may reveal generalised pallor and jaundice. The woman may also appear wasted. Cheilosis (cracks in the corners of the mouth) and glossitis (inflammation of the tongue) may be present. Neurological impairment is present only if the folic acid deficiency anaemia is associated with a vitamin B12 deficiency.

What tests tell you

Typically, blood studies reveal:
- macrocytic RBCs
- decreased reticulocyte count
- increased mean corpuscular volume
- abnormal platelet count
- decreased serum folate levels (below 4 mg/ml).

How it's treated

During pregnancy, treatment consists primarily of folic acid supplements. Supplements may be given orally or parenterally (for women who are severely ill, have malabsorption or can't take oral medication). In addition, a diet high in folic acid is urged. Many women respond favourably to a well-balanced diet.

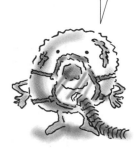

Got oxygen? In folic acid deficiency anaemia, the blood's oxygen-carrying capacity is impaired. No wonder I feel light-headed!

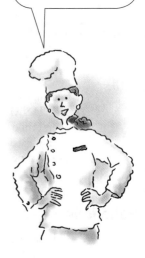

Many women with folic acid deficiency anaemia respond favourably to a well-balanced diet.

Education edge

Foods high in folic acid

If your client is planning to become pregnant or is pregnant, encourage her to eat these foods high in folic acid to help prevent folic acid deficiency anaemia:

- asparagus
- beef liver
- broccoli
- green leafy vegetables such as spring greens
- mushrooms
- oatmeal
- peanut butter
- red beans
- wheat germ
- whole wheat bread.

What to do

- Strongly urge women trying to become pregnant to take a vitamin supplement or eat foods rich in folic acid. (See *Foods high in folic acid*.)
- Instruct the pregnant woman in the use of prescribed folic acid supplements and the need to continue taking them throughout pregnancy.
- Assist with planning a well-balanced diet that includes meals and snacks that are high in folic acid.
- Encourage the woman to eat or drink a rich source of vitamin C at each meal to enhance absorption of folic acid.
- Administer a folic acid supplement as ordered throughout pregnancy, and assess for client compliance.
- If the woman has severe anaemia and requires hospitalisation, plan activities, rest periods and diagnostic tests to conserve energy. Monitor pulse rate often; if tachycardia occurs, the woman's activities are too strenuous.
- Monitor the woman's full blood count (FBC), platelet count and serum folate levels as ordered.
- Assess maternal vital signs and FHR as indicated.

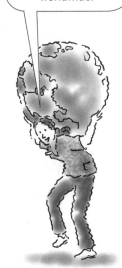

Iron deficiency anaemia is common worldwide.

Iron deficiency anaemia

Iron deficiency anaemia is a disorder in which haemoglobin synthesis is deficient and the body's capacity to transport oxygen is impaired. It's the most common anaemia during pregnancy, affecting up to a quarter of all pregnancies. Iron deficiency anaemia during pregnancy is associated with low fetal birthweight and preterm birth.

What causes it

During pregnancy, maternal iron stores are used for fetal RBC production, thus causing an iron deficiency in the mother. In addition, many women have

deficient iron stores when they enter pregnancy because of factors such as a diet low in iron (inadequate intake), heavy menses (blood loss) or misguided weight-reduction programs. Iron stores also tend to be low in women who have fewer than 2 years between pregnancies and in those from low socioeconomic communities. Other possible causes of iron deficiency anaemia include:
- iron malabsorption
- intravascular haemolysis-induced haemoglobinuria or paroxysmal nocturnal haemoglobinuria
- mechanical trauma to RBCs caused by a prosthetic heart valve or vena caval filter.

No iron, no haemoglobin, no oxygen

Iron deficiency anaemia is considered a microcytic, hypochromic anaemia, meaning that inadequate iron intake results in smaller RBCs that contain less haemoglobin. Cells that aren't as large and rich in haemoglobin as they should be affect the proper transport of oxygen.

> Adequate iron intake helps me grow rich with haemoglobin so I can properly transport oxygen.

What to look for

Typically, the signs and symptoms exhibited by a pregnant woman with iron deficiency anaemia are the same as those for any individual with this disorder. They tend to develop gradually and may include fatigue, listlessness, pallor and exercise intolerance. Some women develop pica (eating of substances such as ice or starch) in response to the body's need for increased nutrients. If the anaemia is severe or prolonged, other signs and symptoms may include:
- dyspnoea on exertion
- inability to concentrate
- susceptibility to infection
- tachycardia
- coarsely ridged, spoon-shaped, brittle, thin nails
- sore, red, burning tongue
- sore, dry skin in the corners of the mouth.

What tests tell you

Diagnosis of iron deficiency anaemia must not precede exclusion of other causes of anaemia, such as thalassaemia minor, cancer and chronic inflammatory, hepatic or renal disease. Blood studies (serum iron, total iron-binding capacity, ferritin levels) and assessment of iron stores in bone marrow may confirm iron deficiency anaemia. However, the results of these tests can be misleading because of complicating factors, such as infection, blood transfusion or use of iron supplements. Characteristic blood test results for women include:
- low haemoglobin (less than 10 g/dl)
- low haematocrit (less than 33%)

- low serum iron (less than 30 mcg/dl) with high binding capacity (greater than 400 mcg/dl)
- low serum ferritin (less than 100 mg/dl)
- low RBC count with microcytic and hypochromic cells (in early stages, RBC count may be normal)
- decreased mean corpuscular haemoglobin (less than 30 g/dl) in severe anaemia
- depleted or absent iron stores (identified by specific staining) and hyperplasia of normal precursor cells (identified by bone marrow studies).

How it's treated

Preventing iron deficiency anaemia with prescription antenatal vitamins is the primary goal. However, if iron deficiency anaemia does develop, an iron supplement (such as ferrous sulphate or ferrous gluconate) is prescribed. Additionally, women should be advised to eat a well-balanced diet that includes foods high in vitamins and iron.

I.V. iron

If the woman's anaemia is severe or she can't comply with the prescribed oral therapy, parenteral iron may be prescribed. Because total dose I.V. infusion of supplemental iron is painless and requires fewer injections, it's usually preferred to I.M. administration. In pregnant women with severe anaemia, total dose infusion (TDI) of iron dextran in normal saline solution is given over 1–8 hours. A test dose of 0.5 ml I.V. is given first to help minimise the risk of allergic reaction.

What to do

- If the woman is hospitalised, administer oral iron with an acid, such as orange juice, to enhance absorption; for outpatients, advise women to take prescribed iron supplements with orange juice or a vitamin C supplement.
- Monitor the woman's FBC and serum iron and ferritin levels regularly.
- Assess the family's dietary habits for iron intake, noting the influence of childhood eating patterns, cultural food preferences and family income on adequate nutrition.
- Monitor the woman's vital signs, especially heart rate, noting tachycardia, which suggests that her activities are too strenuous.
- Evaluate for signs and symptoms of decreased perfusion to vital organs (such as dyspnoea, chest pain and dizziness) and symptoms of neuropathy (such as tingling in the extremities).
- Assess FHR at each visit; if the woman is hospitalised, monitor FHR at least every 8 hours.
- Provide frequent rest periods to decrease physical exhaustion. Assist the woman with planning activities so that she has sufficient rest between them.
- If the anaemia is severe, expect to administer oxygen, as ordered, to help prevent and reduce hypoxia.

• Administer iron supplements as ordered. Use the Z-track injection method when administering iron I.M. to prevent skin discolouration, scarring and irritating iron deposits in the skin. (See *Z-track injection for iron*.)
• If the woman receives iron I.V., monitor the infusion rate carefully. Stop the infusion and begin supportive treatment immediately if she shows

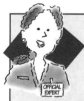

Advice from the experts

Z-track injection for iron

When administering iron using the I.M. route, use the Z-track injection method to displace the skin. This technique blocks the needle pathway after an injection, thereby preventing discomfort and tissue irritation secondary to drug leakage into subcutaneous tissue. To perform a Z-track injection, follow these steps.

• Place your finger on the skin surface, and pull the skin and subcutaneous layers out of alignment with the underlying muscle. You should move the skin approximately 1 cm.

• Insert the needle at a 90-degree angle at the site where you initially placed your finger.

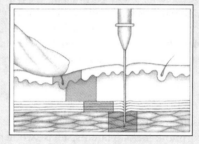

• Aspirate for blood return; if none appears, inject the drug slowly.
• Wait 10 seconds and then withdraw the needle slowly.

• Remove your finger from the skin surface, letting the layers return to normal, thus sealing the needle track. The needle track (as shown by the dotted line in the illustration below) is now broken at the junction of each tissue layer, trapping the drug in the muscle.

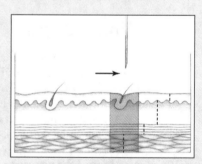

• Don't massage the site or allow the patient to wear a tight-fitting garment over the site because doing so could force medication into the subcutaneous tissue.
• Encourage the patient to walk or move about in bed to facilitate drug absorption from the injection site.

Education edge

Teaching topics on iron supplements

Be sure to cover the following topics when teaching the pregnant woman about iron supplements.

- Reinforcement of the doctor/midwife's explanation of the anaemia.
- Prescribed treatments and possible complications.
- Need for continuing therapy – even if the woman feels better – because replacement of iron stores takes time.
- Foods that interfere with absorption, such as milk and antacids.
- Foods that enhance absorption, such as citrus juices and foods containing vitamin C.
- Administration guidelines, including using a straw when taking the liquid form to prevent staining the teeth, and taking iron on an empty stomach

(if possible) with a vitamin C-rich food or with food if gastric irritation occurs.
- Need to report adverse effects of iron therapy, such as nausea, vomiting, diarrhoea and constipation (dosage adjustment or supplemental stool softeners may be necessary).
- Change in stool appearance.
- Components of a nutritionally balanced diet, including red meats, green vegetables, eggs, whole wheat, iron-fortified bread and milk.
- Intake of high-fibre foods to prevent constipation.
- Infection prevention measures.
- Need to report signs and symptoms of infection, such as fever and chills.
- Need for regular checkups and compliance with prescribed treatments.

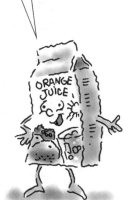

Just a glass full of orange juice helps the iron supplement go down!

signs of an allergic reaction. Also, watch for dizziness and headache and for thrombophlebitis around the I.V. site.
- Assist with planning a well-balanced diet with an increased intake of foods high in vitamins and iron. Consult a nutrition therapist as indicated.
- Document all treatments, observations and medications given as well as all advice offered.
- Provide client teaching about therapy. (See *Teaching topics on iron supplements*.) Offer suggestions for intake of high-fibre foods to prevent possible constipation from iron therapy; also warn the woman that the medication may cause stools to appear black and tarry.

Gestational hypertension

Gestational hypertension is a potentially life-threatening disorder that typically develops after 20 weeks' gestation. It occurs most commonly in nulliparous women.

Gestational hypertension can be classified as pre-eclampsia or eclampsia. Pre-eclampsia, the nonconvulsive form of the disorder, is marked by the onset of hypertension after 20 weeks' gestation. It may be mild or severe and the incidence is significantly higher in women from low socioeconomic groups. Eclampsia, the convulsive form, occurs between 24 weeks' gestation and the end of the first postpartum week. The incidence increases among nulliparous women, women with multiple pregnancy and women with a history of vascular disease. About 5% of women with pre-eclampsia develop eclampsia; of these, about 15% die of eclampsia or its complications. Confidential Enquiry into Maternal and Child Health (CEMACH) stated in their 2002 report that a number of women died from pre-eclampsia/eclampsia but 14 women died due to related conditions arising from pre-eclampsia/eclampsia. They suggest that any women with a systolic blood pressure reading should be treated immediately. The incidence of fetal mortality is high because of the increased incidence of premature delivery. To access the statistics and latest report from CEMACH, use this link http://www.cemach.org.uk/getdoc/26867a99-45e9-46ed-8d16-f2618e626a64/Chapter3.aspx

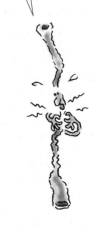

Preexisting vascular disease may contribute to pregnancy-induced hypertension.

Complicating the situation

Generalised arteriolar vasoconstriction associated with gestational hypertension is thought to produce decreased blood flow through the placenta and maternal organs. This can result in intrauterine growth retardation (or restriction), placental infarcts and abruptio placentae. Haemolysis, elevated liver enzyme levels and a low platelet count (HELLP syndrome) are associated with severe pre-eclampsia. Other possible complications include stillbirth of the neonate, seizures, coma, premature labour, renal failure and hepatic damage in the mother.

What causes it

Although the exact cause of gestational hypertension is unknown, systemic peripheral vasospasm occurs and affects every organ system. (See *Changes associated with gestational hypertension*, page 203.) Geographic, ethnic, racial, nutritional, immunological and familial factors may contribute to preexisting vascular disease that, in turn, may contribute to the disorder's occurrence. Age is also a factor; adolescents and primiparas older than age 35 are at higher risk for pre-eclampsia.

Other possible causes include potential toxic sources (such as autolysis of placental infarcts), autointoxication, uraemia, maternal sensitisation to total proteins and pyelonephritis.

What to look for

The classic triad of symptoms in women with gestational hypertension is hypertension, proteinuria and oedema. A woman with mild pre-eclampsia typically reports a sudden weight gain of more than 1.4 kg per week in the second trimester or more than 0.5 kg per week during the third trimester. The woman's history reveals hypertension, as evidenced by high blood

Changes associated with gestational hypertension

This flowchart illustrates the physiological effects of gestational hypertension on the pregnant woman's body.

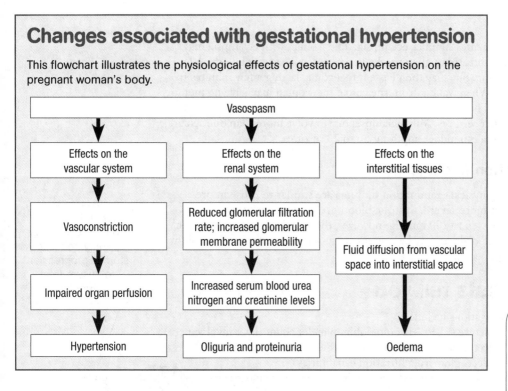

Vasospasm		
Effects on the vascular system	Effects on the renal system	Effects on the interstitial tissues
Vasoconstriction	Reduced glomerular filtration rate; increased glomerular membrane permeability	
Impaired organ perfusion	Increased serum blood urea nitrogen and creatinine levels	Fluid diffusion from vascular space into interstitial space
Hypertension	Oliguria and proteinuria	Oedema

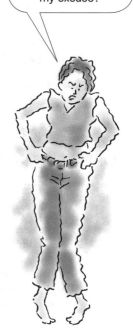

Sudden weight gain during the second or third trimester is a typical finding in a woman with PIH. So, what's my excuse?

pressure readings. The Royal College of Obstetricians and Gynaecologists (RCOG) guidelines suggest that:
- Moderate hypertension is a reading where the diastolic is >100 mmHg
- Severe hypertension is a reading where the diastolic is >110 and the systolic is >170 mmHg on two occasions together with significant proteinuria.

Further examination may reveal generalised oedema, especially of the face. Palpation may reveal pitting oedema of the legs and feet. Deep tendon reflexes may indicate hyper-reflexia and even clonus. As pre-eclampsia worsens, the woman may demonstrate oliguria (urine output of 400 ml/day or less), and blurred vision caused by retinal arteriolar spasms. She could suffer from irritability, emotional tension and may also complain of a severe frontal headache. Epigastric pain or vomiting may result from liver involvement; her liver enzymes will be abnormal and the platelet count will be reduced – she is in great danger of developing HELLP syndrome.

Pressure, spasm, haemorrhage

In severe pre-eclampsia, blood pressure readings increase to 170/110 mmHg or higher on two occasions, 6 hours apart, during bed rest. Ophthalmoscopic examination may reveal vascular spasm, papilledema, retinal oedema or detachment, and arteriovenous nicking or haemorrhage.

Enter eclampsia

The onset of seizures signifies eclampsia. The woman with eclampsia may appear to cease breathing, then suddenly take a deep, gasping breath and resume breathing. She may then lapse into a coma, lasting a few minutes to several hours. When waking from the coma, the woman may have no memory of the seizure. The first seizure is usually self-limiting but often the woman will have further seizures. Mild eclampsia may involve more than one seizure; severe eclampsia can induce anything up to 20 seizures.

Physical examination findings

In eclampsia, physical examination findings are similar to those in pre-eclampsia, but more severe. Systolic blood pressure may increase to 180 mmHg or even to 200 mmHg; however, the blood pressure can also be normal! Marked oedema may be present; some women, however, don't show visible signs of oedema.

What tests tell you

Baseline investigations include:
- full blood picture (FBP) – haemoglobin, platelet count (liver involvement)
- U&E – reflects renal function, could be affected by hypertension
- Urates – reflects glomerula filtration capabilities
- Liver function tests – assesses liver's ability to maintain homoeostasis
- 24 hour urine collection – total protein – assesses renal function.
Additionally, ultrasonography, cardiotocograph (CTG) traces and biophysical profiles are used to evaluate fetal well-being.

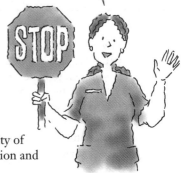

When it comes to pre-eclampsia, priority one is to stop its progression to ensure fetal survival.

How it's treated

Adequate nutrition, good antenatal care and control of preexisting hypertension during pregnancy help decrease the incidence and severity of pre-eclampsia. However, if pre-eclampsia does develop, early recognition and prompt treatment can prevent progression to eclampsia.

Suppress the progress

Therapy for women with pre-eclampsia is intended to stop the disorder's progression and ensure fetal survival. Some doctors advocate the prompt inducement of labour, especially if the mother is near term; others follow a more conservative approach. Therapy may include:
- bed rest in the preferred left lateral recumbent position to enhance venous return
- administration of anti-hypertensive drugs, such as nifedipine orally, hydralazine (apresolin) I.V. or labetalol orally or I.V. (should be avoided in asthmatic women)

• administration of magnesium to promote diuresis, reduce blood pressure and prevent seizures if blood pressure fails to respond to bed rest and anti-hypertensives (persistently rising above 160/100 mmHg) or central nervous system (CNS) irritability increases.

Plan B

If these measures fail to improve the woman's condition, or if fetal life is endangered (as determined by CTG tests and biophysical profiles), caesarean delivery or labour induction may be required. If the woman develops seizures, emergency treatment consists of immediate I.V. administration of magnesium and oxygen therapy along with electronic fetal monitoring. After the woman's condition stabilises, caesarean delivery may be indicated.

What to do

• Monitor the woman regularly for changes in blood pressure, pulse rate, respiratory rate, FHR, vision, level of consciousness and deep tendon reflexes as well as headache unrelieved by medication.
• Report changes immediately to doctor. Record all clinical observations and any action taken. Assess these signs and symptoms before administering medications. (See *Emergency interventions for gestational hypertension*.)
• If the woman is receiving I.V. magnesium sulphate, administer the loading dose over 15–30 minutes and then maintain the infusion at a rate of 1–2 g/hour.
• Monitor the extent and location of oedema. Elevate affected extremities to promote venous return. Avoid constricting clothing, slippers and bed linens.

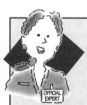

Advice from the experts

Emergency interventions for gestational hypertension

When caring for a woman with gestational hypertension, be prepared to perform these nursing interventions.

• Observe for signs of fetal distress by closely monitoring the results of stress and nonstress tests.
• Keep emergency resuscitative equipment and anticonvulsant drugs readily available in case of seizures and cardiac or respiratory arrest.
• Maintain a patent airway and have oxygen and suction readily available.
• Carefully monitor the I.V. infusion of magnesium sulphate, observing for signs and symptoms of

toxicity, such as absence of patellar reflexes, flushing, muscle flaccidity, decreased urine output, a significant drop in blood pressure (more than 15 mmHg) and respiratory rate less than 12 breaths/minute.
• Keep calcium gluconate readily available at the bedside to counteract the toxic effects of magnesium sulphate.
• Prepare for emergency caesarean delivery if indicated.
• Maintain seizure precautions to protect the woman from injury. Never leave an unstable woman unattended.

Advice from the experts

Administering magnesium sulphate safely

If the woman requires I.V. magnesium therapy, use caution when administering the drug because magnesium toxicity may occur. Follow these guidelines to ensure maternal and fetal safety during administration.

- Always administer the drug as a piggyback infusion so that it can be discontinued immediately if the woman develops signs and symptoms of toxicity.
- Obtain a baseline serum magnesium level before initiating therapy and monitor levels frequently thereafter.
- Keep in mind that for I.V. magnesium to be effective as an anticonvulsant, serum magnesium levels should be between 5 and 8 mg/dl. Levels above 8 mg/dl indicate toxicity and place the patient at risk for respiratory depression, cardiac arrhythmias and cardiac arrest.

- Assess the woman's patellar reflex. If she has received epidural anaesthesia, test the biceps or triceps reflex. Diminished or hypoactive reflexes suggest magnesium toxicity.
- Assess for ankle clonus (alternating contractions and relaxations of the muscles) by rapidly dorsiflexing the woman's ankle three times, then removing your hand and observing the foot's movement. If no further motion is noted, ankle clonus is absent; if the foot continues to move involuntarily, clonus is present. Moderate (three to five movements) or severe (six or more movements) suggests possible magnesium toxicity.
- Have calcium gluconate readily available at the bedside. Anticipate administering this antidote for I.V. magnesium.

- Assess fluid balance by measuring intake and output and checking daily weight. Insert an indwelling urinary catheter, if necessary, to provide a more accurate measurement of output.
- Provide a quiet, darkened room, limit visitation by friends and family members until the woman's condition stabilises, and enforce complete bed rest.
- Provide emotional support for the woman and her family. Encourage them to verbalise their feelings. If the woman's condition requires preterm delivery, point out that infants of mothers with gestational hypertension are usually small for gestational age, but sometimes fare better than other premature infants of the same weight, possibly because they have developed adaptive responses to stress in utero.
- Encourage the woman to eat a well-balanced, high-protein diet; limit high-sodium foods, include high-fibre foods and drink at least eight 8 oz glasses of noncaffeinated beverages each day.
- Teach the woman to report signs and symptoms that indicate worsening gestational hypertension, which include headache, vision disturbances (blurring, flashes of light, 'spots' before the eyes), GI symptoms (nausea, pain), worsening oedema (especially of the face and fingers) and a noticeable decrease in urine output.
- Help the woman and her family develop effective coping strategies.
- Prepare to administer betamethasone I.M. as indicated. (This is a steroid which is given I.M. to mothers where premature delivery is expected – it matures fetal lungs, reducing the need for ventilation of the baby after birth.)

Women with PIH should avoid constricting bed linens, so keep 'em loose!

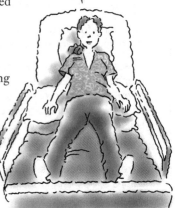

Access the RCOG website for further information on managing pre-eclampsia and eclampsia in pregnancy: http://www.rcog.org.uk/resources/Public/pdf/management_pre_eclampsia_mar06.pdf

Gestational trophoblastic disease

Gestational trophoblastic disease, also called *hydatidiform mole or molar pregnancy*, is the rapid deterioration of trophoblastic villi cells. Trophoblast cells are located in the outer ring of the blastocyst (the structure that develops around the third or fourth day after fertilisation) and eventually become part of the structure that forms the placenta and fetal membranes. As trophoblast cells begin to deteriorate, they fill with fluid. The cells become oedematous, appearing as grapelike clusters of vesicles. As a result of these cell abnormalities, the embryo fails to develop past the early stages.

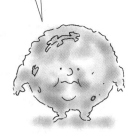

As trophoblast cells deteriorate, they fill with fluid. I'm pretty full already!

Leading to bleeding

Gestational trophoblastic disease is a major cause of second trimester bleeding. It's also associated with choriocarcinoma (a fast-growing, highly invasive malignant tumour that develops in the uterus), which is why early detection is important.

All or some

Chromosomal analysis helps classify gestational trophoblastic disease as a complete or partial mole. A complete mole is characterised by swelling and cystic formation of all trophoblastic cells. No fetal blood is present. If an embryo does develop, it's most likely only 1–2 mm in size and will probably die early in development. This form is associated with the development of choriocarcinoma.

A partial mole is characterised by oedema of some of the trophoblastic villi with some of the normal villi. Fetal blood may be present in the villi, and an embryo up to the size of 9 weeks' gestation may be present. Typically, a partial mole has 69 chromosomes in which there are 3 chromosomes for every one pair.

Hard to recognise

Gestational trophoblastic disease is reported to occur in about 1 in every 2,000 pregnancies. Recent research indicates that the incidence would be much higher if all cases of the disorder were identified. Some cases aren't recognised because the pregnancy is aborted early and the products of conception aren't available for analysis. The incidence is higher in women from low socioeconomic groups, older women and multiparous women. The incidence is highest in Asian women, especially those from Southeast Asia.

What causes it

The cause of gestational trophoblastic disease is unknown. Several unconfirmed theories relate gestational trophoblastic disease to chromosomal abnormalities, hormonal imbalances or deficiencies in protein and folic acid. About one-half of women with choriocarcinoma have had a preceding molar pregnancy. In the remaining women, the disease is usually preceded by a spontaneous or induced abortion, an ectopic pregnancy or a normal pregnancy.

What to look for

A woman with gestational trophoblastic disease may report vaginal bleeding, ranging from brownish red spotting to bright red haemorrhage. She may report passing tissue that resembles grape clusters. Her history may also include hyperemesis, lower abdominal cramps (such as those that accompany spontaneous abortion) and signs and symptoms of pre-eclampsia.

On inspection, a uterus that's exceptionally large for the woman's gestational date is detected. Vaginal examination may reveal grapelike vesicles in the vagina. Palpation may detect ovarian enlargement caused by cysts. Auscultation of the uterus may reveal the absence of fetal heart tones that had been noted at a previous visit.

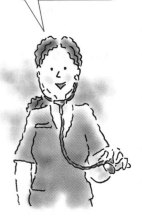

Hmmm ... an exceptionally large uterus, the presence of grapelike vesicles and absence of fetal heart tones. Sounds like gestational trophoblastic disease.

What tests tell you

Differential diagnosis is necessary to rule out normal pregnancy, imminent spontaneous abortion, uterine leiomyomas, multiple pregnancy and incorrect gestational date. These diagnostic test results suggest the presence of gestational trophoblastic disease:
• Radioimmunoassay detects extremely elevated hCG levels for early pregnancy.
• Histologic examination confirms the presence of vesicles.
• Ultrasonography performed after the third month shows grapelike clusters instead of a fetus.
• Amniography (a procedure that introduces a water-soluble dye into the uterus) reveals the absence of a fetus. (This test is done only when the diagnosis is in question.)
• Doppler ultrasonography shows the absence of fetal heart tones.
• Haemoglobin level and haematocrit, RBC count, prothrombin time, partial thromboplastin time, fibrinogen levels and hepatic and renal function findings are abnormal.
• White blood cell (WBC) count and erythrocyte sedimentation rate (ESR) are increased.

How it's treated

Gestational trophoblastic disease necessitates uterine evacuation by dilatation and suction curettage. Labour induction with oxytocin or prostaglandins is contraindicated because of the increased risk of haemorrhage.

Postoperative treatment varies, depending on the amount of blood lost and complications. If no complications develop, hospitalisation is usually brief and normal activities can be resumed quickly as tolerated.

Monitoring for malignancy

Because of the possibility that choriocarcinoma will develop following gestational trophoblastic disease, scrupulous follow-up care is essential. Such care includes monitoring hCG levels weekly until titres are negative for 3 consecutive weeks, then monthly for 6 months, then every 2 months for the next 6 months.

Follow-up also includes monthly chest x-rays to check for lung metastasis until hCG titres are negative. Chest x-rays are then obtained once every 2 months for 1 year. Contraceptive methods are used to prevent another pregnancy until at least 1 year after all titres and x-ray findings are negative.

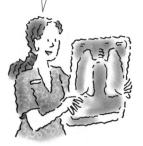

There's no sign of lung metastasis and hCG titres are negative. This woman hasn't developed choriocarcinoma.

What to do

- Assess the woman's vital signs to obtain a baseline for future comparison.
- Preoperatively, observe for signs of complications, such as haemorrhage and uterine infection, and vaginal passage of vesicles. Save any expelled tissue for laboratory analysis.
- Prepare the woman for surgery.
- Postoperatively, monitor vital signs and fluid intake and output, and check for signs of haemorrhage.
- Encourage the woman and her family to express their feelings about the disorder. Offer emotional support and help them through the grieving process.
- Help the woman and her family develop effective coping strategies. Refer them for additional grief and loss counselling if needed.
- Assist with obtaining baseline information – including a pelvic examination, chest x-ray and serum hCG levels – and with ongoing monitoring. (See *Monitoring hCG levels*.)
- Stress the need for regular monitoring (hCG levels and chest x-rays) to detect malignant changes.
- Instruct the woman to report new symptoms promptly (for example, haemoptysis, cough, suspected pregnancy, nausea, vomiting and vaginal bleeding).

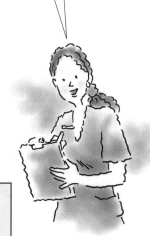

Explain to the woman, the importance of reporting new symptoms promptly.

Monitoring hCG levels

When evaluating serum human chorionic gonadotropin (hCG) levels in a woman previously diagnosed with gestational trophoblastic disease, gradually declining levels suggest no further disease. However, if hCG levels plateau three times or increase at any time during the monitoring period, suspect the development of a malignancy.

- Explain to the woman that she must use contraceptives to prevent pregnancy for at least 1 year after hCG levels return to normal and her body reestablishes regular ovulation and menstrual cycles.

HELLP syndrome

HELLP is an acronym that stands for haemolysis, elevated liver enzymes and low platelets. HELLP syndrome is a category of gestational hypertension that involves changes in blood components and liver function.

Temporary HELLP

HELLP syndrome develops in 12% of women with gestational hypertension. It can occur in primigravidas and multigravidas. When it occurs, maternal and infant mortality is high; approximately a quarter of women and a third of infants die from this disorder. However, after birth, laboratory results return to normal – usually within 1 week – and the mother experiences no further problems.

What causes it

Although the exact cause of HELLP is unknown, theories have been proposed about the development of its signs and symptoms. Haemolysis is believed to result because RBCs are damaged by their travel through small, impaired blood vessels. Elevated liver enzymes are believed to result from obstruction in liver flow by fibrin deposits. Low platelets are believed to be the result of vascular damage secondary to vasospasm. Women with severe pre-eclampsia are at high risk for developing HELLP syndrome.

What to look for

Typically, the woman complains of pain, most commonly in the right upper quadrant, epigastric area or lower chest. Additional signs and symptoms include nausea, vomiting, general malaise and severe oedema. The right upper quadrant may be tender on palpation because of a distended liver. In addition, the woman exhibits signs and symptoms of pre-eclampsia.

What tests tell you

Laboratory studies reveal:
- haemolysis of RBCs (appearing fragmented and irregular on a peripheral blood smear)
- thrombocytopenia (a platelet count below 100,000/mm^3)
- elevated levels of alanine aminotransferase and serum aspartate aminotransferase.

How it's treated

Treatment involves intensive care management for the woman and her fetus. Drug therapy, such as with magnesium sulphate, is instituted to reduce blood pressure and prevent seizures. Transfusions of fresh frozen plasma or platelets may be used to reverse thrombocytopenia. Delivery of the fetus may occur vaginally or by caesarean birth and generally resolves the condition.

What to do

• Assess maternal vital signs and FHR frequently; be alert for signs and symptoms of complications, including haemorrhage, hypoglycaemia, hyponatraemia, subcapsular liver haematoma and renal failure.
• Maintain a quiet, calm, dimly lit environment to reduce the risk of seizures; limit visitation.
• Avoid palpating the abdomen because this increases intraabdominal pressure, which could lead to rupture of a subcapsular liver haematoma.
• Institute bleeding precautions, and monitor the woman for signs and symptoms of bleeding. Administer blood transfusions and medications as ordered.
• If the woman develops hypoglycaemia, expect to administer I.V. dextrose solutions.
• Prepare the woman for delivery; explain all events and procedures being done; assist with evaluations for fetal maturity.
• Record all treatments and drugs given.
• Be aware that because of the increased risk of bleeding due to thrombocytopenia the woman may not be a candidate for epidural anaesthesia.
• Assess the woman carefully throughout labour and delivery for possible haemorrhage.

A quiet, dimly lit environment with limited visitors reduces the risk of seizures.

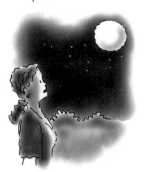

Hyperemesis gravidarum

Unlike the transient nausea and vomiting that's normally experienced until about the 12th week of pregnancy, hyperemesis gravidarum is severe and unremitting nausea and vomiting persist after the first trimester. It usually occurs with the first pregnancy and commonly affects women with conditions that produce high levels of hCG, such as gestational trophoblastic disease or multiple pregnancy.

This disorder occurs in about 7 out of 1,000 pregnancies and the prognosis is usually good. However, if untreated, hyperemesis gravidarum produces substantial weight loss, starvation with ketosis and acetonuria, dehydration with subsequent fluid and electrolyte imbalance (hypokalaemia), and acid-base disturbances (acidosis and alkalosis). Retinal, neurological and renal damage may also occur.

What causes it

The specific cause of hyperemesis gravidarum is unknown. Possible causes include pancreatitis (elevated serum amylase levels are common), biliary tract disease, decreased secretion of free hydrochloric acid in the stomach, decreased gastric motility, drug toxicity, inflammatory obstructive bowel disease and vitamin deficiency (especially B6). In some women, this disorder may be related to psychological factors.

What to look for

The woman typically complains of unremitting nausea and vomiting. The vomitus initially contains undigested food, mucus and small amounts of bile. Later, it contains only bile and mucus. Finally, the vomitus includes blood and material that resembles coffee grounds.

Enough is enough!

The woman may report thirst, hiccups, oliguria, vertigo and headache as well as substantial weight loss and eventual emaciation caused by persistent vomiting. She may appear confused or delirious. Lassitude, stupor and, possibly, coma may occur. Additional findings may include:
- pale, dry, waxy and, possibly, jaundiced skin with decreased skin turgor
- dry, coated tongue
- subnormal or elevated temperature
- rapid pulse
- foetid, fruity breath (from acidosis).

> Unremitting nausea and vomiting should be enough! But there's more – headache, weight loss, vertigo, lassitude and so on, and so on . . . Stop me any time!

What tests tell you

Diagnostic tests are used to rule out other disorders, such as gastroenteritis, cholecystitis, peptic ulcer and pancreatic or liver disorders, which produce similar clinical effects. Differential diagnosis also rules out gestational trophoblastic disease, hepatitis, inner ear infection, food poisoning, emotional problems and eating disorders.

Urine test results show ketonuria and slight proteinuria. The following results of serum analysis support a diagnosis of hyperemesis gravidarum:
- decreased protein, chloride, sodium and potassium levels
- increased blood urea nitrogen levels
- elevated haemoglobin levels
- elevated WBC count.

How it's treated

The woman with hyperemesis gravidarum may require hospitalisation to correct electrolyte imbalances and prevent starvation. I.V. infusions are used to maintain nutrition until she can tolerate an oral diet.

An infusion of 3,000 ml of I.V. fluid over 24 hours will usually cause a reduction in symptoms. Oral fluids and food are usually withheld until there's no vomiting for 24 hours, after which clear liquids can be initiated. Antiemetics such as ondansetron (Zofran) may be administered to control vomiting. The woman progresses slowly to a clear liquid diet, then a full liquid diet and, finally, small, frequent meals of high-protein solid foods. A midnight snack helps stabilise blood glucose levels. Parenteral vitamin supplements and potassium replacements are used to help correct deficiencies if the problem becomes long term.

Antihistamines (promethazine, prochlorperazine) have been studied as a possible line of treatment and have shown promising results, although some drowsiness was reported. These have now been recommended in the NICE guidelines for treatment of hyperemesis.

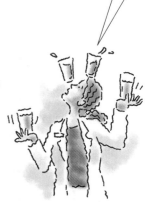

When a woman with hyperemesis gravidarum can tolerate oral feedings, she'll start with a clear liquid diet.

Easy does it

If persistent vomiting jeopardises the woman's health, antiemetic medications may be prescribed. Antiemetics must be prescribed with caution and the benefits must outweigh the risks to the mother and her fetus.

After vomiting stops and the woman's electrolyte balance has been restored, the pregnancy usually continues without recurrence of hyperemesis gravidarum. Most women feel better as they begin to regain normal weight, but some continue to vomit throughout the pregnancy, requiring extended treatment and total parenteral nutrition.

What to do

• Administer I.V. fluids as ordered until the woman can tolerate oral feedings.
• Monitor fluid intake and output, vital signs, skin turgor, daily weight, serum electrolyte levels and urine for ketones; anticipate the need for electrolyte replacement therapy.
• Provide frequent mouth care.
• Consult a dietitian to provide a diet high in dry, complex carbohydrates. Suggest decreased liquid intake during meals. Provide company and encourage diversionary conversation at mealtime.
• Instruct the woman to remain upright for 45 minutes after eating to decrease reflux.
• Suggest that the woman eat two or three dry crackers before getting out of bed in the morning to alleviate nausea.
• Provide reassurance and a calm, restful atmosphere. Encourage the woman to discuss her feelings about her pregnancy and the disorder.
• Document all care given, medications administered and any additional information relating to the woman's care.
• Help the woman to develop effective coping strategies. Refer her to a mental health professional for additional counselling if necessary (hyperemisis may be an extreme response to psychosocial problems). Refer her to the social service department for help in caring for other children at home if appropriate.

- Teach the woman protective measures to conserve energy and promote rest. Include relaxation techniques, fresh air and moderate exercise (if tolerated), and activities scheduled appropriately to prevent fatigue.

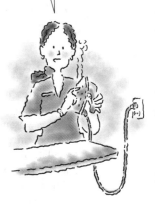

It takes time to restock the iron stores. That's why mothers should be encouraged to stick with their treatment, even when they're feeling better.

Isoimmunisation

Isoimmunisation, also called *Rh incompatibility*, refers to a condition in which the pregnant woman is Rh-negative but her fetus is Rh-positive. This condition, if left untreated, can lead to haemolytic disease in the neonate. Before the development of anti-D, this condition was a major cause of kernicterus (nerve cell deterioration) and neonatal death.

Prevention

Routine antenatal anti-D prophylaxis (RAADP) is currently a dose of anti-D immunoglobulin of at least 500 international units (IU) at 28 and 34 weeks' gestation or a single dose of at least 1,500 IU at weeks 28–30 and is offered to all RhD-negative women. If the woman has had, or is believed to have had, a sensitising event early in her pregnancy, antenatal anti-D prophylaxis (AADP) can be offered earlier, the dose depending on the gestation period.

Technology

Anti-D immunoglobulin is made from the plasma (liquid part of blood) of blood donors.

Anti-D immunoglobulin (D-Gam; Bio Products Laboratory) available as 250, 500, 1,500, 2,500 IU vials for intramuscular use (preferably into the deltoid muscle) only to Rh-negative woman for prevention of Rh(D) sensitisation:

- Antenatal prophylaxis is given at weeks 28 and 34 of pregnancy; a further dose may still needed immediately or within 72 hours of delivery.

Current NICE guidance

- It's recommended that RAADP is offered to all nonsensitised pregnant women who are RhD-negative.
- The clinician (obstetrician, midwife or general practitioner) responsible for the antenatal care of a nonsensitised RhD-negative woman should discuss RAADP with her and the options available allowing the woman can make an informed choice about treatment. The clinician should talk to the woman about circumstances where RAADP would be neither necessary nor cost-effective. Such circumstances might include those where the woman:

    has opted to be sterilised after the birth of the baby

    is in a stable relationship with the father of the child, and he is known or found to be RhD-negative

    is certain that she will not have another child after her current pregnancy.

- The difference between RAADP (routine prophylaxis at 28 and 34 weeks) and prophylactic anti-D given because of likely sensitisation should be clearly explained to the woman.
- A woman's consent for RAADP at 28 and 34 weeks should not be affected by whether she has already had AADP for a potentially sensitising event early in pregnancy.

Access the NICE guidelines for prophylactic administration of anti-D to pregnant women on http://www.nice.org.uk/guidance/TA41

What causes Rh isoimmunisation?

During her first pregnancy, an Rh-negative woman may become sensitised to Rh antigens by:
- being exposed to Rh-positive fetal blood antigens inherited from the father
- receiving alien Rh antigens from a blood transfusion, causing agglutinins (antibodies in the woman's blood) to develop
- receiving inadequate doses of anti-D or failing to receive anti-D after significant fetal–maternal leakage from abruptio placentae.

Subsequent pregnancy with an Rh-positive fetus provokes increasing amounts of maternal agglutinating antibodies to cross the placental barrier, attach to Rh-positive cells in the fetus and cause haemolysis and anaemia. To compensate for this, the fetus steps up the production of RBCs, and erythroblasts (immature RBCs) appear in the fetal circulation. Extensive haemolysis results in the release of large amounts of unconjugated bilirubin, which the liver can't conjugate and excrete, causing hyperbilirubinaemia and haemolytic anaemia. (See *Pathogenesis of Rh isoimmunisation*, page 216.)

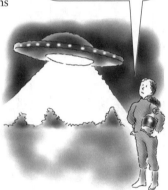

Alien Rh antigens from a blood transfusion may sensitise an Rh-negative woman to Rh antigens during her first pregnancy. It's a close encounter of the Rh kind!

What to look for

Typically, the pregnant woman doesn't exhibit signs or symptoms of this disorder. The fetus – and subsequently the neonate – are affected.

What tests tell you

At the first antenatal visit, an anti-D antibody titre should be performed on all women with Rh-negative blood.

A sensitive situation

Antenatal screening is ongoing throughout pregnancy. An anti-D antibody titre of 1:16 or greater indicates Rh sensitisation. If this is the case, titre monitoring continues every 2 weeks for the remainder of the pregnancy.

Amniocentesis is performed to evaluate the status of the fetus. During amniocentesis, the fluid density of the amniotic fluid is determined using spectrophotometry. The results are plotted on a graph and correlated with

Pathogenesis of Rh isoimmunisation

Rh isoimmunisation progresses throughout pregnancies in Rh-negative mothers who give birth to Rh-positive babies. The illustrations below outline the process of isoimmunisation.

A nonpregnant woman has Rh-negative blood.

She becomes pregnant with an Rh-positive fetus. Normal antibodies appear.

Placental separation occurs.

After delivery, the mother develops anti–Rh-positive antibodies.

With the next Rh-positive fetus, antibodies enter fetal circulation, causing haemolysis.

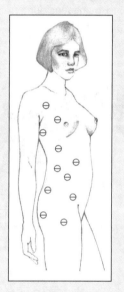 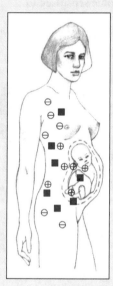 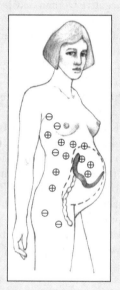 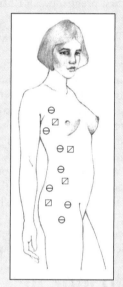 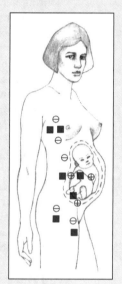

⊖ Rh− blood　　⊕ Rh+ blood　　■ Normal antibodies

gestational age to determine the extent of involvement and the amount of bilirubin present. Amniotic fluid analysis may show increased bilirubin levels (indicating possible haemolysis) and increased anti-Rh titres.

Radiologic studies may show oedema and, in those with hydrops fetalis (oedema of the fetus), the halo sign (oedematous, elevated subcutaneous fat layers).

How it's treated

Treatment focuses on preventing Rh isoimmunisation by administering anti-D to any unsensitised Rh-negative woman as soon as possible after the birth of an Rh-positive neonate or after spontaneous or elective abortion.

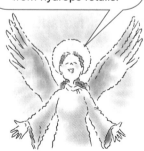

Believe me, I'm no angel! The halo sign refers to oedematous, elevated subcutaneous fat layers from hydrops fetalis.

In addition, screening for Rh isoimmunisation or irregular antibodies is indicated for the following women:
• Rh-negative women during their first antenatal visit and at 24, 28, 32 and 36 weeks' gestation
• Rh-positive women with a history of transfusion, a neonate with jaundice, stillbirth, caesarean birth, induced abortion, placenta praevia or abruptio placentae.

Towering titre

If the pregnant woman's Rh antibody titre is high, she may be given high doses of anti-D to help reduce fetal involvement; the goal is to interfere with the rapid destruction of fetal RBCs. The fetus may receive a blood transfusion in utero via an injection of RBCs directly into a vessel in the fetal cord or instillation in the fetal abdomen via amniocentesis. After birth, the neonate may receive an exchange transfusion to remove haemolysed RBCs and replace them with healthy blood cells.

Bilirubin levels in amniotic fluid are monitored for early delivery intervention or intrauterine fetal transfusion if needed. Repeated transfusions may be needed in the neonate.

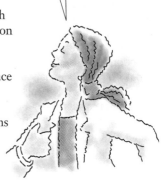

I'm positive that anti-D should be administered to an unsensitised Rh-negative woman as soon as possible after delivery of an Rh-positive baby.

What to do

• Assess all pregnant women for possible Rh incompatibility.
• Expect to administer anti-D, I.M. as ordered, to all Rh-negative women at 28 weeks' and 34 weeks' gestation and after transfusion reaction, ectopic pregnancy, spontaneous or induced abortion, or during the second and third trimesters to women with abruptio placentae, placentae praevia or amniocentesis.
• If sensitisation has occurred and the fetus has been affected, prepare the woman for a planned delivery, usually 2–4 weeks before term date depending on maternal history, serologic tests and amniocentesis. Delivery may be much earlier, depending on the fetal RBC count and serum bilirubin levels.

For more information on NICE guidelines on prophylactic anti-D therapy, visit the website: www.nice.org.uk/guidance/index

Placenta praevia

Placenta praevia occurs when the placenta implants in the lower uterine segment obstructing the internal cervical os and failing to provide as much nourishment as implantation in the fundus would supply. The placenta tends to spread out, seeking the blood supply it needs, and it becomes larger and thinner than normal. Haemorrhage occurs as the internal cervical os effaces and dilates, tearing the uterine vessels. One of the most common causes of bleeding during the second half of pregnancy, this disorder occurs in about 1 in 200 pregnancies and more commonly in multigravidas than primigravidas.

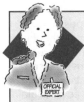

Advice from the experts

Administering anti-D

Anti-D is a concentrated solution of human immune globulin containing Rh(D) antibodies. An I.M. injection of anti-D keeps the Rh-negative woman from producing active antibody responses and forming anti-Rh(D) to Rh-positive fetal blood cells and endangering future Rh-positive fetuses.

Anti-D should be administered to an Rh-negative woman after abortion, ectopic pregnancy, delivery of a neonate with Rh(D)-positive blood and cord blood that's direct Coombs' negative, accidental transfusion of Rh-positive blood, amniocentesis, placental abruption or abdominal trauma. It's given within 72 hours to prevent future maternal sensitisation. Administration at approximately 28 and 34 weeks' gestation can also protect the fetus of an Rh-negative mother.

Anti-D is given I.M. into the gluteal site. When administering anti-D, the same steps are followed as for any I.M. injection, but be sure to include these steps:

- Check the vial's identification numbers with another midwife, and stick the label that comes with the anti-D into the mother's notes. Both midwives sign the mother's notes and the medicine kardex after administering the anti-D. Usually there will be another record kept in the ward.
- Send the remaining two copies, along with the empty anti-D vial, to the laboratory or blood bank.
- Give the woman a card indicating her Rh-negative status, and instruct her to carry it with her or keep it in a convenient location.

It's a cover-up!

The placenta may cover all or part of the internal cervical os, or it may gradually overlap the os as the cervix dilates. Complete obstruction is known as *total*, *complete* or *central placenta praevia*. Partial obstruction is known as *incomplete* or *partial placenta praevia*. When a small placental edge is felt through the maternal os, the placenta praevia is referred to as *low marginal*. (See *Three types of placenta praevia*, page 219.) Obstruction that occurs as the cervix dilates is caused by marginal implantation or a low-lying placenta.

The apparent degree of placenta praevia may depend largely on the extent of cervical dilation at the time of examination. Maternal prognosis is good if haemorrhage can be controlled. Fetal prognosis depends on gestational age and the amount of blood lost.

What causes it

The specific cause of placenta praevia is unknown. Factors that may affect the site of the placenta's attachment to the uterine wall include:
- defective vascularisation of the decidua
- multiple pregnancy (the placenta requires a larger surface for attachment)

Three types of placenta praevia

There are three basic types of placenta praevia: low marginal, partial and complete.

Low marginal

In low-marginal placenta praevia, a small placental edge can be felt through the maternal os.

Partial

In partial placenta praevia, the placenta partially caps the internal os.

Complete

In complete placenta praevia, the placenta completely covers the internal os.

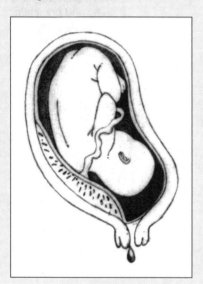
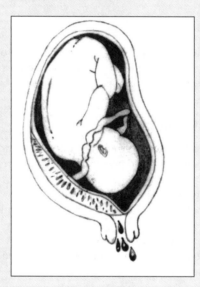
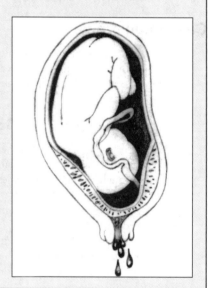

- previous uterine surgery
- multiparity
- advanced maternal age.

What to look for

Typically, a woman with placenta praevia reports the onset of painless, bright red vaginal bleeding after the 20th week of pregnancy. Such bleeding, beginning before the onset of labour, tends to be episodic; it starts without warning, stops spontaneously and resumes later.

About 7% of women with placenta praevia are asymptomatic. In these women, ultrasound examination reveals the disorder incidentally.

Palpation may reveal a soft, nontender uterus. Deep pelvic palpation abdominal examination reveals various malpresentations because the placenta's abnormal location has interfered with descent of the fetal head. Minimal descent of the fetal presenting part may indicate placenta praevia. The fetus remains active, however, with a heart rate audible on auscultation.

What tests tell you

A differential diagnosis is necessary to exclude genital lacerations, excessive bloody show, abruptio placentae and cervical lesions. Laboratory studies may reveal decreased maternal haemoglobin levels (due to blood loss).

Ultrasound is most sound

Transvaginal ultrasonography is used to determine placental position.

Caesarean ready

Vaginal examination should be performed only in a surgical suite or a birthing room that's equipped for caesarean birth in the event that haemorrhage necessitates immediate delivery.

How it's managed

Treatment of placenta praevia focuses on assessing, controlling and restoring blood loss; delivering a viable neonate and preventing coagulation disorders. Immediate therapy includes:
- starting an I.V. infusion using a large-bore catheter
- drawing blood for haemoglobin levels, haematocrit, typing and crossmatching
- initiating external electronic fetal monitoring
- monitoring maternal blood pressure, pulse rate and respirations
- assessing the amount of vaginal bleeding.

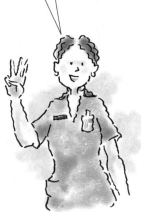

Treatment of placenta praevia focuses on controlling and restoring blood loss, delivering the baby and preventing coagulation disorders.

When the fetus is premature

If the fetus is premature (following determination of the degree of placenta praevia and necessary fluid and blood replacement), treatment consists of careful observation to allow the fetus more time to mature. If clinical evaluation confirms complete placenta praevia, the woman is usually hospitalised because of the increased risk of haemorrhage. As soon as the fetus is sufficiently mature, or in cases of severe haemorrhage, immediate caesarean delivery may be necessary.

The woman may have had the advantage of steroid treatment (to mature fetal lungs) if her baby is <34 weeks' gestation. Vaginal delivery is considered only when the bleeding is minimal and the placenta praevia is marginal, or when the labour is rapid.

Have hands on hand

Because of possible fetal blood loss through the placenta, a paediatric team should be on hand during such a delivery to immediately assess and treat neonatal shock, blood loss and hypoxia.

What to do

- If the woman with placenta praevia shows active bleeding, continuously monitor her blood pressure, pulse rate, respirations, intake and output and amount of vaginal bleeding in the fetus; continuously monitor the FHR and rhythm.
- Anticipate the need for electronic fetal monitoring, and assist with application as indicated.
- Have oxygen readily available in case fetal distress occurs. (Many facilities will administer oxygen continuously in labour and delivery to increase the amount of oxygen delivered to the fetus.) Evidence of fetal distress includes bradycardia, tachycardia or late or variable decelerations.
- If the woman is Rh-negative, administer anti-D after every bleeding episode.
- Institute complete bed rest.
- Prepare the woman and her family for a possible caesarean delivery and the birth of a premature baby. Thoroughly explain postpartum care so the mother and her family know which measures to expect.
- If the fetus isn't mature, expect to administer an initial dose of betamethasone I.M. to the mother to aid in promoting fetal lung maturity. Explain that additional doses may be given again in 24 hours and, possibly, 1–2 weeks.
- Provide emotional support during labour as well as pain relief. Reassure her of her progress throughout labour, and keep her informed of the fetus's condition.
- Make sure that all clinical observations and care are documented throughout and all treatments and medications are recorded.
- Assess for signs of infection (fever, chills). The woman is at increased risk of infection because of the proximity of vaginal organisms to the placenta and the susceptibility of the placental environment to the growth of microorganisms.
- Teach the woman to identify and report signs of placenta praevia (bleeding, cramping) immediately.
- During the postpartum period, monitor the mother for signs of haemorrhage and shock caused by the uterus's diminished ability to contract.
- Tactfully discuss the possibility that her baby could require intensive care after delivery.
- Encourage the woman and her family to verbalise their feelings, and help them develop effective coping strategies. Refer them for counselling if necessary.

Placental abruption

Placental abruption – also called *Abruptio placentae* – occurs when the placenta separates from the uterine wall prematurely, usually after 20 weeks' gestation, producing haemorrhage. This disorder may be classified according to the degree of placental separation and the severity of maternal and fetal symptoms.

More births, more risk

Abruption is most common in multigravidas and is a common cause of bleeding during the second half of pregnancy. The fetal prognosis depends on gestational age and the amount of blood lost. The maternal prognosis is good if haemorrhage can be controlled.

What causes it

The cause of placental abruption is unknown. Predisposing factors include:
- traumatic injury such as a direct blow to the uterus
- placental site bleeding caused by a needle puncture during amniocentesis
- chronic hypertension or gestational hypertension, which raises pressure on the maternal side of the placenta
- multiparity (more than 5)
- short umbilical cord
- dietary deficiency
- smoking
- pressure on the venae cavae from an enlarged uterus.

(See *Understanding placental abruption*.)

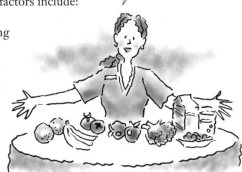

Dietary deficiency is thought to be a predisposing factor in placental abruption. So, encourage your mothers to eat up!

What to look for

Placental abruption produces a wide range of signs and symptoms, depending on the extent of placental separation and the amount of blood lost from maternal circulation. In addition to the major complications of abruption – haemorrhage and shock – it may also cause renal failure, pituitary necrosis (Sheehan's syndrome), disseminated intravascular coagulation (DIC) and maternal and fetal death.

Understanding placental abruption

With placental abruption, lack of resiliency or abnormal changes in uterine vasculature cause blood vessels at the placental bed to rupture spontaneously. Hypertension and an enlarged uterus that can't contract sufficiently to seal off the torn blood vessels further complicate the situation. As a result, bleeding continues unchecked, potentially shearing off part or all of the placenta.

External versus internal

About 80% of bleeding is external (marginal), meaning that a peripheral portion of the placenta separates from the uterine wall. The bleeding is internal (concealed) if

the central portion of the placenta becomes detached and the still-intact peripheral portions trap the blood. This occurs in about 20% of cases.

Effects of bleeding

As blood enters the muscle fibres, detached and still-intact peripheral portions of the placenta trap the blood. Complete relaxation of the uterus becomes impossible. Uterine tone and irritability increase. If bleeding into the muscle fibres is profuse, the uterus turns blue or purple and the accumulated blood prevents its normal contractions after delivery.

Three degrees of separation

Three degrees of separation can occur with placental abruption.

1. *Mild* abruption (marginal separation) develops gradually and produces mild-to-moderate bleeding, vague lower abdominal discomfort, mild-to-moderate abdominal tenderness and uterine irritability. FHR remain strong and regular.
2. *Moderate* abruption (about 50% placental separation) may develop gradually or abruptly and produces continuous abdominal pain, moderate dark red vaginal bleeding, a tender uterus that remains firm between contractions, barely audible or irregular and bradycardic FHR and, possibly, signs of shock. Labour typically starts within 2 hours and usually proceeds rapidly.
3. *Severe* abruption (70% placental separation) develops abruptly and causes agonising, unremitting uterine pain (described as tearing or knifelike); a boardlike, tender uterus; moderate vaginal bleeding; rapidly progressive shock and absence of FHR (related to fetal cardiac distress).

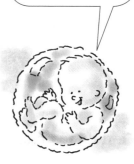

As placental abruption becomes more severe, I'm at greater risk for cardiac distress.

Placental separation in placental abruption

Here are descriptions and illustrations of the three degrees of placental separation in placental abruption.

Mild separation

Mild separation begins with small areas of separation and internal bleeding (concealed haemorrhage) between the placenta and uterine wall.

Moderate separation

Moderate separation may develop abruptly or progress from mild to extensive separation with external haemorrhage.

Severe separation

With severe separation, external haemorrhage occurs, along with shock and, possibly, fetal cardiac distress.

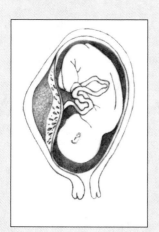
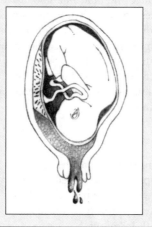
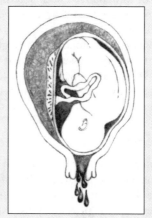

What tests tell you

Vaginal examination (in preparation for emergency caesarean delivery) and ultrasonography are performed to rule out placenta praevia. Decreased haemoglobin levels and platelet counts support the diagnosis. Periodic assays for fibrin split products aid in monitoring the progression of placental abruption and in detecting DIC. Differential diagnosis excludes placenta praevia, ovarian cysts, appendicitis and degeneration of leiomyomas.

How it's treated

Treatment of placental abruption focuses on assessing, controlling and restoring the amount of blood lost; delivering a viable neonate and preventing coagulation disorders.

First things first!

Immediate measures for treatment of placental include:
* call for help – get the appropriate professionals to the ward – call for a doctor in the first instance
* starting an I.V. infusion (through a large-bore catheter) to combat hypovolaemia
* taking blood for haemoglobin level, haematocrit, coagulation studies and grouping and crossmatching
* external electronic fetal monitoring and monitoring of maternal vital signs and vaginal bleeding
* administering blood replacement as necessary
* insert a self-retaining urinary catheter to monitor output and keep bladder empty
* document all events and treatments as soon as they happen.

Delivery details

After the severity of abruption has been determined and fluid and blood have been replaced, prompt caesarean delivery is necessary if the fetus is in distress or if heavy bleeding continues. If the fetus isn't in distress, monitoring continues.

Because of possible fetal blood loss through the placenta, a paediatric team should be ready at delivery to assess and treat the neonate for shock, blood loss and hypoxia. If placental separation is severe and no signs of fetal life are present, vaginal delivery may be performed unless it's contraindicated by uncontrolled haemorrhage or other complications.

What to do

* Assess the woman's extent of bleeding and monitor fundal height every 30 minutes for changes. Count the number of perineal pads used by the woman, weighing them as needed to determine the amount of blood loss.
* Monitor maternal blood pressure, pulse rate, respirations, intake and output and amount of vaginal bleeding every 10–15 minutes.

- Begin electronic fetal monitoring to assess FHR continuously.
- Have equipment for emergency caesarean delivery readily available.
- If vaginal delivery is elected, provide emotional support during labour. Because of the baby's prematurity, the mother may not receive analgesics during labour and may experience intense pain. Reassure the mother of her progress through labour, and keep her informed of the fetus's condition.
- Prepare the woman and her family for the possibility of an emergency caesarean delivery of a premature neonate and the changes to expect in the postpartum period. Offer emotional support and an honest assessment of the situation.
- Tactfully discuss the possibility of her baby being in a poor condition. Let the mother know in a sensitive manner that the baby's survival depends primarily on gestational age, the amount of blood lost and associated hypertensive disorders. Assure her that frequent monitoring and prompt management greatly reduce the risk of morbidity/mortality.
- Encourage the woman and her family to verbalise their feelings

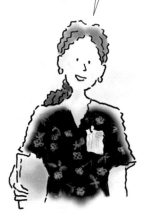

In premature labour, fetal prognosis depends on birthweight and length of gestation.

Premature labour

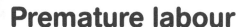

Premature labour, also known as *preterm labour*, is the onset of rhythmic uterine contractions that produce cervical changes after fetal viability but before fetal maturity. It usually occurs between weeks 20 and 37 of gestation – between 5% and 10% of pregnancies end prematurely.

Weighing in

Fetal prognosis depends on birthweight and length of gestation. Fetuses born before 26 weeks' gestation and weighing less than 737 g (1 lb, 10 oz) have a survival rate of about 10%. Fetuses born at 27–28 weeks' gestation and weighing between 737 and 992 g have a survival rate of more than 50%. Those born after 28 weeks' gestation and weighing 992 g to 1.21 Kg have a 70–90% survival rate.

What causes it

Causes of premature labour include PROM (in 30–50% of cases), gestational hypertension, chronic hypertensive vascular disease, hydramnious, multiple pregnancy, placenta praevia, placental abruption, incompetent cervix, abdominal surgery, trauma, structural anomalies of the uterus, infections (such as group B streptococci) and fetal death.

What to look for

The woman reports the onset of rhythmic uterine contractions, possible rupture of membranes, passage of the cervical mucus plug (operculum) and a bloody discharge. Her history indicates that she's in week 20–37 of pregnancy. Vaginal examination shows cervical effacement and dilation.

What tests tell you

Premature labour is confirmed by the combined results of antenatal history, physical examination, presenting signs and symptoms and ultrasonography (if available), showing the position of the fetus in relation to the mother's pelvis.

How it's treated

Treatment is designed to suppress preterm labour when tests show immature fetal pulmonary development, cervical dilation of less than 4 cm and the absence of factors that contraindicate continuation of pregnancy. Such treatment consists of bed rest and, when necessary, tocolytic drug therapy. Steroids may be administered to mature fetal lungs.

> Steps to prevent premature labour begin with good antenatal care, nutrition and proper rest.

Prevention first

Taking steps to prevent premature labour is important. This requires good antenatal care, adequate nutrition and proper rest. Inserting a purse-string suture (cerclage) to reinforce an incompetent cervix at 14–18 weeks' gestation may prevent premature labour in a woman with a history of incompetent cervix.

Slow to a stop

Atosiban is widely used as the drug of choice in slowing down or halting premature labour. The theory is that if delivery is delayed, even for a few days, it allows time for the mother to be given corticosteroids to mature the fetal lungs, and perhaps allow the transfer of the mother to a regional maternity hospital with a neonatal unit.

Atosiban is recommended by the RCOG for treatment of preterm labour. The initial bolus dose is 6.75 mg over 1 minute, followed by an infusion of 18 mg/hour for 3 hours and then 6 mg/hour for up to 45 hours. It is recommended that it should not be used for more than 48 hours.

Ritrodine is also popular, but like all beta-agonists, it has a high frequency of adverse effects.

Indomethacin (Indocin), a prostaglandin synthesis inhibitor, may be given, but its use has been associated with premature closure of ductus arteriosus if given after 34 weeks' gestation (used more in US).

Weighing the risks

Sometimes preterm delivery is the lesser risk if maternal factors, such as intrauterine infection, placental abruption, placental insufficiency and severe pre-eclampsia, jeopardise the fetus. Fetal problems, particularly isoimmunisation and congenital anomalies, can become more perilous as pregnancy nears term and may require preterm delivery.

Treatment and delivery require intensive team effort. The fetus's health requires continuous assessment through fetal monitoring.

Close at hand

Ideally, treatment of active premature labour should take place in a regional maternity unit, where the staff are specially trained to handle this situation. In such settings, the baby can remain close to his parents. (Community hospitals commonly lack the facilities for special neonatal care and this may result in mother and baby being separated when the baby is transferred to a regional neonatal unit.)

Sedatives and narcotics, which may harm the fetus, shouldn't be used – they depress CNS function and may cause fetal respiratory depression; therefore, they should be administered in the smallest doses possible and only when absolutely necessary.

Amniotomy (rupture of the amniotic fluid membranes) should be avoided, if possible, to prevent cord prolapse or damage to the fetus's tender skull. Adequate hydration is maintained with I.V. fluids.

What to do

• Closely observe the woman in premature labour for signs of fetal or maternal distress and provide comprehensive supportive care.
• Make sure the woman maintains bed rest during attempts to suppress premature labour.
• Administer medications as ordered.
• Give sedatives and analgesics sparingly because they may be harmful to the fetus. Minimise the need for these drugs by providing comfort measures, such as frequent repositioning and good perineal and back care.
• Monitor blood pressure, pulse rate, respirations, FHR and uterine contraction pattern when administering a beta-adrenergic stimulant, sedative or narcotic. Minimise adverse reactions by keeping the woman in a side-lying position as much as possible to ensure adequate placental perfusion.
• Administer fluids as ordered to ensure adequate hydration.
• Assess deep tendon reflexes frequently when administering magnesium sulphate. Monitor the neonate for signs of magnesium toxicity, including neuromuscular and respiratory depression.
• During active premature labour, remember that the preterm fetus has a lower tolerance for the stress of labour and is more likely to become hypoxic than a full-term fetus. If necessary, administer oxygen to the woman through a nasal cannula. Encourage the mother to lie on her left side or sit up during labour; this position prevents vena caval compression, which can cause supine hypotension and subsequent fetal hypoxia.
• Observe fetal response to labour through continuous monitoring. Prevent maternal hyperventilation; use a rebreathing bag as necessary. Continually reassure the woman throughout labour to help reduce her anxiety.
• Prepare to administer I.M. betamethasone as indicated.
• Help the mother proceed through labour with as little analgesia and anaesthesia as possible. To minimise fetal CNS depression, avoid administering an analgesic when delivery seems imminent. Monitor fetal and maternal response to local and regional anaesthetics.

Further information on management of premature labour is available on the RCOG website:http://www.rcog.org.uk/resources/public/pdf/tocolytic_drugs_no1(b).pdf

Premature rupture of membranes

PROM is a spontaneous break or tear in the amniotic sac before onset of regular contractions. It results in progressive cervical dilation. This common abnormality of parturition occurs in nearly 16% of all pregnancies longer than 20 weeks' gestation; more than 80% of babies are mature. Labour usually starts within 24 hours – 91% of these women will go into labour within 48 hours.

In labour limbo

The latent period (between membrane rupture and labour onset) is generally brief when membranes rupture near term. When the fetus is premature, the latent period is prolonged, which increases the risk of mortality from maternal infection (amnionitis, endometritis), fetal infection (pneumonia, septicaemia) and prematurity.

If membranes rupture when the fetus isn't near term, the baby is then at increased risk for mortality from maternal infection (amnionitis, endometritis), fetal infection (pneumonia, septicaemia) and prematurity.

Mum's PROM problems

Maternal complications associated with PROM include:
- endometritis
- amnionitis
- septic shock and death if amnionitis goes untreated.

Baby's PROM predicament

Neonatal complications of PROM include:
- increased risk of respiratory distress syndrome
- asphyxia
- pulmonary hypoplasia
- congenital anomalies
- malpresentation
- cord prolapse
- severe fetal distress that can result in neonatal death.

What causes it

Although the cause of PROM is unknown, malpresentation and a contracted pelvis commonly accompany the rupture.

Usual suspects

Predisposing factors include:
- lack of proper antenatal care
- poor nutrition and hygiene
- smoking
- incompetent cervix
- increased intrauterine tension from hydramnios or multiple gestation
- reduced amniotic membrane tensile strength
- uterine infection.

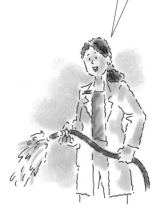

Blood-tinged amniotic fluid is a sure sign of PROM.

What to look for

Typically, PROM causes blood-tinged amniotic fluid containing vernix caseosa particles to gush or leak from the vagina. Maternal fever, fetal tachycardia and foul-smelling vaginal discharge indicate infection.

What tests tell you

Differential diagnosis is used to exclude urinary incontinence or vaginal infection as the underlying cause. Passage of amniotic fluid confirms the rupture. Slight fundal pressure may expel fluid through the cervical os. Ultrasound examination or vaginal examination is performed to determine if multiple pregnancy is involved. Abdominal palpation determines fetal presentation and size. Mother's history and physical examination findings determine gestational age.

Diagnosis of PROM can be confirmed by the following test results:
- On insertion of a speculum, it may be possible to see a pool of liquor in the posterior fornix of the vagina
- If fluid is amniotic, a smear of the fluid placed on a slide and allowed to dry takes on a fernlike pattern (because of the high sodium and protein content of amniotic fluid). Verification of amniotic fluid leakage confirms PROM.
- Vaginal probe ultrasonography allows visualisation of the amniotic sac to detect tears or ruptures.
- Avoid digital vaginal examinations due to the high risk of introducing infection.

How it's treated

Treatment of PROM depends on fetal age and the risk of infection. In a term pregnancy, if spontaneous labour and vaginal delivery don't result within a relatively short time (usually within 24 hours after the membranes rupture), induction of labour with oxytocin usually follows; then, if induction fails, caesarean delivery is performed.

Heed the signs

Management of a preterm pregnancy of less than 34 weeks is controversial. Treatment of preterm pregnancy between 28 and 34 weeks includes hospitalisation and observation for signs of infection while the fetus matures.

A high white cell count, a raised temperature or fetal tachycardia could indicate chorioamnionitis.

All mothers with PROM should have their temperatures taken 4 hourly, a high vaginal swab taken weekly and a full blood picture, including a C-reactive protein (CRP), done weekly also. Regular CTG traces should be performed as per unit policy. Biophysical profile of the fetus may also be done.

Treatment

Once a mother's membranes rupture, she requires antibiotic therapy: erythromycin 250 mg orally, 6 hourly for 10 days. Antenatal corticosteroids should also be given if the woman is less than 34 weeks pregnant.

The RCOG guidelines suggest that the woman may be allowed to stay at home – but only after she has been hospitalised for at least 48–72 hours and her observations have been stable. She will be required to take her temperature twice daily and arrange for follow-up checks at the antenatal clinic.

Suspect infection – induce to reduce

If the presence of infection is suspected, baseline cultures and sensitivity tests are appropriate. If these tests confirm infection, labour must be induced, followed by I.V. administration of an antibiotic. Blood cultures may be taken from the newborn infant to rule out infection, as antibiotic therapy may be indicated for him as well. During such a delivery, resuscitative equipment must be readily available to manage neonatal distress.

What to do

- Prepare the woman for a vaginal examination. Before physically examining a woman who's suspected of having PROM, explain all diagnostic tests and clarify any misunderstandings she may have.
- During the examination, stay with the woman and offer reassurance.
- Provide sterile gloves and sterile lubricating jelly. Some lubricants can affect results when testing for amniotic fluid.
- After the examination, provide proper perineal care – ideally the woman should wear sterile sanitary towels after PROM.
- Send fluid specimens to the laboratory promptly because bacteriologic studies require immediate evaluation.
- Anticipate administering I.V. prophylactic antibiotics to the woman who's positive for streptococcal B infection to reduce the risk of this infection in the neonate.
- If labour starts, observe the contractions and monitor vital signs.
- Watch for signs and symptoms of maternal infection (fever, abdominal tenderness, changes in amniotic fluid such as purulence and foul odour) and fetal tachycardia. Fetal tachycardia may precede maternal fever. Report such signs and symptoms immediately.
- Provide maternal teaching. (See *Teaching about PROM*, page 231.)

Education edge

Teaching about PROM

Here are some guidelines to follow when teaching a woman about premature rupture of membranes (PROM).

- Inform her about PROM, including its signs and symptoms, during the early stages of pregnancy.
- Make sure the woman understands that amniotic fluid doesn't always gush; it sometimes leaks slowly in PROM.
- Stress the importance of immediately reporting PROM (prompt treatment may prevent dangerous infection).
- Warn the woman not to engage in sexual intercourse, use the bidet, or take a bath after her membranes rupture.
- Advise the woman to refrain from orgasm and breast stimulation after rupture of membranes, which can stimulate uterine contractions.
- Tell the woman to report to her midwife or doctor a temperature above 38°C, which may indicate the onset of infection.

- Encourage the woman and her family to express their feelings and concerns related to the fetus's health and survival.
- Tell the mother to record fetal kick counts and to report fewer than 10 kicks in a 12-hour period. A decrease in fetal kick counts may indicate fetal distress.
- Document all clinical observations, care and any medications that are given to the mother.
- Tell the mother to report uterine contractions, reduced fetal activity or signs of infection (fever, chills and foul-smelling discharge).

Access further information from the RCOG guidelines: http://www.rcog .org.uk/index.asp?PageID=1813

Multiple pregnancy

Multiple pregnancy, or *multiple gestation*, refers to a pregnancy involving more than one fetus. It's considered a complication of pregnancy because the woman's body must adjust to the effects of carrying multiple fetuses.

Baby boom

Multiple pregnancies may be single-ovum conceptions (monozygotic twins) or multiple-ova conceptions (dizygotic twins and greater). The higher a woman's parity and age, the more likely she is to have a multiple pregnancy. Inheritance, based on the mother's family pattern, also appears to play a role in natural dizygotic twinning.

Memory jogger

To remember the difference between monozygotic (identical) and dizygotic (fraternal) twins, picture the 'i' in 'identical' as the roman numeral one (I). One egg fertilised by one spermatozoan makes an identical twin.

Types of twins

There are two types of twins: monozygotic and dizygotic.

Monozygotic

Monozygotic (identical) twins begin with one ovum and one spermatozoan. In the process of fusion, or in one of the first cell divisions, the zygote divides into two identical individuals. Single-ovum twins usually have one placenta, one chorion, two amnions and two umbilical cords. The twins are always the same sex.

Dizygotic

Dizygotic (fraternal) twins are the result of the fertilisation of two separate ova by two separate spermatozoa. Double-ova twins have two placentas, two chorions, two amnions and two umbilical cords. The twins may be of the same or different sex.

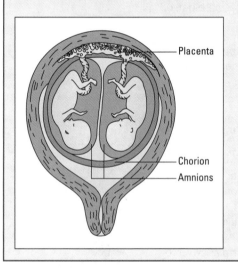

Placenta

Chorion

Amnions

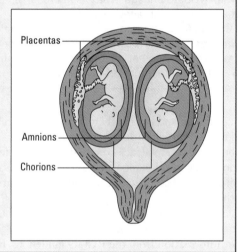

Placentas

Amnions

Chorions

Double, triple or quadruple the risks

The risks of such complications as gestational hypertension, hydramnios, placenta praevia, preterm labour and anaemia are higher in women with multiple pregnancy. Additionally, postpartum bleeding is more common because the uterus is stretched more. Multiple pregnancies also tend to end before normal term, meaning that the fetuses are at risk for premature birth.

It's a twin thing

With twins, the risk of congenital anomalies, such as spinal cord defect, is higher. The incidence of velamatous cord insertion (the cord inserted into the fetal membranes) is also higher and increases the risk of bleeding during delivery due to a torn cord. With monozygotic twins, fetuses share the placenta, which may lead to a condition known as twin-to-twin transfusion. In this condition, one fetus overgrows while the other undergrows. Additionally, if a single amnion is present, the umbilical cords can become knotted or twisted, leading to fetal distress or difficulty with birth.

Best to be first

In addition, the second fetus (twin B) is at more risk for birth-related complications, such as umbilical cord prolapse, malpresentation and placental abruption.

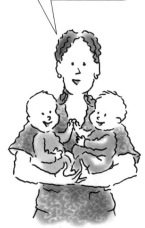

The risk of congenital anomalies is higher with twins than with single births.

What causes it?

Multiple pregnancy is the result of the fertilisation of one ova forming one zygote that divides into two identical zygotes, or the simultaneous fertilisation of two or more ova. The increasing use of fertility drugs has led to a rise in the number of multiple pregnancies because these drugs stimulate the ovaries to release multiple ova to increase chances of fertilisation.

What to look for

When the uterus begins to grow at a rate faster than usual, a multiple pregnancy is suspected. In addition, the woman may report that with quickening she feels fluttering actions at different areas of her abdomen rather than at one specific and consistent spot. She also may report an increased amount of fetal activity than expected for the date. Auscultation may reveal multiple sets of fetal heart sounds.

The woman may report an increase in fatigue and backache. Resting or sleeping may be difficult because of the increased discomfort and fetal activity level. Appetite and intake may decrease because the enlarging uterus is compressing her stomach.

What tests tell you

Diagnostic test results that help determine multiple pregnancy may include:
• elevated AFP levels
• evidence of multiple gestational sacs on ultrasound and, possibly, evidence of multiple amniotic sacs early in pregnancy.

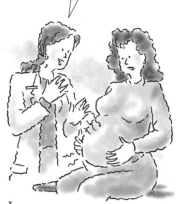

If you're experiencing this much fetal activity at this stage of your pregnancy, you may be expecting more than one baby!

How it's managed

Multiple gestation pregnancies put the mother at risk for developing many complications of pregnancy, such as preterm labour, intrauterine growth retardation, PROM, gestational hypertension and placental abruption. Management is concentrated on complications that may arise. In addition, the mother may be ordered to go on complete bed rest for a period of her pregnancy to prevent such complications as preterm labour. Depending on the number of fetuses, their gestational age and their position, the manner of delivery will vary. Vaginal delivery is possible for a mature twin gestation at term when both twins are in the head down, or vertex, position. If the first, or presenting, twin is vertex and the second is breech, it's possible to proceed with a vaginal birth; however, because this situation is more complicated, a caesarean delivery would most probably be the method of choice.

What to do

Other than more frequent monitoring, midwifery care for the woman with multiple pregnancy is similar to that for any pregnancy.
• Help the woman understand her current condition and stress the need for close, frequent follow-up visits.
• Encourage frequent rest periods throughout the day to help relieve fatigue.
• Urge the woman to rest in the side-lying position to prevent supine hypotension syndrome.
• Monitor maternal vital signs, weight gain and fundal height at every visit.
• Assess FHR and position at every visit.
• Arrange for follow-up testing, such as ultrasounds and nonstress test monitoring, as well as 24-hour fetal monitoring if the woman is on complete bed rest during the third trimester of her pregnancy.
• Urge the woman to comply with her antenatal vitamin regimen and to eat a well-balanced diet high in vitamins and iron.
• Explain danger signs and symptoms to report immediately, especially those related to preterm labour.
• Provide emotional support to the woman and her family; allow the pregnant woman to verbalise her fears and anxieties about the pregnancy and fetuses. Correct any misconceptions that the woman verbalises.
• During labour, provide separate electronic fetal monitoring for each fetus (listen-in with Pinard's stethoscope as well!).
• Maintain the woman in the side-lying position to aid breathing during labour.
• Be alert for hypotonic labour, which might necessitate labour augmentation or caesarean delivery.
• At delivery, have all medication readily accessible for each baby.
• During delivery, make sure that one midwife is available for each baby and one for the mother; in most cases, an anaesthetist and a paediatrician or an advanced neonatal nurse practitioner should be present in anticipation of maternal or neonatal problems.

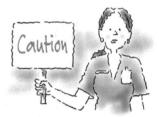

A multiple gestation pregnancy puts the mother at risk for preterm labour and PROM.

Sickle cell anaemia

Sickle cell anaemia is a congenital haematologic disease that causes impaired circulation, chronic ill health and premature death. It results from an inherited mutation in the formation of haemoglobin, the blood component that carries oxygen to body tissues. Women who suffer from this disease inherit the sickling gene from both parents, although some parents may be only carriers and don't experience symptoms. If both parents are carriers, chances are that one in four of their children will be affected. (See *Sickle cell anaemia and ethnicity*.)

Viral blockage

The sickle cell trait doesn't appear to influence the course of pregnancy; however, women with the trait tend to experience bacteriuria (which commonly produces no symptoms), which leads to pyelonephritis. Sickle cell anaemia can threaten the woman's life if such vital blood vessels as those to the liver, kidneys, heart, lungs or brain become blocked. During pregnancy, placental circulation may become blocked, causing low fetal birthweight and, possibly, fetal death.

What causes it

Sickle cell anaemia results from homozygous inheritance of an autosomal recessive gene that produces a defective haemoglobin molecule (haemoglobin S). The defect is caused by a structural change in the gene that encodes the beta chain of haemoglobin. The amino acid valine is substituted for glutamic acid in the sixth position of the beta chain, causing the haemoglobin's structure to change.

Haemoglobin S causes RBCs to become sickle shaped. The sickle cells start to build up in the capillaries and smaller blood vessels, making the blood more viscous. Normal circulation is impaired, causing pain, tissue infarctions and swelling. The level of oxygen deficiency in sickle cell anaemia and the factors that trigger a sickle cell crisis differ in each woman. (See *Sickle cell crisis*, page 236.)

Sickle cell trait, which results from heterozygous inheritance of this gene, causes few or no symptoms. However, people with this trait are carriers who may pass the gene to their offspring.

What to look for

The disease begins to manifest in the later part of the first year of life. Signs and symptoms include unusual swelling of the fingers and toes, chronic anaemia, pallor, fatigue and decreased appetite. Signs and symptoms of sickle cell crisis include severe abdominal pain, muscle spasms, leg pains, painful and swollen joints, fever, vomiting, haematuria, seizures, stiff neck, coma and paralysis.

What tests tell you

Diagnosis of sickle cell anaemia is based on:
- positive family history and the presence of typical clinical features
- haemoglobin electrophoresis revealing haemoglobin S
- stained blood smear showing sickled cells
- haemoglobin level of 6–8 mg/dl or less, possibly decreasing to as low as 5–6 mg/dl during a crisis

Bridging the gap

Sickle cell anaemia and ethnicity

Sickle cell anaemia is an inherited disease that's most common in people of African or Mediterranean descent. About 1 in 10 black people carry the abnormal gene, and 1 in every 400–600 black children has sickle cell anaemia.

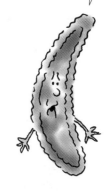

It's a family affair – unfortunately. Sickle cell trait is passed on from parents.

Sickle cell crisis

Infection, exposure to cold, high altitudes, overexertion or other situations that cause cellular oxygen deprivation may trigger a sickle cell crisis. The deoxygenated, sickle-shaped red blood cells stick to the capillary wall and one another, blocking blood flow and causing cellular hypoxia. The crisis worsens as tissue hypoxia and acidic waste products cause more sickling and cell damage. With each new crisis, organs and tissues (especially the kidneys and spleen) are slowly destroyed.

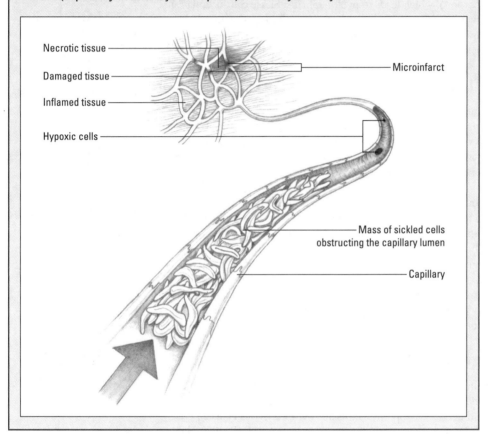

Necrotic tissue

Damaged tissue

Inflamed tissue

Hypoxic cells

Microinfarct

Mass of sickled cells obstructing the capillary lumen

Capillary

- decreased RBC count and ESR
- increased indirect bilirubin level (during a crisis)
- clean-catch urine specimen positive for bacteria.

How it's treated

Although sickle cell anaemia can't be cured, treatments can alleviate symptoms and prevent painful crises. A pregnant woman who's considered at risk for this disease but hasn't been tested should be screened for sickle cell anaemia at the first antenatal visit.

Drugs for bugs

Anti-infectives (such as low-dose oral penicillin) and certain vaccines (such as polyvalent pneumococcal vaccine and *Haemophilus influenzae* B vaccine) can minimise complications of sickle cell disease and transfusion therapy. Analgesics may be used to relieve the pain of crisis.

Selected supplements

For pregnant women, it's crucial to maintain adequate fluid intake and administer folic acid supplements. Iron supplements typically aren't prescribed because the woman's cells can't absorb iron in the usual manner; taking supplements can lead to iron overload.

Sickle stock exchange

Periodic exchange transfusions throughout the pregnancy may be used to replace sickle cells with normal cells. This procedure also helps reduce the high levels of bilirubin produced from the breakdown of RBCs.

What to do

- Monitor the woman's FBC regularly.
- Assess the woman's hydration status. Monitor her intake and output, and check for signs of dehydration.
- Urge the woman to drink at least eight 8 oz glasses of fluid each day.
- Monitor the woman's vital signs and the FHR as indicated. Monitor weight gain, and assess fundal height for changes indicating adequate fetal growth.
- Assess the woman for signs and symptoms of sickle cell crisis and chronic complications. Administer analgesics and I.V. fluids as ordered if crisis develops.
- Expect to administer hypotonic saline solution I.V. for fluid replacement because the kidneys have difficulty concentrating urine to remove large amounts of fluid.
- Obtain a clean-catch urine specimen for culture to assess for possible bacteriuria.
- Assess lower extremities for venous pooling. Encourage the woman to avoid standing for long periods and to rest in a chair with her legs elevated in a side-lying position to promote venous return to the heart.
- Prepare the woman for ultrasound at 16–24 weeks' gestation and for weekly nonstress tests beginning at approximately 30 weeks' gestation.
- Be aware that blood flow velocity tests may be ordered to evaluate blood flow through the uterus and placenta. Reduced blood flow may suggest intrauterine growth retardation.
- Anticipate the woman's desire to determine if the fetus has the disease. Assist with percutaneous umbilical blood sampling to obtain a sample for RBC electrophoresis.
- Watch for signs and symptoms of infection, such as fever, chills and purulent drainage.

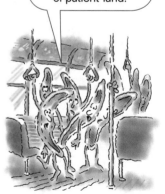

Thanks to periodic exchange transfusions, we're on a one-way trip out of patient-land.

- Assess the woman's respiratory status. Perform regular respiratory assessments, including auscultation of breath sounds. Expect to administer oxygen if sickle cell crisis develops.
- Provide comfort and emotional support to the woman and her family.
- Assist with measures to maintain hydration during labour and delivery.
- Document all care and treatments given.

In the UK, newborn babies are tested for sickle cell disease as part of their heel prick at 6 days of age.

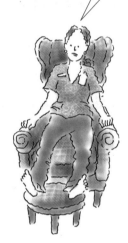

Ah, that feels better! Resting in a chair with the legs elevated promotes venous return to the heart.

Spontaneous abortion

Abortion refers to the spontaneous expulsion of the products of conception from the uterus before fetal viability. Up to 15% of all pregnancies and about 30% of first pregnancies end in spontaneous abortion (miscarriage). At least 75% of spontaneous abortions occur during the first trimester. (See *Types of spontaneous abortion.*)

What causes it

Spontaneous abortion may result from abnormal fetal, placental or maternal factors.

Types of spontaneous abortion

Spontaneous abortions occur without medical intervention and in various ways.

- In *complete abortion*, the uterus passes all products of conception. Minimal bleeding usually accompanies complete abortion because the uterus contracts and compresses the maternal blood vessels that feed the placenta.
- *Habitual abortion* refers to the spontaneous loss of three or more consecutive pregnancies.
- In *incomplete abortion*, the uterus retains part or all of the placenta. Before 10 weeks' gestation, the fetus and placenta are usually expelled together; after the 10th week, they're expelled separately. Because part of the placenta may adhere to the uterine wall, bleeding continues. Haemorrhage is possible because the uterus doesn't contract and seal the large vessels that feed the placenta.

- In *inevitable abortion*, the membranes rupture and the cervix dilates. As labour continues, the uterus expels the products of conception.
- In *missed abortion*, the uterus retains the products of conception for 2 months or more after the fetus has died. Uterine growth ceases; uterine size may even seem to decrease. Prolonged retention of the dead products of conception may cause coagulation defects such as disseminated intravascular coagulation.
- In *septic abortion*, infection accompanies abortion. This may occur with spontaneous abortion but usually results from a lapse in sterile technique during therapeutic abortion.
- In *threatened abortion*, bloody vaginal discharge occurs during the first half of pregnancy. About 20% of pregnant women have vaginal spotting or actual bleeding early in pregnancy. Of these, about 50% abort.

Small flaws

When caused by fetal factors, spontaneous abortion usually occurs at 6–10 weeks' gestation. Such factors include defective embryologic development from abnormal chromosome division (the most common cause of fetal death), faulty implantation of the fertilised ovum and failure of the endometrium to accept the fertilised ovum.

Poor placenta performance

When placental factors are responsible, spontaneous abortion usually occurs around the 14th week, when the placenta takes over the hormone production needed to maintain the pregnancy. Placental factors include premature separation of the normally implanted placenta, abnormal placental implantation and abnormal platelet function.

Maternal mechanical difficulties

When caused by maternal factors, spontaneous abortion usually occurs between weeks 11 and 19. Such factors include maternal infection, severe malnutrition and abnormalities of the reproductive organs (especially incompetent cervix, in which the cervix dilates painlessly and without blood in the second trimester). Other maternal factors include endocrine problems (such as thyroid dysfunction and lowered oestriol secretion), trauma (including any type of surgery that requires manipulation of the pelvic organs), ABO blood group incompatibility and Rh isoimmunisation, and drug ingestion.

What to look for

Prodromal symptoms of spontaneous abortion include a pink discharge for several days or a scant brown discharge for several weeks before the onset of cramps and increased vaginal bleeding. For a few hours, the cramps intensify and occur more frequently; then, the cervix dilates for expulsion of uterine contents. If the entire contents are expelled, cramps and bleeding subside. However, if contents remain, cramps and bleeding continue.

What tests tell you

Diagnosis of spontaneous abortion is based on evidence of expulsion of uterine contents, vaginal examination and laboratory studies. If the blood or urine contains hCG, pregnancy is confirmed; decreased hCG levels suggest spontaneous abortion. Vaginal examination determines the size of the uterus and whether that size is consistent with the stage of the pregnancy. Expelled tissue cytology provides evidence of products of conception. Laboratory tests reflect decreased haemoglobin levels and haematocrit from blood loss. Ultrasonography confirms the presence or absence of fetal heartbeats or an empty amniotic sac.

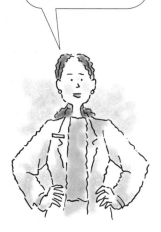

If the uterine contents are expelled completely during spontaneous abortion, cramps and bleeding subside. Cramps and bleeding continue if there are remnants in the uterus.

How it's treated

An accurate evaluation of uterine contents is necessary before planning treatment. Spontaneous abortion can't be stopped, except in those cases attributed to an incompetent cervix. Control of severe haemorrhage requires hospitalisation. Severe bleeding requires transfusion with packed RBCs or whole blood. Initially, I.V. administration of oxytocin stimulates uterine contractions. If there are remnants in the uterus, the preferred treatment is dilatation and vacuum extraction or dilatation and curettage.

The Rh factor

After an abortion, an Rh-negative female with a negative indirect Coombs' test should receive anti-D to prevent future Rh isoimmunisation.

Habitual abortion

Habitual abortion can result from an incompetent cervix. Treatment involves surgical reinforcement of the cervix (cerclage) about 14–16 weeks after the woman's last menses. A few weeks before the estimated delivery date, the sutures are removed and the woman waits for the onset of labour. An alternative procedure – used particularly for women wanting to have more children – involves leaving the sutures in place and delivering the baby by caesarean birth.

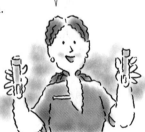

Decreased hCG levels suggest spontaneous abortion.

What to do

• Discourage the woman from using the bathroom as she may expel uterine contents without knowing it. After she uses a bedpan, inspect the contents carefully for intrauterine material.
• Note the amount, colour and odour of vaginal bleeding. Save all pads the woman uses for evaluation.
• Place the woman's bed in Trendelenburg's position as ordered.
• Administer analgesics and oxytocin as ordered.
• Assess vital signs every 4 hours for 24 hours (or more frequently depending on the extent of bleeding).
• Monitor urine output closely.
• Provide good perineal care by keeping the area clean and dry.
• Check the woman's blood type and administer anti-D as ordered.
• Provide emotional support and counselling during the grieving process; refer the woman and her family to loss or grief counsellors as appropriate.
• Encourage the woman and her partner to express their feelings. Some couples may want to talk to a member of the clergy or, depending on their religion, may wish to have the fetus baptised.
• Help the woman and her partner develop effective coping strategies.
• Explain all procedures and treatments to the woman and provide teaching about aftercare and follow-up. (See *After spontaneous abortion*, page 241.)
• Document all care given and any medications or treatments administered to the woman.

Education edge

After spontaneous abortion

If the woman experiences a spontaneous abortion, be sure to include these instructions in your advice to the woman.

- Expect vaginal bleeding or spotting to continue for several days.
- Immediately report bleeding that lasts longer than 8–10 days, or bleeding that's excessive or appears as bright red blood.
- Watch for signs of infection, such as a temperature higher than 37.8°C and foul-smelling vaginal discharge.

- Gradually increase daily activities to include whatever tasks are comfortable to perform, as long as the activities don't increase vaginal bleeding or cause fatigue.
- Abstain from sexual intercourse for approximately 2 weeks.
- Use a contraceptive when you and your partner resume intercourse.
- Avoid the use of tampons for 1–2 weeks.
- Schedule a follow-up visit with her general practitioner or obstetrician in 2–4 weeks.

HIV infection

HIV is the organism that causes acquired immunodeficiency syndrome (AIDS). HIV infection can have serious implications for a pregnant woman and her fetus.

Women on the rise

Currently, women are the fastest growing segment of the population infected with HIV. Research also shows that women are diagnosed with HIV infection later in the course of the disease than men are. There is, however, a screening programme in the UK that includes all pregnant women and through this, counselling, further screening and treatment can be offered.

Don't lose hope

Studies demonstrate that pregnancy doesn't accelerate progression of the infection in the mother. In addition, women who stay healthy during pregnancy reduce the risk of transmitting the virus to the fetus because the placenta provides a barrier to disease transmission. Even so, if HIV is contracted concurrently or close to the time of conception or the mother suffers from disorders that affect placental health (such as infections unrelated to HIV or complications of advanced HIV infection [malnutrition]), the placenta may not be an effective barrier.

Suspending transmission

Before advances in drug therapy, the risk of a neonate becoming infected via maternal virus transmission ranged from 25% to 35%. However, with appropriate antiviral drug therapy during and after pregnancy, the rate of possible infection has dropped to nearly 5%. Unfortunately, if infection occurs in the fetus or neonate, it progresses more quickly than in an adult.

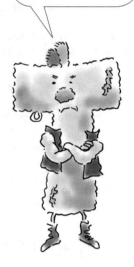

I'm a target for the retrovirus that causes HIV infection.

What causes it

HIV infection is caused by a retrovirus that targets helper T-cells containing the CD4+ antigen (cells that regulate normal immune response). The virus integrates itself into the cells' genetic makeup, causing cellular dysfunction that disrupts immune response. This makes women vulnerable to opportunistic infections.

HIV is transmitted in several ways:
• through sexual intercourse
• through contact with infected blood
• across the placenta to the fetus during pregnancy (in cases of active disease, medication noncompliance and placental inflammation)
• through contact during labour and delivery
• through breast milk.

For women, heterosexual contact and use of injectable drugs are the two major modes of HIV transmission. Other risk factors for contracting HIV include:
• a history of multiple sexual partners (either in the woman or her partner)
• having bisexual partners
• use of injectable drugs by the woman's partner
• blood transfusions (rare).

What to look for

Signs and symptoms of HIV infection include lymphadenopathy, bacterial pneumonia, fevers, night sweats, weight loss, dermatologic problems, thrush, thrombocytopenia and diarrhoea. In addition, women commonly experience severe vaginal yeast infections that are difficult to treat.

Other manifestations specific to women may include:
• abnormal Papanicolaou tests
• frequent human papilloma virus infections
• frequent and recurrent bacterial vaginosis, trichomonas and genital herpes infections
• severe PID.

Pneumocystis carinii pneumonia is the most common opportunistic infection associated with female HIV infection. Cervical cancer ranks second in prevalence. Kaposi's sarcoma may also occur in women, although it's rare.

What tests tell you

In some cases, a woman doesn't know that she's HIV-positive until it's discovered at an antenatal visit, after pregnancy has begun. Positive results from two enzyme-linked immunosorbent assays that are then further confirmed by the Western blot test classify a woman as HIV-positive. Positive status means that the woman has developed antibodies to the virus after having been exposed. In addition, a CD4[+] T-cell count of less than 200 cells/µl and the presence of one or more opportunistic infections confirm the diagnosis.

Load up on viral load

Viral load testing measures the level of HIV in the blood. Although blood levels don't reflect all possible areas of HIV infection, research suggests that these levels effectively demonstrate virus levels throughout the body. This testing relies on the detection of ribonucleic acid (RNA) in HIV molecules. This RNA is responsible for replication of the virus. Scientists have a good idea of what some parts of HIV RNA look like. With this image, they can find HIV RNA in the blood of a potentially infected person. Two techniques are used to detect HIV RNA strands in a blood sample:

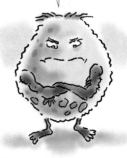

Viral load measures HIV levels in the bloodstream, which effectively indicates levels throughout the body.

Branched chain DNA sets off a chemical reaction in the HIV RNA; the RNA gives off light and the amount of light is measured to determine the levels of HIV RNA in a sample.

The quantitative polymerase chain reaction technique encourages the HIV RNA to replicate in a test tube. This replication makes it easier to measure the amount of HIV RNA that was originally in the blood sample.

How it's treated

Treatment involves medicating the pregnant woman who's HIV-positive with combination antiretroviral therapy. This treatment is aimed at reducing the mother's viral load and minimising the risk of transmitting the infection to the fetus.

Risky delivery

Caesarean delivery provides the lowest risk of HIV transmission from mother to fetus – lowest if performed before labour begins or membranes are ruptured (usually at 37 weeks' gestation). If vaginal delivery is unavoidable, episiotomy is contraindicated as is amniocentesis and fetal monitoring via scalp electrodes. For every hour of labour after membranes rupture, the risk of transmission from mother to fetus increases by 2%.

When breast isn't best

Risk of transmission during breastfeeding depends on the mother's health, including her nutritional and immune status and viral load, as well as the length of time the infant feeds each time and whether the mother breastfeeds exclusively. In addition, the duration of breastfeeding impacts the likelihood of transmission. About 15% of infected mothers who breastfeed for 24 months or longer transmit the infection to their infants.

Shutting the door on opportunity

Zidovudine (AZT) and didanosine (Videx) are used to slow progression of opportunistic infections such as *P. carinii* pneumonia, the most common. These drugs are given orally during pregnancy, I.V. during labour and then to the neonate in syrup form. Cotrimoxazole (Bactrim) is also used but may be teratogenic in early pregnancy. Additionally, sulfamethoxazole (Gantanol) may cause increased bilirubin levels in the neonate if administered late in pregnancy.

What to do

- Provide emotional support and guidance for the woman who's HIV-positive and considering pregnancy.
- Institute standard precautions when caring for the mother throughout the pregnancy, after delivery and when caring for the neonate.
- Teach the pregnant woman measures to minimise the risk of virus transmission.
- Encourage the pregnant woman who's HIV-positive to verbalise her feelings; provide support.
- Monitor CD4$^+$ T-cell counts and viral loads as indicated.
- Assess the woman for signs and symptoms of opportunistic infections, such as *P. carinii* pneumonia (fever, dry cough, chest discomfort, fatigue, shortness of breath on exertion and later at rest) and Kaposi's sarcoma (slightly raised, painless lesions on the skin or oral mucous membranes that are reddish or purple in fair-skinned women and bluish or brown in dark-skinned women; painful swelling, especially in the lower legs; nausea, vomiting and bleeding if the GI tract is involved; difficulty breathing if the lungs are involved).
- Encourage the woman to keep antenatal follow-up appointments to evaluate the status of her pregnancy.
- Administer antiretroviral therapy as ordered, and instruct the woman about this regimen. Assist with scheduling medications and evaluate for compliance on return visits.
- Institute measures during labour and delivery to minimise the fetus's risk of exposure to maternal blood or body fluids. Avoid the use of internal fetal monitors, scalp blood sampling, forceps and vacuum extraction to prevent the creation of an open lesion on the fetal scalp.
- Advise the mother that breastfeeding isn't recommended because of the risk of transmitting the virus.
- Delay blood sampling and injections in the neonate until maternal blood has been removed with the first bath.
- Educate the mother about the mode of HIV transmission and safer sex practices.
  The Royal College of Obstetricians & Gyanecologists' Guidelines for management of HIV in pregnancy are available on their website: http://www.rcog.org.uk/resources/Public/pdf/RCOG_Guideline_39_low.pdf

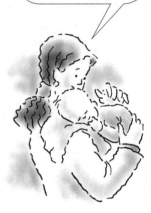

Mothers with HIV who breastfeed increase the risk of transmission to their infants.

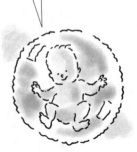

Special precautions must be taken during pregnancy to reduce my risk of contracting HIV.

Sexually transmitted infections

Sexually transmitted infections (STIs) are those conditions spread through sexual contact with an infected partner. Although all STIs can be serious, certain STIs place the pregnant woman at greater risk for problems because of their potential effect on the pregnancy, fetus or neonate. (See *Selected STIs and pregnancy*.)

Selected STIs and pregnancy

This chart lists some common sexually transmitted infections (STIs) along with their causative organisms and assessment findings, appropriate treatments for pregnant women and special considerations.

STI	Causative organism	Assessment findings	Treatment	Special considerations
Chlamydia	*Chlamydia trachomatis*	• Commonly produces no symptoms; suspicion raised if partner treated for nongonococcal urethritis	• Amoxicillin (Amoxil)	• Screening for infection at first antenatal visit because it's one of the most common types of vaginal infection seen during pregnancy
		• Heavy, gray-white vaginal discharge		• Repeated screening in the third trimester if the woman has multiple sexual partners
		• Painful urination		• Doxycycline (Vibramycin) – drug of choice for treatment if the woman isn't pregnant – contraindicated during pregnancy due to association with fetal long-bone deformities
		• Positive vaginal culture using special chlamydial test kit		• Concomitant testing for gonorrhoea due to high incidence of concurrent infection
				• Possible premature rupture of the membranes, preterm labour and endometritis in the postpartum period resulting from infection
				• Possible development of conjunctivitis or pneumonia in baby born to mother with infection present in the vagina
Condyloma acuminata	Human papillomavirus	• Discrete papillary structures that spread, enlarge and coalesce to form large lesions; increase in size during pregnancy	• Topical application of trichloroacetic acid or bichloroacetic acid to lesions	• Serious infections associated with the development of cervical cancer later in life

(continued)

Selected STIs and pregnancy (continued)

STI	Causative organism	Assessment findings	Treatment	Special considerations
		• Possible secondary ulceration and infection with foul odour	• Lesion removal with laser therapy, cryocautery, or knife excision; lesions left in place during pregnancy unless bothersome and removed during the postpartum period	
Genital herpes	Herpes simplex virus, type 2	• Painful, small vesicles with erythematous base on vulva or vagina rupturing within 1–7 days to form ulcers	• Acyclovir (Zovirax) orally or in ointment form	• Reduction or suppression of symptoms, shedding or recurrent episodes only with drug therapy (not a cure for infection)
		• Low-grade fever		• Abstinence urged until vesicles completely heal
		• Dyspareunia		• Primary infection transmission possible across the placenta, resulting in congenital infection
		• Positive viral culture of vesicular fluid		• Transmission to neonate possible at birth if active lesions are present in the vagina or on the vulva (can be fatal)
		• Positive enzyme-linked immunosorbent assay		• Caesarean delivery recommended if woman has active lesions
Gonorrhoea	*Neisseria gonorrhoeae*	• May not produce symptoms	• Cefixime (Suprax) as a one-time I.M. injection	• Associated with spontaneous miscarriage, preterm birth and endometritis in the postpartum period
		• Yellow-green vaginal discharge		• Treatment of sexual partners required to prevent re-infection
		• Male partner who experiences severe pain on urination and purulent, yellow penile discharge		• Major cause of pelvic infectious disease and infertility
		• Positive culture of vaginal, rectal or urethral secretions		• Severe eye infection leading to blindness in the neonate (ophthalmia neonatorum) if infection present at birth

Selected STIs and pregnancy *(continued)*

STI	Causative organism	Assessment findings	Treatment	Special considerations
Group B streptococci infection	Spirochaete	• Usually no symptoms	• Broad-spectrum penicillin such as ampicillin	• Occurs in as many as 15–35% of pregnant women
				• May lead to urinary tract infection, intra-amniotic infection leading to preterm birth, and postpartum endometritis
				• Screening for all pregnant women recommended
Group B streptococci infection (continued)				• Infection rate of approximately 40–70% in babies of actively infected mothers due to placental transfer or direct contact with the organisms at birth, possibly leading to severe pneumonia, sepsis, respiratory distress syndrome or meningitis
Syphilis	*Treponema pallidum*	• Painless ulcer on vulva or vagina (primary syphilis)	• Penicillin G benzathine (Bicillin L-A) I.M. (single dose)	• Possible transmission across placenta after approximately 18 weeks' gestation, leading to spontaneous miscarriage, preterm labour, stillbirth or congenital anomalies
		• Hepatic and splenic enlargement, headache, anorexia and maculopapular rash on the palms of the hands and soles of the feet occurring about 2 months after initial infection (secondary syphilis)		• Standard screening for syphilis at the first antenatal visit, screening at 36 weeks' gestation for women with multiple partners and possible re-screening at beginning of labour for any women considered high risk (with babies subsequently tested for congenital syphilis using a sample of cord blood)
		• Cardiac, vascular and central nervous system changes occurring after an undetermined latent phase (tertiary syphilis)		• Jarisch–Herxheimer reaction (sudden hypotension, fever, tachycardia and muscle aches) after medication administration, lasting for about 24 hours, and then fading because spirochaetes are destroyed

(continued)

Selected STIs and pregnancy (continued)

STI	Causative organism	Assessment findings	Treatment	Special considerations
		• Positive Venereal Disease Research Laboratory serum test; confirmed with positive rapid plasma reagin and fluorescent treponemal antibody absorption tests		
		• Dark-field microscopy positive for spirochaete		
Trichomoniasis	Single-cell protozoa	• Yellow-gray, frothy, odorous vaginal discharge	• Topical clotrimazole (Gyne-Lotrimin) instead of metronidazole (Flagyl) because of the latter drug's possible teratogenic effects if used during the first trimester of pregnancy	• Possibly associated with preterm labour, premature rupture of membranes and postcaesarean infection
		• Vulvar itching, oedema and redness		• Treatment of partner required, even if asymptomatic
		• Vaginal secretions on a wet slide treated with potassium hydroxide positive for organism		

What causes it

STIs can be caused by infection with various organisms, including:
• fungi
• bacteria
• protozoa
• parasites
• viruses.

What to look for

The signs and symptoms exhibited by the woman with an STI typically involve some type of vaginal discharge or lesion. Vulvar or vaginal irritation, such as itching and pruritus, commonly accompany the discharge or lesion.

How it's treated

Treatment focuses on the underlying causative organism. Typically, antimicrobial or antifungal agents are prescribed.

Preventing the spread

In addition, education about the mode of transmission and safer sex practices are important to prevent the spread of infection.

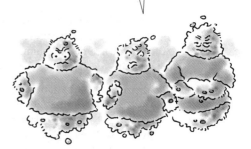

Some STIs can cause serious problems for the pregnant woman – and her baby!

What to do

• Explain the mode of transmission of the STI and instruct the woman in measures to reduce the risk of transmission.
• Administer drug therapy, as ordered, and teach the woman about the drug therapy regimen. Advise her to comply with therapy, completing the entire course of medication even if she feels better.
• Urge the woman to refrain from sexual intercourse until the active infection is completely gone.
• Instruct the woman to have her partner arrange to be examined so that treatment can be initiated, thus preventing the risk of re-infection.
• Provide comfort measures to reduce vulvar and vaginal irritation; encourage the woman to keep the vulvar area clean and dry and to avoid using strong soaps, creams or ointments unless prescribed. Avoid sprays, talcum or any perfumed products in that area.
• Suggest the use of cool or tepid baths or use the bidet to relieve itching.
• Encourage the woman to wear cotton underwear and avoid tight-fitting clothing as much as possible.
• Instruct the woman in safer sex practices, including the use of condoms and spermicides such as nonoxynol 9.
• Encourage follow-up to ensure complete resolution of the infection (if possible).

Quick quiz

1. The risks for a pregnant woman with cardiac disease and her fetus are greatest between gestation weeks:
    A. 8 and 12.
    B. 16 and 24.
    C. 28 and 32.
    D. 36 and 40.

Answer: C. Although the risks for the pregnant woman with cardiac disease and her fetus are always present, the most dangerous time is between weeks 28 and 32, when blood volume peaks and the woman's heart may be unable to compensate adequately for this change.

2. Screening for gestational diabetes in women is usually performed at:
    A. 4–8 weeks' gestation.
    B. 12–16 weeks' gestation.
    C. 24–28 weeks' gestation.
    D. 32–36 weeks' gestation.

Answer: C. All women are typically screened for gestational diabetes at 24–28 weeks' gestation.

3. The ovum of an ectopic pregnancy most commonly lodges in the:
    A. fallopian tube.
    B. abdominal viscera.
    C. ovary.
    D. cervical os.

Answer: A. The most common site of an ectopic pregnancy is the fallopian tube, either in the fimbria, ampulla or isthmus.

4. After a spontaneous abortion, a woman who's Rh-negative would be given:
    A. magnesium sulphate.
    B. anti-D.
    C. terbutaline.
    D. betamethasone.

Answer: B. A woman who's Rh-negative would receive anti-D after a spontaneous abortion to reduce the risk of possible isoimmunisation of the fetus in a future pregnancy.

5. A major factor contributing to the increased incidence of multiple pregnancy is:
    A. increased use of fertility drugs.
    B. women becoming pregnant at a younger age.
    C. previous pregnancy.
    D. underlying iron deficiency anaemia.

Answer: A. The increased use of fertility drugs has led to a doubling of the incidence of multiple pregnancy.

6. Assessment of a woman with placenta praevia would most likely reveal:
   A. absence of fetal heart.
   B. boardlike abdomen.
   C. painless, bright red vaginal bleeding.
   D. signs of shock.

Answer: C. A woman with placenta praevia would most likely report the onset of painless, bright red vaginal bleeding after week 20 of gestation.

7. The drug of choice for treating a pregnant woman with chlamydia is:
   A. doxycycline (Vibramycin).
   B. azithromycin (Zithromax).
   C. acyclovir (Zovirax).
   D. miconazole (Monistat).

Answer: B. Chlamydia infection in the pregnant woman is treated with azithromycin or amoxicillin.

Scoring

☆☆☆ If you answered all seven questions correctly, congratulations! You've laboured long and hard to optimise your knowledge!

☆☆ If you answered five or six questions correctly, great job! You've delivered the goods on this labour-intensive topic.

☆ If you answered fewer than five questions correctly, don't panic – give the material a quick review and keep on kickin'!

7 Labour and birth

Just the facts

In this chapter, you'll learn:

♦ types of fetal presentations and positions

♦ ways in which labour can be stimulated

♦ signs and symptoms of labour

♦ stages and mechanisms of labour

♦ midwifery responsibilities during labour and birth, including ways to provide comfort and support.

The midwife's role

The midwife has a huge part to play in providing individualised, holistic care for the labouring woman and her partner. She must:

- act as an advocate for the woman
- empower the woman to believe that she is capable of delivering her baby
- facilitate the mother through the stages of labour and the delivery
- do her best to make sure that the mother has as normal a labouring experience as possible with minimal intervention or medicalisation
- provide physical and psychological care at all times
- utilise all of her skills and knowledge in making sure that birth for mother and baby is safe.

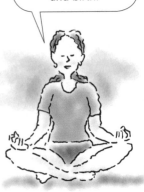

Meditate on this: relaxation is key during labour and birth.

A look at labour and birth

Labour and birth is physically and emotionally straining for a woman. As the woman's body undergoes physical changes to help the fetus pass through the cervix, she may also feel discomfort, pain, panic, irritability and loss of control. To ensure the safest outcome for the mother and child, you must fully understand the stages of labour as well as the factors affecting its length and difficulty. With an understanding of the labour and birth process, you'll be better able to provide supportive measures that promote relaxation and help increase the woman's sense of control.

Fetal presentation

Fetal presentation is the relationship of the fetus to the cervix. It can be assessed through abdominal inspection and palpation, vaginal examination and sonography. By knowing the fetal presentation, you can anticipate which part of the fetus will first pass through the cervix during delivery.

How long and how hard

Fetal presentation can affect the length and difficulty of labour as well as how the fetus is delivered. For example, if the fetus is in a breech presentation (the fetus's soft buttocks are presenting first), the force exerted against the cervix by uterine contractions is less than it would be if the fetus's firm head presented first. The decreased force against the cervix decreases the effectiveness of the uterine contractions that help open the cervix and push the fetus through the birth canal.

Presenting difficulties

Sometimes, the fetus's presenting part is too large to pass through the mother's pelvis or the fetus is in a position that's undeliverable. In such cases, caesarean birth may be necessary. In addition to the usual risks associated with surgery, an abnormal fetal presentation increases the risk of complications for the mother and fetus.

The primary factors that can affect fetal presentation during birth are fetal attitude, lie and position.

Fetal attitude
Fetal attitude (degree of flexion) is the relationship of the fetal body parts to one another. It indicates whether the presenting parts of the fetus are in flexion or extension.

Complete flexion
The most common fetal attitude is *complete flexion*. This attitude results in a vertex (top of the head) presentation of the fetus through the birth canal. Commonly called 'the fetal position', complete flexion is the traditional attitude referred to when describing a fetus in utero.

Tucked, folded and crossed

In complete flexion, the head of the fetus is tucked down onto the chest, with the chin touching the sternum. The fetus's arms are folded over the chest with the elbows flexed. The lower legs are crossed, and the thighs are drawn up onto the abdomen. The calf of each leg is pressed against the thigh of the opposite leg.

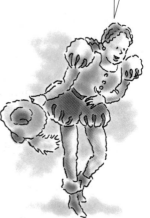

Hail Caesar! Caesarean birth may be necessary when the fetus's presenting part is too large to pass through the mother's pelvis.

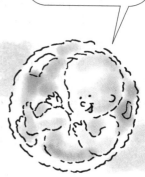

Hey mum! For once, I bet you won't mind me giving you some attitude.

All about attitude

Complete flexion is the ideal attitude for gestation and birth because the fetus occupies as little space as possible in the uterus. Birth of a fetus in complete flexion is easier because the smallest anteroposterior diameter of the fetal skull is presented to pass through the pelvis first.

Moderate flexion

Moderate flexion (military position) is the second most common fetal attitude. It tends to result in a sinciput (forehead) presentation through the birth canal. Many fetuses assume this attitude early in labour but convert into complete flexion as labour progresses.

Ten-hut!

In moderate flexion, the head of the fetus is slightly flexed but held straighter than in complete flexion. The chin doesn't touch the chest. This attitude is commonly called the *military position* because the straightness of the head makes the fetus appear to be at attention.

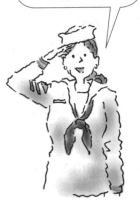

Give a salute to the military position – moderate flexion where the fetal head looks as if it's at attention.

Low rank of difficulty

The birth of a fetus in moderate flexion usually isn't difficult because the second smallest anteroposterior diameter of the skull is presented through the pelvis first. Hopefully further flexion will occur during labour, decreasing the diameter of the fetal skull.

Partial extension

Partial extension is an uncommon fetal attitude that results in a brow presentation through the birth canal. The head of the fetus is extended, with the head pushed slightly backward so that the brow becomes the first part of the fetus to pass through the pelvis during birth. Partial extension of the fetus can make birth difficult because the anteroposterior diameter of the skull may be the same size as or larger than the opening in the woman's pelvis.

Complete extension

Complete extension is a relatively rare and abnormal fetal attitude that results in a face presentation through the birth canal.

Extended and arched

In complete extension, the head and neck of the fetus are hyperextended and the occiput touches the fetus's upper back. The back is usually arched, which increases the degree of hyperextension. The occipitomental diameter of the head presents first to pass through the pelvis. Commonly, this skull diameter is too large to pass through the pelvis, but much depends on whether the fetal head is mentoanterior or mentoposterior.

Complete extension may be caused by:

- oligohydramnios (less than normal amniotic fluid)
- neurological abnormalities

- multiparity
- a large abdomen with decreased uterine tone
- a nuchal cord with multiple coils around the fetus's neck
- fetal malformation (found in up to 60% of cases).

Fetal lie

The relationship of the long axis of the fetal spine to the maternal spine is referred to as *fetal lie*. Fetal lie can be described as longitudinal, transverse or oblique.

Longitudinal lie

When the fetal spine is parallel to the maternal spine, the fetus is in a longitudinal lie. This means that the fetus is lying vertically (top to bottom) in the uterus. Most fetuses are in longitudinal lie at the onset of labour.

Heads or tails?

Longitudinal lie can be further classified as *cephalic* or *breech*. In cephalic longitudinal lie, an area of the fetal head – determined by attitude and position – is the presenting part. In a breech longitudinal lie, the fetal buttocks or foot (possibly feet) is the presenting part.

Transverse lie

When the fetal spine and the maternal spine are at 90° angles to each other, the fetus is in transverse lie. This means that the fetus is lying horizontally (side to side) in the uterus. Transverse lie is considered abnormal, and it occurs in less than 1% of deliveries. If labour progresses while the fetus is in transverse lie, the presenting part may be a shoulder, iliac crest, hand or elbow.

Oblique lie

When the fetal spine and the maternal spine are at 45° angles to each other – midway between the transverse and the longitudinal lies – the fetus is in an oblique lie. This lie is rare and is considered abnormal if the fetus remains in this position after the onset of labour.

Fetal position

Fetal position is the relationship of the presenting part of the fetus to a specific quadrant of the mother's pelvis. It's important to define fetal position because it influences the progression of labour and whether surgical intervention is needed.

Spelling it out

Fetal position is defined using three letters. The first letter designates whether the presenting part is facing the woman's right (R) or left (L) side. The second letter or letters refer to the presenting part of the fetus: the occiput (O), mentum (M) and sacrum (S). The third letter designates whether

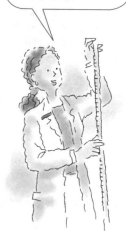

It all measures up! A caesarean birth may be necessary if the fetus is in complete extension because occipitomental skull diameter makes it impossible for the fetus to pass through the pelvis.

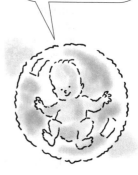

I wouldn't lie to you. When I'm in line with my mum's spine, I'm in longitudinal lie.

Fetal position abbreviations

Here's a list of abbreviations, organised according to variations in presentation, that are used when documenting fetal position.

Vertex presentations (occiput)	Breech presentations (sacrum)	Face presentations (mentum)	Shoulder presentations (acromion process)
LOA, left occipitoanterior	LSaA, left sacroanterior	LMA, left mentoanterior	LAA, left scapuloanterior
LOP, left occipitoposterior	LSaP, left sacroposterior	LMP, left mentoposterior	LAP, left scapuloposterior
LOT, left occipitotransverse	LSaT, left sacrotransverse	LMT, left mentotransverse	RAA, right scapuloanterior
ROA, right occipitoanterior	RSaA, right sacroanterior	RMA, right mentoanterior	RAP, right scapuloposterior
ROP, right occipitoposterior	RSaP, right sacroposterior	RMP, right mentoposterior	
ROT, right occipitotransverse	RSaT, right sacrotransverse	RMT, right mentotransverse	

the presenting part is pointing to the anterior (A), posterior (P) or transverse (T) section of the mother's pelvis. The occiput typically presents first when the fetus is in the vertex fetal presentation; the mentum, in face presentation; the sacrum, in breech presentation and the scapula, in shoulder presentation.

The most common fetal positions are left occipitoanterior (LOA) and right occipitoanterior (ROA). (See *Fetal position abbreviations*.)

Duration determinant

Commonly, the duration of labour and birth is shortest when the fetus is in the LOA or ROA position. When the fetal position is posterior, such as left occipitoposterior (LOP), labour tends to be more painful for the woman because the fetal head puts pressure on her sacral nerves. (See *Determining fetal position*, page 257.)

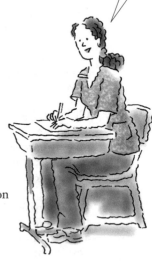

I love writing letters. Like LOA – meaning an ideal fetal position!

Types of fetal presentation

Fetal presentation refers to the part of the fetus that presents into the birth canal first. It's determined by fetal attitude, lie and position. Fetal presentation should be determined in the early stages of labour in case an abnormal presentation endangers the mother and the fetus. (See *Classifying fetal presentation*, pages 258 and 259.)

The four main types of fetal presentation are:

 cephalic

 breech

 shoulder

 compound.

Determining fetal position

Fetal position is determined by the relationship of a specific presenting part (occiput, sacrum, mentum [chin] or sinciput [deflected vertex]) to the four quadrants (anterior, posterior, right or left) of the maternal pelvis. For example, a fetus whose occiput (O) is the presenting part and who's located in the right (R) and anterior (A) quadrant of the maternal pelvis is identified as ROA.

These illustrations show the possible positions of a fetus in vertex presentation.

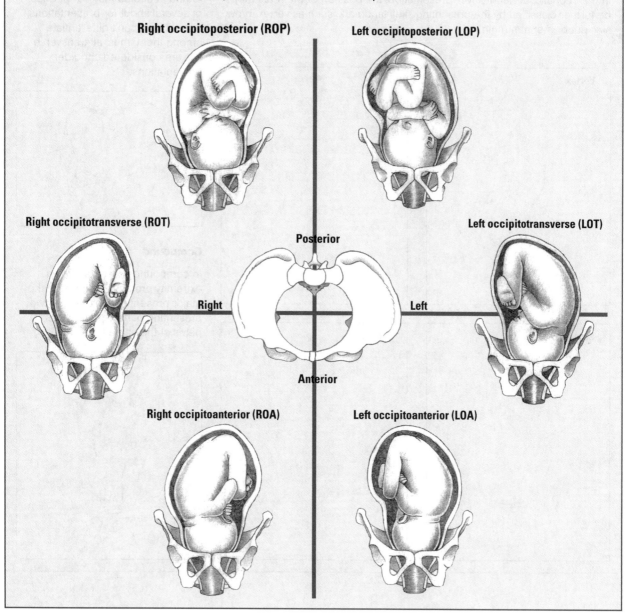

Right occipitoposterior (ROP)

Left occipitoposterior (LOP)

Right occipitotransverse (ROT)

Left occipitotransverse (LOT)

Posterior

Right

Left

Anterior

Right occipitoanterior (ROA)

Left occipitoanterior (LOA)

Classifying fetal presentation

Fetal presentation may be broadly classified as cephalic, shoulder, compound or breech. Almost all births are cephalic presentations. Breech births are the second most common type.

Cephalic

In the cephalic, or head-down, presentation, the position of the fetus may be further classified by the presenting skull landmark, such as vertex, brow, sinciput or mentum (chin).

Shoulder

Although a fetus may adopt one of several shoulder presentations, examination can't differentiate among them; thus, all transverse lies are considered shoulder presentations.

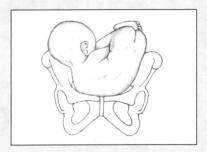

Compound

In compound presentation, an extremity prolapses alongside the major presenting part so that two presenting parts appear in the pelvis at the same time.

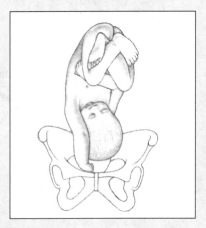

Vertex

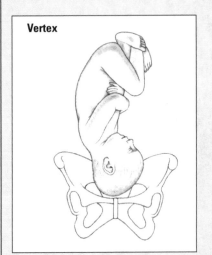

Brow

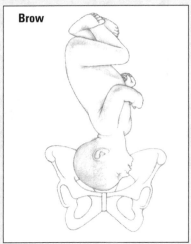

Sinciput

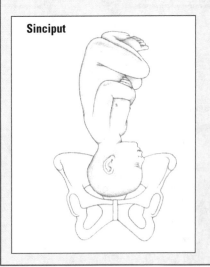

Mentum

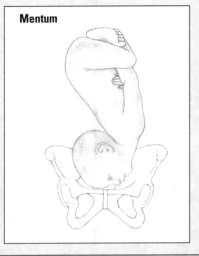

Classifying fetal presentation *(continued)*

Breech

In the breech, or head-up, presentation, the position of the fetus may be further classified as *frank*, where the hips are flexed and knees remain straight; *complete*, where the knees and hips are flexed; *kneeling*, where the knees are flexed and the hips remain extended; and *incomplete*, where one or both hips remain extended and one or both feet or knees lie below the breech or *footling*, where one or both feet extend below the breech.

Frank
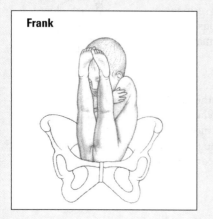

Complete
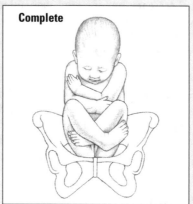

Footling
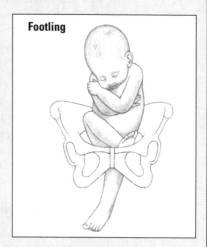

Kneeling
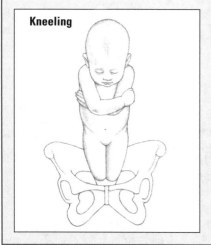

Incomplete
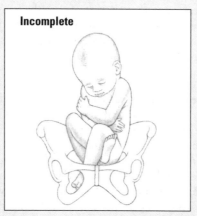

Cephalic presentation

When the fetus is in cephalic presentation, the head is the first part to contact the cervix and expel from the uterus during delivery. Most fetuses are in cephalic presentation at birth.

The four types of cephalic presentation are vertex, brow, face and mentum (chin).

Vertex

In the vertex cephalic presentation, the most common presentation overall, the fetus is in a longitudinal lie with an attitude of complete flexion. The parietal bones (between the two fontanelles) are the presenting part of the fetus. This presentation is considered optimal for fetal descent through the pelvis.

Brow

In brow presentation, the fetus's brow or forehead is the presenting part. The fetus is in a longitudinal lie and exhibits an attitude of moderate flexion. Although this isn't the optimal presentation for a fetus, few suffer serious complications from the delivery. Although some brow presentations convert into vertex presentations during descent through the pelvis, they may still be in an unfavourable for a normal vaginal delivery.

Face

The face type of cephalic presentation is unfavourable for the mother and the fetus; however, a lot will depend on the position of the chin, whether it is anterior or posterior. In this presentation, the fetus is in a longitudinal lie and exhibits an attitude of partial extension. Because the face is the presenting part of the fetal head, severe oedema and facial distortion may occur from the pressure of uterine contractions during labour.

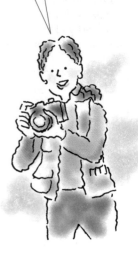

Picture this. Vertex presentation is considered optimal for delivery.

Faced with potential complications

If labour is allowed to progress, careful monitoring of both the fetus and the mother is necessary to reduce the risk of compromise. Labour may be prolonged and ineffective in some instances, and vaginal birth may not be possible because the presenting part has a larger diameter than the pelvic outlet.

Mentum

The mentum, or chin, type of cephalic presentation is also unfavourable for the mother and the fetus. In this presentation, the fetus is in a longitudinal lie with an attitude of complete extension. The presenting part of the fetus is the chin, which may lead to severe oedema and facial distortion from the pressure of the uterine contractions during labour. The widest diameter of the fetal head is presenting through the pelvis because of the extreme extension of the head. If labour is allowed to progress, careful monitoring of both the fetus and the mother is necessary to reduce the risk of compromise. Labour is usually prolonged and ineffective. Vaginal delivery can be difficult if the head is posterior because the fetus may get stuck at the ischial spines.

Let's face it, for fetuses in the mentum cephalic presentation, pressure from uterine contractions may cause severe oedema and facial distortion.

Breech presentation

Although 25% of all fetuses are in breech presentation at week 30 of gestation, most turn spontaneously at 32–34 weeks' gestation. However, breech presentation occurs at term in about 3% of births. Labour is usually prolonged with breech presentation because of ineffective cervical dilation caused by decreased pressure on the cervix and delayed descent of the fetus.

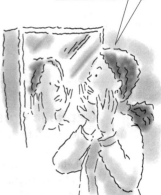

It gets complicated

In addition to prolonging labour, the breech presentation increases the risk of complications. In the fetus, cord prolapse; anoxia; intracranial haemorrhage caused by rapid moulding of the head; neck trauma and shoulder, arm, hip and leg dislocations or fractures may occur. If the baby's abdomen is squeezed too tightly, rupture of the spleen, liver or kidneys can result – hence the phrase – 'Hands off the breech!'

Complications that may occur in the mother include perineal tears and cervical lacerations during delivery and infection from premature rupture of the membranes.

How will I know?

A breech presentation can be identified by abdominal and vaginal examination. The signs of breech presentation include:
- fetal head is felt at the uterine fundus during an abdominal examination
- breech may be palpated during the deep pelvic palpation
- fetal heart sounds are heard above the umbilicus
- soft buttocks or feet are palpated during vaginal examination.

Once, twice, three types more

The three types of breech presentation are complete, frank and incomplete.

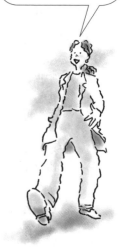

Don't be defeated by a complete breech, where the presenting parts of the fetus are the buttocks and the feet.

Complete breech
In a complete breech presentation, the fetus's buttocks and the feet are the presenting parts. The fetus is in a longitudinal lie and is in complete flexion. The fetus is sitting cross-legged and both legs are drawn up (hips flexed) with the anterior of the thighs pressed tightly against the abdomen; the lower legs are crossed with the calves pressed against the posterior of the thighs and the feet are tightly flexed against the outer aspect of the posterior thighs. Although considered an abnormal fetal presentation, complete breech is the least difficult of the breech presentations.

Frank breech
In a frank breech presentation, the fetus's buttocks are the presenting part. The fetus is in a longitudinal lie and is in moderate flexion. Both legs are drawn up (hips flexed) with the anterior of the thighs pressed against the body; the knees are fully extended and resting on the upper body with the lower legs stretched upward; the arms may be flexed over or under the legs and the feet are resting against the head. The attitude is moderate.

Incomplete breech
In an incomplete breech presentation, also called a *footling breech*, one or both of the knees or legs are the presenting parts. If one leg is extended, it's called a *single-footling breech* (the other leg may be flexed in the normal attitude); if both legs are extended, it's called a *double-footling breech*. The fetus is in

a longitudinal lie. At least one of the thighs and one of the lower legs are extended with little or no hip flexion.

Perhaps expect prolapse

A footling breech is the most difficult of the breech deliveries. Cord prolapse is common in a footling breech because of the space created by the extended leg. A caesarean birth is necessary to reduce the risk of fetal or maternal mortality.

Shoulder presentation

Although common in multiple pregnancies, the shoulder presentation of the fetus is an abnormal presentation that occurs in less than 1% of deliveries. In this presentation, the shoulder, iliac crest, hand or elbow is the presenting part. The fetus is in a transverse lie, and the attitude may range from complete flexion to complete extension.

Lacking space and support

In the multiparous woman, shoulder presentation may be caused by the relaxation of the abdominal walls. If the abdominal walls are relaxed, the unsupported uterus falls forward, causing the fetus to turn horizontally. Other causes of shoulder presentation may include pelvic contraction (the vertical space in the pelvis is smaller than the horizontal space) or placenta praevia (the low-lying placenta decreases the vertical space in the uterus).

Early identification and intervention are critical when the fetus is in a shoulder presentation. Abdominal and vaginal examination, and ultrasound are used to confirm whether the mother's abdomen has an abnormal or distorted shape. Attempts to turn the fetus may be unsuccessful unless the fetus is small or preterm. A caesarean delivery may be necessary to reduce the risk of fetal or maternal death.

Compound presentation

In a compound presentation, an extremity presents with another major presenting part, usually the head. In this type of presentation, the extremity prolapses alongside the major presenting part so that they present simultaneously.

Engagement

Engagement occurs when the presenting part of the fetus passes into the pelvis to the point where, in cephalic presentation, the biparietal diameter of the fetal head is at the level of the midpelvis (or at the level of the ischial spines). Abdominal and/or vaginal examination is used to assess the degree of engagement before and during labour.

A good sign

Because the ischial spines are usually the narrowest area of the female pelvis, engagement of the presenting part indicates that the pelvic inlet is large

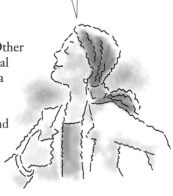

Ahem! A compound presentation compounds the difficulty of birth because an extremity presents with the major presenting part. Whew! There, I said it.

enough for the fetus to pass through (because the widest part of the fetus has already passed through the narrowest part of the pelvis).

Floating away

In the primipara, nonengagement of the presenting part at the onset of labour may indicate a complication, such as cephalopelvic disproportion, abnormal presentation or position or an abnormality of the fetal head. The nonengaged presenting part is described as 'high'. In the multipara, nonengagement is common at the onset of labour; however, the presenting part quickly becomes engaged as labour progresses.

Station

Station is the relationship of the presenting part of the fetus to the mother's ischial spines. If the fetus is at station 0, the fetus is considered to be at the level of the ischial spines. The fetus is considered engaged when it reaches station 0.

Grand central stations

Fetal station is measured in centimetres. The measurement is called *minus* when it's above the level of the ischial spines and *plus* when it's below that level. (See *Assessing fetal engagement and station*.)

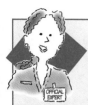

Advice from the experts

Assessing fetal engagement and station

During a vaginal examination, you'll assess the extent of the fetal presenting part into the pelvis. This is referred to as fetal engagement.

After you have determined fetal engagement, palpate the presenting part and grade the fetal station (where the presenting part lies in relation to the ischial spines of the maternal pelvis). If the presenting part isn't fully engaged into the pelvis, you won't be able to assess station.

Station grades range from −3 (3 cm above the maternal ischial spines) to +4 (4 cm below the maternal ischial spines, causing the perineum to bulge). A zero grade indicates that the presenting part lies at level with the ischial spines.

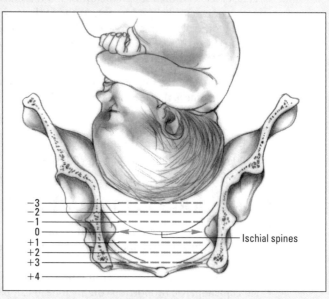

Induction of labour

Induced labour has an impact on the birth experience of women. It may be less efficient and is usually more painful than spontaneous labour, and epidural analgesia and assisted delivery are more likely to be required. Induction of labour is a relatively common procedure with approximately one in every five labours in the UK being induced. This includes induction for medical reasons also.

Can I assist you?

For some women, it's necessary to stimulate labour. The stimulation of labour may involve induction (artificially starting labour) or augmentation (assisting a labour that started spontaneously).

Although induction and augmentation involve the same methods and risks, they're performed for different reasons. Many high-risk pregnancies must be induced because the safety of the mother or fetus is in jeopardy. Medical problems that justify induction of labour include pre-eclampsia, eclampsia, severe hypertension, diabetes, Rh sensitisation, prolonged rupture of the membranes (over 24 hours) and a postmature fetus (a fetus that's 42 weeks' gestation or older). Augmentation of labour may be necessary if the contractions are too weak or infrequent to be effective.

Past your dates!

Women with uncomplicated pregnancies should usually be offered induction of labour between 41 and 42 weeks to avoid the risks of prolonged pregnancy. The exact timing should take into account the woman's preferences and local circumstances. Women should be informed that most mothers would go into labour spontaneously by 42 weeks. At the 38th week antenatal visit, all women should be offered information about the risks associated with pregnancies that last longer than 42 weeks, and their options. The information should cover:

1. membrane sweeping:
   * that membrane sweeping may make spontaneous labour more likely, and so reduces the need for formal induction of labour to prevent prolonged pregnancy
   * what a membrane sweep is
   * that discomfort and vaginal bleeding are possible from the procedure
2. induction of labour between 41 and 42 weeks
3. expectant management.

Conditions for induction of labour

Before stimulating labour, the fetus must be:
* in longitudinal lie (the long axis of the fetus is parallel to the long axis of the mother)
* engaged, especially the presenting part
* in cephalopelvic proportion (the fetal head can pass through the pelvis).

The ripe type

In addition to the above fetal criteria, the mother must have a ripe cervix before labour is induced. A ripe cervix is soft and supple to the touch rather than firm. Softening of the cervix allows for cervical effacement, dilation and effective coordination of contractions. Using Bishop's score, you can determine whether a cervix is ripe enough for induction. (See *Bishop's score*, page 266.)

Here's something interesting. A ripe cervix allows for effacement and dilation.

When it isn't so great to stimulate

Stimulation of labour should be done with caution in women with grand parity or uterine scars.

Labour shouldn't be stimulated if:
- vaginal birth is too risky
- stimulation of the uterus increases the risk of such complications as placenta praevia, abruptio placenta, uterine rupture and decreased fetal blood supply caused by the increased intensity or duration of contractions
- multiple pregnancy is involved
- the woman has an active genital herpes infection
- evidence of fetal distress exists
- the fetus is in an unusual presentation (such as a footling breech presentation)
- the uterus is unusually large (which increases the risk of uterine rupture).

Recommended methods for induction of labour

Membrane sweeping

Membrane sweeping involves the examining finger passing through the cervix to rotate against the wall of the uterus, to separate the chorionic membrane from the decidua. If the cervix will not admit a finger, massaging around the cervix in the vaginal fornices may achieve a similar effect. For the purpose of this text, membrane sweeping is regarded as an adjunct to induction of labour rather than an actual method of induction. All women are offered membrane sweeping postdates.

Vaginal PGE$_2$

When offering PGE$_2$ for induction of labour, health care professionals should inform women about the associated risks of uterine hyperstimulation. Vaginal PGE$_2$ is the preferred method of induction of labour, unless there are specific clinical reasons for not using it (in particular the risk of uterine hyperstimulation). It should be administered as a gel, tablet or controlled-release pessary.

Success half the time

The success of the induction method varies with the agent used. After just a single insertion of a ripening agent, about 50% of women go into labour

Bishop's score

Bishop's score is a tool that you can use to assess whether a woman is ready for labour. A score ranging from 0 to 3 is given for each of five factors: cervical dilation, length (effacement), consistency, position and station.

If the woman's score exceeds 8, the cervix is considered suitable for induction.

Factor	Score
Cervical dilation	
• Cervix dilated < 1 cm	0
• Cervix dilated 1–2 cm	1
• Cervix dilated 2–4 cm	3
• Cervix dilated > 4 cm	2
Cervical length (effacement)	
• Cervical length > 4 cm (0% effaced)	0
• Cervical length 2–4 cm (0–50% effaced)	1
• Cervical length 1–2 cm (50–75% effaced)	2
• Cervical length < 1 cm (> 75% effaced)	3
Cervical consistency	
• Firm cervical consistency	0
• Average cervical consistency	1
• Soft cervical consistency	2
Cervical position	
• Posterior cervical position	0
• Middle or anterior cervical position	1
Zero station notation (presenting part level)	
• Presenting part at ischial spines –3 cm	0
• Presenting part at ischial spines –1 cm	1
• Presenting part at ischial spines +1 cm	3
• Presenting part at ischial spines +2 cm	2

Modifiers

Add 1 point to score for:

• Pre-eclampsia
• Each prior vaginal delivery

Subtract 1 point from score for:

• Postdates pregnancy
• Nulliparity
• Premature or prolonged rupture of membranes

Adapted with permission from Bishop, E.H. 'Pelvic Scoring for Elective Induction', *Obstetrics and Gynecology* 24:266–168, August 1964.

spontaneously and deliver within 24 hours. Those women who don't go into labour require a different method of labour stimulation.

Prostaglandin should be used with caution in women with asthma, glaucoma and renal or cardiac disease.

Not to be ignored

When the pessary is inserted, carefully monitor the mother's uterine activity. If uterine hyperstimulation occurs or if labour begins, the prostaglandin agent should be removed. The woman should also be monitored for adverse effects of prostaglandin application, including headache, vomiting, fever, diarrhoea, hypertension, painful contractions, hyperstimulation and fetal distress. Fetal heart rate (FHR) should be monitored continuously for at least 30 minutes after each application and up to 2 hours after vaginal insertion.

Misoprostol and *mifepristone* should only be offered as a method of induction of labour to women who have intrauterine fetal death, or in the context of a clinical trial. (Misoprostol has not yet been licensed for use in the UK.)

Amniotomy (artificial rupture of membranes – ARM)

Amniotomy, alone or with oxytocin (Syntocinon), should not be used as a primary method of induction of labour unless there are specific clinical reasons for not using vaginal PGE_2, in particular, the risk of uterine hyperstimulation. Amniotomy is performed to augment or induce labour when the membranes haven't ruptured spontaneously. This procedure allows the fetal head to contact the cervix more directly, thus increasing the efficiency of contractions. Amniotomy is virtually painless for both the mother and the fetus because the membranes don't have nerve endings.

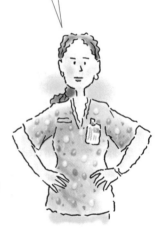

Amniotomy allows the fetal head to contact the cervix more directly, increasing the efficiency of contractions.

System requirements

To perform amniotomy, the fetus must be in the vertex presentation with the fetal head well into the pelvis. In addition, the mother must have a Bishop's score of at least 8.

Let it flow, let it flow, let it flow

During amniotomy, the woman is placed in a dorsal recumbent position. An amniohook (a long, thin instrument similar to a crochet hook) is inserted into the vagina to puncture the membranes. If puncture is properly performed, amniotic fluid gushes out.

Persevere if it isn't clear

Normal amniotic fluid is clear. Bloody or meconium-stained amniotic fluid is considered abnormal and requires careful, continuous monitoring of the mother and fetus. Bloody amniotic fluid may indicate a bleeding problem.

Advice from the experts

Complications of amniotomy (ARM)

Umbilical cord prolapse – a life-threatening complication of amniotomy – is an emergency that requires immediate caesarean birth to prevent fetal death. It occurs when amniotic fluid, gushing from the ruptured sac, sweeps the cord down through the cervix. Prolapse risk is higher if the fetal head isn't engaged in the pelvis before rupture occurs.

Cord prolapse can lead to cord compression as the fetal presenting part presses the cord against the pelvic brim. Immediate action must be taken to relieve the pressure and prevent fetal anoxia and fetal distress. Here are some options:

- Insert a gloved hand into the vagina and gently push the fetal presenting part away from the cord.

- Place the woman in Trendelenburg's position to tilt the presenting part backward into the pelvis and relieve pressure on the cord.
- Administer oxygen to the mother by face mask to improve oxygen flow to the fetus.

If the cord has prolapsed to the point that it's visible outside the vagina, don't attempt to push the cord back in. This can add to the compression and may cause kinking. Cover the exposed portion with a compress soaked with sterile saline solution to prevent drying, which could result in atrophy of the umbilical vessels.

Meconium-stained amniotic fluid may indicate fetal distress. If the fluid is meconium stained, note whether the staining is thin, moderate, thick or particulate. When meconium-stained amniotic fluid is present, a paediatrician should be present at delivery where possible because of the increased risk of meconium aspiration by the baby.

Prolapse potential

Amniotomy increases the risk to the fetus because there's a possibility that a portion of the umbilical cord will prolapse with the amniotic fluid. FHR should be monitored during and after the procedure to make sure that umbilical cord prolapse didn't occur. (See *Complications of amniotomy*.)

Oxytocin administration

Synthetic oxytocin (Syntocinon) is used to induce or augment labour. It may be used in women with gestational hypertension, prolonged gestation, maternal diabetes, Rh sensitisation, premature or prolonged rupture of membranes and incomplete or inevitable abortion. Syntocinon is also used to control bleeding and enhance uterine contractions after the placenta is delivered.

Syntocinon should be prescribed by the obstetric registrar or consultant and is always administered I.V. with an infusion pump. Syntocinon should not be administered unless 6 hours have elapsed since the last PGE_2 pessary was given. ARM should have been performed or spontaneous rupture of membranes should be imminent. Throughout administration, uterine contractions should be assessed and monitored to ensure that they're occurring in a 20-minute span and extra attention should be paid to the FHR. Extreme caution should be exercised if the woman has had a previous caesarean section or she is a multipara.

Midwifery interventions
Here's how to administer Syntocinon:
* Start a primary I.V. line.
* Prepare the Syntocinon by adding 5 IU to 500 ml of Hartmann's solution.
* Insert the tubing of the administration set through the infusion pump, and set the drip rate to administer the Syntocinon at a starting infusion rate of 6 ml/hour. The infusion is increased every 30 minutes if the mother's condition allows it. So the rate is increased at 6, 12, 24, 48, 96 and 190 ml/hour.
  The maximum dosage of Syntocinon is 190 ml/hour.

Piggyback ride

* The Syntocinon solution is then piggybacked to the primary I.V. line.
* If a problem occurs, such as decelerations of FHR or fetal distress, stop the piggyback infusion immediately and resume the primary line.

Immediate action

* Because Syntocinon begins acting immediately, be prepared to start monitoring uterine contractions.
* Increase the Syntocinon dosage as ordered – but never increase the dose more than the required regimen every 30 minutes. Typically, the dosage continues at a rate that maintains a regular pattern (uterine contractions occur every 2–3 minutes).
  Each maternity unit should have strict protocols drawn up for staff to use as guidance.

If more is in store

* Before each increase, be sure to assess contractions, maternal vital signs, fetal heart rhythm and FHR. If you're using an external fetal monitor, the uterine activity strip should show contractions occurring every 2–3 minutes – always record any increase in dose/rate of Syntocinon on the trace. The contractions should last for about 60 seconds and be followed by uterine relaxation.
* Assist with comfort measures, such as repositioning the woman on her other side, as needed.

Following through

- Continue assessing maternal and fetal responses to the Syntocinon.
- Review the infusion rate to prevent uterine hyperstimulation.

To manage hyperstimulation, reduce the rate or discontinue the infusion and administer oxygen. (See *Complications of oxytocin administration*.)

- Drugs such as Utopar, GTN spray or Terbutaline 2.5 milligrams S.C. can be used.

Advice from the experts

Complications of oxytocin administration

Oxytocin can cause uterine hyperstimulation. This, in turn, may progress to tetanic contractions, which last longer than 2 minutes. Signs of hyperstimulation include contractions that are less than 2 minutes apart and last 90 seconds or longer, uterine pressure that doesn't return to baseline between contractions and intrauterine pressure that rises over 75 mmHg.

What else to watch for

Other potential complications include fetal distress, placental abruption, uterine rupture and water intoxication. Water intoxication, which can cause maternal seizures or coma, can result because the antidiuretic effect of oxytocin causes decreased urine flow.

Stop signs

Watch for the following signs of oxytocin administration complications. If any indication of any potential complications exists, stop the oxytocin administration, administer oxygen via face mask and notify the doctor immediately.

Fetal distress

Signs of fetal distress include:

- late decelerations
- bradycardia.

Placental abruption

Signs of placental abruption include:

- sharp, stabbing uterine pain
- pain over and above the uterine contraction pain
- heavy bleeding
- hard, boardlike uterus.

Also watch for signs of shock, including rapid, weak pulse; falling blood pressure; cold and clammy skin and dilation of the nostrils.

Uterine rupture

Signs of uterine rupture include:

- sudden, severe pain during uterine contractions
- tearing sensation
- absent fetal heart sounds.

Also watch for signs of shock, including rapid, weak pulse; falling blood pressure; cold and clammy skin and dilation of the nostrils.

Water intoxication

Signs and symptoms of water intoxication include:

- headache and vomiting (usually seen first)
- hypertension
- peripheral oedema
- shallow or laboured breathing
- dyspnoea
- tachypnoea
- lethargy
- confusion
- change in level of consciousness.

- To reduce uterine irritability, try to increase uterine blood flow. Do this by changing the woman's position and increasing the infusion rate of the primary I.V. line. After hyperstimulation resolves, resume the Syntocinon infusion per your unit's policy.

Visit the NICE website (https://www.nice.org.uk/nicemedia/pdf/inductionoflabourrcogrep.pdf) and the RCOG website (http://www.rcog.org.uk/index.asp?PageID=1046) for more information on induction of labour.

Failed induction

If induction fails, health care professionals should discuss this with the woman and provide support. The woman's condition and the pregnancy in general should be fully reassessed, and fetal well-being should be assessed using electronic fetal monitoring. The subsequent management options include a further attempt to induce labour (the timing should depend on the clinical situation and the woman's wishes), or a caesarean section (refer to 'Caesarean section' [NICE clinical guideline 13] and this section should be read in conjunction with 'Antenatal care: routine care for the healthy pregnant woman' [NICE clinical guideline 62], available from www.nice.org.uk/CG062, and 'Intrapartum care: care of healthy women and their babies during childbirth' [NICE clinical guideline 55], available from www.nice.org.uk/CG055).

Previous caesarean section

If delivery is indicated, women who have had a previous caesarean section may be offered induction of labour with vaginal PGE_2, caesarean section or expectant management on an individual basis, taking into account the woman's circumstances and wishes. Women should be informed of the following risks with induction of labour:
- increased risk of need for emergency caesarean section during induced labour
- increased risk of uterine rupture.

Special request?

Induction of labour should not routinely be offered on maternal request alone. However, under exceptional circumstances (for example if the woman has been traumatised by a previous delivery), induction may be considered at or after 40 weeks.

> Ah ha! As I suspected, prostaglandin application may cause uterine hyperstimulation. Monitor the woman's uterine activity.

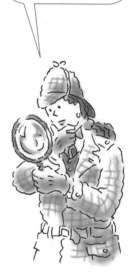

Onset of labour

True labour begins when the woman has bloody show, her membranes rupture and she has painful contractions of the uterus that cause effacement and dilation of the cervix. The actual mechanism that triggers this process is unknown.

Before the onset of true labour, preliminary signs appear that indicate the beginning of the birthing process. Although not considered to be a true stage of labour, these signs signify that true labour isn't far away.

Preliminary signs and symptoms of labour

Preliminary signs and symptoms of labour include lightening, increased level of activity, Braxton Hicks contractions and ripening of the cervix. Subjective signs, such as restlessness, anxiety and sleeplessness, may also occur. (See *Labour: True or false?*)

Lightening
Lightening is the descent of the fetal head into the pelvis. The uterus lowers and moves into a more anterior position, and the contour of the abdomen changes. In primiparas, these changes commonly occur about 2 weeks before birth. In multiparas, these changes can occur on the day labour begins or after labour starts.

More pressure here, less pressure there

Lightening increases pressure on the bladder, which may cause urinary frequency. In addition, leg pain may occur if the shifting of the fetus and

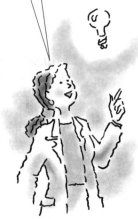

To illuminate, lightening is the descent of the fetal head into the pelvis.

Advice from the experts

Labour: True or false?

Use this chart to help differentiate between the signs and symptoms of true labour and those of false labour.

Signs and symptoms	True labour	False labour
Cervical changes	Cervix softens and dilates	No cervical dilation or effacement
Level of discomfort	Intense	Mild
Location of contractions	Start in the back and spread to the abdomen	Abdomen or groin
Uterine consistency when palpated	Hard as a board; can't be indented	Easily indented with a finger
Regularity of contractions	Regular with increasing frequency and duration	Irregular; no discernible pattern; tends to decrease in intensity and frequency with activity
Frequency and duration of contractions affected by position or activity	No	Yes
Ruptured membranes	Possible	No

The pregnant woman

As a result of hormonal activity, the breasts may double in size during pregnancy. During this time, fatty tissue is largely replaced by glandular tissue and the mammary glands become capable of secreting milk.

During the third trimester, the fundus reaches the xiphoid process. In addition, the uterus remains oval in shape. Its muscular walls become progressively thinner as it enlarges. In some women, the uterus becomes large enough that the maternal umbilicus everts and protrudes.

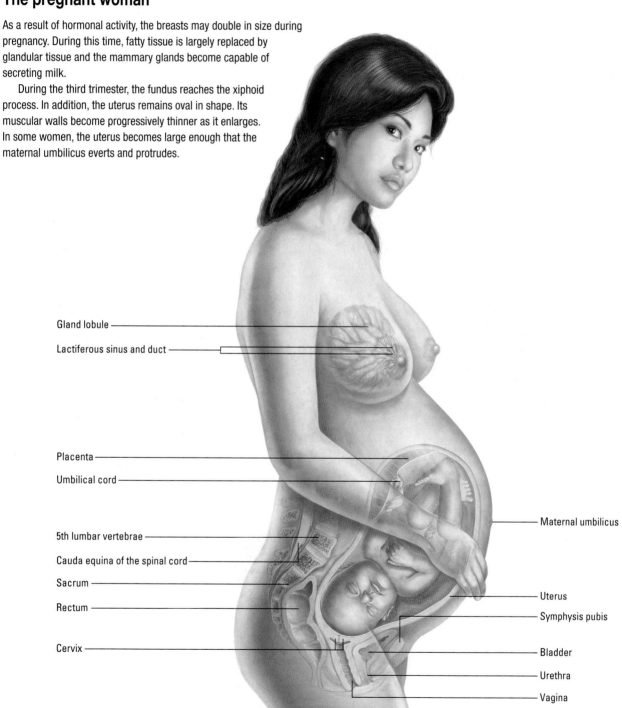

Gland lobule

Lactiferous sinus and duct

Placenta

Umbilical cord

5th lumbar vertebrae

Cauda equina of the spinal cord

Sacrum

Rectum

Cervix

Maternal umbilicus

Uterus

Symphysis pubis

Bladder

Urethra

Vagina

Conditions for caesarean birth

A caesarean birth is removal of the fetus through an abdominal incision. It's a surgical procedure that's performed in certain instances when a vaginal birth would pose a problem to either the mother or the fetus. Conditions that may necessitate caesarean birth include fetal malpresentation, cephalopelvic disproportion (CPD), placenta praevia, selected cases of placental abruption and umbilical cord prolapse. A caesarean birth may also be performed in cases of fetal distress.

Fetal malpresentation

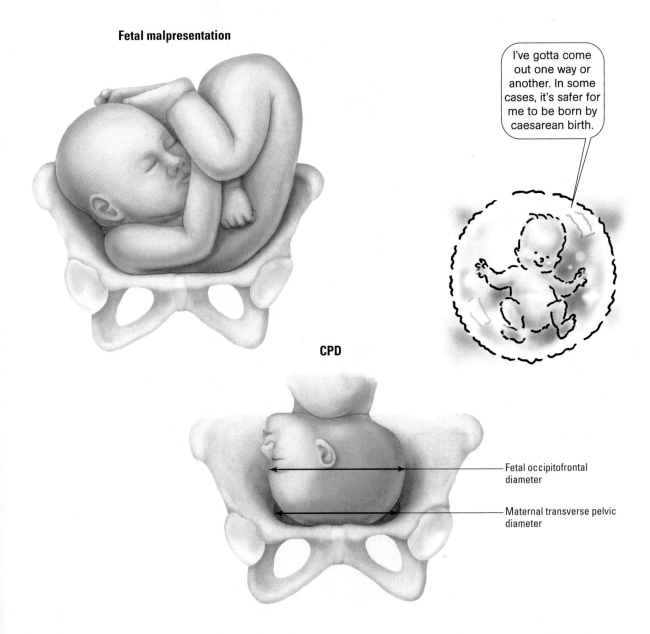

I've gotta come out one way or another. In some cases, it's safer for me to be born by caesarean birth.

CPD

Fetal occipitofrontal diameter

Maternal transverse pelvic diameter

Placenta praevia

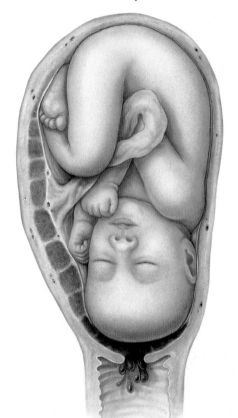

Placental abruption

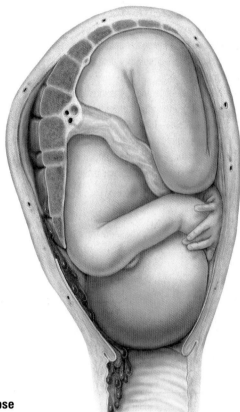

Umbilical cord prolapse

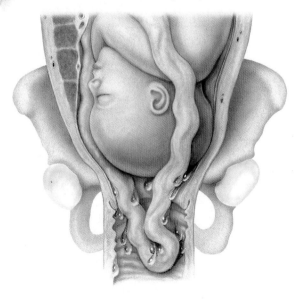

Fetal circulation

Because fetal lungs don't function until after birth, fetal blood is oxygenated by the placenta. Fetal circulation differs from neonatal circulation in that three shunts bypass the liver and the lungs and separate the systemic and pulmonary circulation. These shunts include:

• ductus venosus—circulatory pathway that allows blood to bypass the liver
• foramen ovale—opening in the interstitial septum that directs blood from the right atrium to the left atrium
• ductus arteriosus—tubular connection that shunts blood away from the pulmonary circulation.

   Because of these shunts, the umbilical vein carries oxygenated blood and the umbilical arteries carry deoxygenated blood.

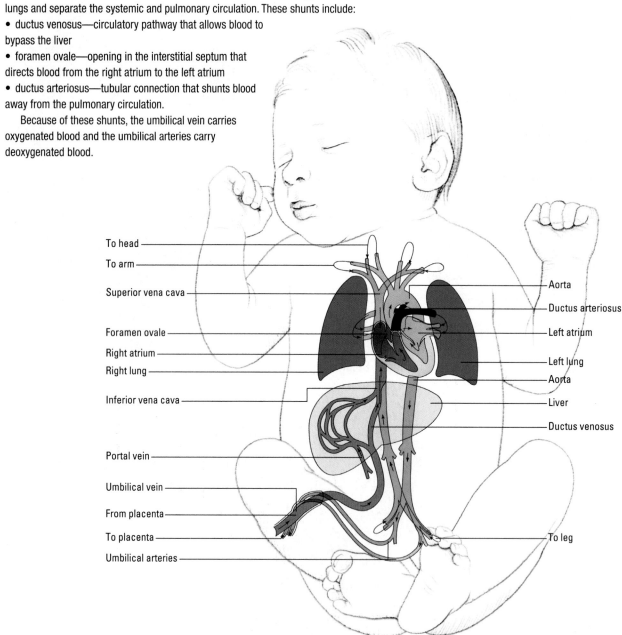

To head
To arm
Superior vena cava
Foramen ovale
Right atrium
Right lung
Inferior vena cava
Portal vein
Umbilical vein
From placenta
To placenta
Umbilical arteries

Aorta
Ductus arteriosus
Left atrium
Left lung
Aorta
Liver
Ductus venosus
To leg

uterus increases pressure on the sciatic nerve. The mother may also notice an increase in vaginal discharge because of the pressure of the fetus on the cervix. However, breathing becomes easier for the woman after lightening because pressure on the diaphragm is decreased.

Increased level of activity

After having endured increased fatigue for most of the third trimester, it's common for a woman to experience a sudden increase in energy before true labour starts. This phenomenon is sometimes referred to as 'nesting' because, in many cases, the woman directs this energy towards last-minute activities, such as organising the baby's room, cleaning and decorating her home and preparing other children in the household for the new arrival.

A built-in energy source

The woman's increase in activity may be caused by a decrease in placental progesterone production (which may also be partly responsible for the onset of labour) that results in an increase in the release of epinephrine. This epinephrine increase gives the woman extra energy for labour.

Braxton Hicks contractions

Braxton Hicks contractions are mild contractions of the uterus that occur throughout pregnancy. They may become extremely strong a few days to a month before labour begins, which may cause some women, especially a primipara, to misinterpret them as true labour. Several characteristics, however, distinguish Braxton Hicks contractions from labour contractions.

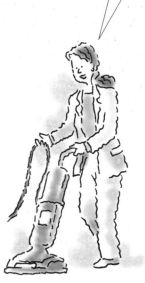

Experiencing an increased energy level before true labour starts can induce a different kind of labour – like cleaning the house.

Patternless

Braxton Hicks contractions are irregular. There's no pattern to the length of time between them and they vary widely in their strength. They gradually increase in frequency and intensity throughout the pregnancy, but they maintain an irregular pattern. In addition, Braxton Hicks contractions can be diminished by increasing activity or by eating, drinking or changing position. Labour contractions can't be diminished by these activities.

Painless

Braxton Hicks contractions are commonly painless – especially early in pregnancy. Many women feel only a tightening of the abdomen in the first or second trimester. If the woman does feel pain from these contractions, it's felt only in the abdomen and the groin – usually not in the back. This is a major difference from the contractions of labour.

No softening or stretching

Probably the most important differentiation between Braxton Hicks contractions and true labour contractions is that Braxton

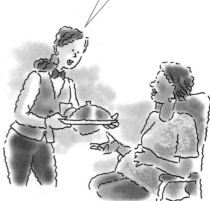

Bon appetit! Eating can help calm Braxton Hicks contractions.

Hicks contractions don't cause progressive effacement or dilation of the cervix. The uterus can still be indented with a finger during a contraction, which indicates that the contractions aren't efficient enough for effacement or dilation to occur.

Ripening of the cervix

Ripening of the cervix refers to the process in which the cervix softens to prepare for dilation and effacement. It's thought to be the result of hormone-mediated biochemical events that initiate breakdown of the collagen in the cervix, thus causing it to soften and become flexible. As the cervix ripens, it also changes position by tipping forward in the vagina.

Ripening of the cervix doesn't produce outwardly observable signs or symptoms. The ripeness of the cervix is determined during a vaginal examination, usually in the last weeks of the third trimester.

Signs of true labour

Signs of true labour include uterine contractions, cervical dilation, show and spontaneous rupture of membranes.

Uterine contractions

The involuntary uterine contractions of true labour help effacement and dilation of the cervix and push the fetus through the birth canal. Although uterine contractions are irregular when they begin, as labour progresses they become regular with a predictable pattern.

Early contractions occur anywhere from 5 to 30 minutes apart and last about 30–45 seconds. The interval between the contractions allows blood flow to resume to the placenta, which supplies oxygen to the fetus and removes waste products. As labour progresses, the contractions increase in frequency, duration and intensity. During the transition phase of the first stage of labour – when contractions reach their maximum intensity, frequency and duration – they each last 60–90 seconds and recur every 2–3 minutes.

Sweeping waves

Uterine contractions are painful and wavelike – they build and recede – beginning in the lower back and moving around to the abdomen and, possibly, the legs. They're stronger in the upper uterus than in the lower uterus so they can push the fetus downward and allow for dilation. These contractions cause a palpable hardening of the uterus that can't be indented with a finger.

Efface it!

Most important, the uterine contractions of labour cause progressive effacement and dilation of the cervix. As labour progresses, a visible bulging of intact membranes can be observed.

Show

Bloody show occurs as the cervix thins and begins to dilate, allowing passage of the mucus plug (operculum) that seals the cervical canal during pregnancy. Mucus from the plug mixes with blood from the cervical capillaries because of the pressure of the fetus on the canal and other changes in the cervix. Consequently, show may appear pinkish, blood tinged or brownish. Occasionally, in primiparas it may be passed up to 2 weeks before labour begins.

Spontaneous rupture of membranes

Twenty-five percent of all labours begin with spontaneous rupture of the membranes. The membranes – consisting of the amniotic and chorionic membranes – cover the fetal surface of the placenta and form a sac that contains and supports the fetus and the amniotic fluid. This fluid, produced by the amniotic membrane, acts as a cushion throughout gestation, protects the fetus from temperature changes, protects the umbilical cord from pressure and is believed to aid in fetal muscular development by allowing the fetus to move freely.

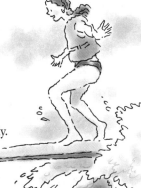

Uterine contractions are like, wavelike, you know?

Fluid facts

Spontaneous rupture of the membranes may occur as a sudden gush of fluid or as a steady or intermittent, slow leakage of fluid. Rupture isn't painful because the membranes don't have a nerve supply. Even though much of the amniotic fluid is lost when the membranes rupture, the fetus is still protected. The amniotic membrane continues to produce more fluid that surrounds and protects the fetus until it's delivered.

Colour-coded

The amniotic fluid that's lost after the rupture of the membranes should be odourless and clear. Coloured fluid usually indicates a problem. Yellow fluid indicates that the amniotic fluid is bilirubin stained from the breakdown of red blood cells, which may be caused by blood incompatibility. Green fluid indicates meconium staining, possibly from a breech presentation or fetal anoxia, and needs immediate evaluation.

Rupture or be ruptured

If a woman's membranes haven't ruptured spontaneously before the transition phase of the first stage of labour, they may rupture when the cervix becomes fully dilated at 10 cm or amniotomy may be performed. Membrane rupture aids in the dilation of the cervix; however, the mother may experience more painful contractions following the procedure. Membranes that remain intact delay full dilation and lengthen the duration of labour because the amniotic fluid cushions the pressure of the fetal head against the cervix, preventing the contractions from exerting their full impact. It is important that you fully explain to the mother, the disadvantages of having artificial rupture performed!

A little premature

Premature rupture of membranes (rupture that occurs more than 24 hours before labour begins) is associated with a risk of infection and umbilical cord prolapse.

Stages of labour

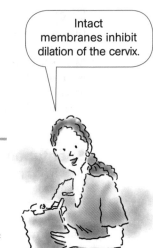

Intact membranes inhibit dilation of the cervix.

Labour is typically divided into three stages:

The first stage, when effacement and dilation occur, begins with the onset of true uterine contractions and ends when the cervix is fully dilated.

The second stage, which encompasses the actual birth, begins when the cervix is fully dilated and ends with the delivery of the fetus.

The third stage, also called the *placental stage*, begins immediately after the baby is delivered and ends when the placenta is delivered. During this stage, homeostasis is reestablished.

First stage

The first stage of labour begins with the onset of contractions and ends when the cervix is dilated to 10 cm (full dilation). It's divided into three phases: latent, active and transition.

Latent phase

The latent phase of labour begins with the onset of regular contractions. Usually, the contractions during this phase are mild. They last about 20–40 seconds and recur every 5–30 minutes. Initially, the contractions may vary in intensity and duration, but they become consistent within a few hours.

Waiting for dilation

The latent phase lasts about 6 hours in the primipara and 4 hours in the multipara and ends when rapid cervical dilation begins. During this phase, the cervix dilates from 0 to 3 cm and becomes fully effaced; however, there's minimal fetal descent through the pelvis. The contractions usually cause little discomfort if the woman remains relaxed and continues to walk around. A warm bath can help too.

Lasting longer than expected?

Poor fetal position, cephalopelvic disproportion and a cervix that hasn't softened sufficiently may increase the duration of the latent phase.

Keep her calm, moving or voiding

Midwifery care during the latent phase is mainly supportive. Provide the woman with a calm environment and psychological support for the conflicting emotions – such as excitement, anxiety and, possibly, depression – that she's experiencing. If possible, the woman could try and stay at home during much of this stage. If she is in hospital, give a clear liquid diet or light snacks as tolerated, and encourage the woman to move about and empty her bladder frequently. A warm bath or relaxing in a recliner chair might ease her discomfort. Be sure to involve the woman's partner or support person in her care as much as possible.

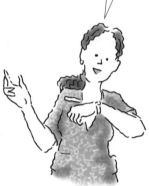

During the latent phase, start timing the frequency and length of contractions. OK? Ready, set go!

Technical stuff

Obtain the required blood sample and urine specimen, monitor the woman's vital signs and monitor FHR by intermittent auscultation. For a high-risk mother, explain and initiate electronic monitoring if necessary.

It's all about timing and intensity

During the latent phase, start timing the frequency and length of the contractions and assessing their intensity. To time the frequency of contractions, gently rest a hand on the woman's abdomen at the fundus of the uterus. Count from the beginning of one contraction to the beginning of the next. Begin timing at the start of the gradual tensing and upward rising of the fundus (initially, these sensations may not be felt by the woman); end timing when the uterus has fully relaxed.

Do you feel a nose, a chin or a forehead?

The intensity of contractions can be determined by assessing the uterus. With mild contractions, the uterus is minimally tense. It may be easily indented with a fingertip and feel similar to pressing on the tip of the nose. With moderate contractions, the uterus feels firmer. It can't be indented with a finger, and it feels similar to pressing on the chin. With strong contractions, the uterus feels extremely hard – it feels similar to pressing on the forehead.

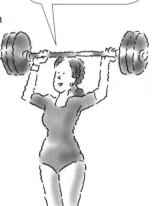

The strength of contractions increases in the active phase of labour.

Active phase

During the active phase of labour, the release of show increases and the membranes may rupture spontaneously. The contractions are stronger, each lasting about 40–60 seconds and recurring about every 3–5 minutes. The increased strength of the contractions commonly causes pain. Cervical dilation occurs more rapidly, increasing from about 3 to 7 cm, and the fetus begins to descend through the pelvis at an increased rate.

Whole lot of changing going on

The active phase is an emotionally charged time for the woman. She may be feeling excitement as well as fear. The woman also undergoes many systemic changes. (See *Systemic changes in the active phase of labour*, page 278.)

Systemic changes in the active phase of labour

This chart shows the systemic changes that occur during the active phase of labour.

System	Change
Cardiovascular	• Increased blood pressure • Increased cardiac output • Supine hypotension
Respiratory	• Increased oxygen consumption • Increased rate • Possible hyperventilation leading to respiratory alkalosis, hypoxia and hypercapnia (if breathing isn't controlled)
Neurological	• Increased pain threshold and sedation caused by endogenous endorphins • Anaesthetised perineal tissues caused by constant intense pressure on nerve endings
GI	• Dehydration • Decreased motility • Slow absorption of solid food • Nausea • Diarrhoea
Musculoskeletal	• Diaphoresis • Fatigue • Backache • Joint pain • Leg cramps
Endocrine	• Decreased progesterone level • Increased oestrogen level • Increased prostaglandin level • Increased oxytocin level • Increased metabolism • Decreased blood glucose
Renal	• Difficulty voiding • Proteinuria (1+ normal)

How long must this go on?

The active phase of labour lasts about 3 hours in a primipara and 2 hours in a multipara. If analgesics are given at this time, they won't slow labour. Poor fetal position and a full bladder may prolong this phase.

Shower her with comfort and support

Midwifery care during the active phase focuses on the psychological status of the woman as well as her physical care. Expect the woman to have mood swings and difficulty coping. Offer support, and encourage the woman to use proper breathing techniques. In addition, continue to involve the woman's partner or labour support person in her care. Placing the woman in an upright or side-lying position may provide additional comfort – moving about can be a distraction for her.

Other measures that may be necessary include:
* monitoring intake and output
* monitoring vital signs
* auscultating FHR (with a Pinard's stethoscope and if mother requests it, a sonicaid) every 30 minutes for a low-risk mother – a high-risk mother should have a cardiotocograph (CTG) trace done on a regular basis
* performing perineal care frequently to reduce the risk of infection, especially after each voiding and bowel movement
* recording all observations made, care given, medications administered and any interventions by midwifery or medical staff.

Transition phase

During the transition phase, contractions reach maximum intensity. They each last 60–90 seconds, and they occur every 2–3 minutes. The cervix dilates from about 7 to 10 cm to become fully dilated and effaced. If the membranes aren't already ruptured, they usually rupture when the woman's cervix is 10 cm dilated and the remainder of the mucus plug is expelled.

The transition phase peaks when cervical dilation slows slightly at 9 cm. This slowdown signifies the end of the first stage of labour – it gives the woman's body a chance to summon the strength for the hard work that is about to begin. Some women draw 'into themselves' and appear distant and noncommunicative for a short period. For multiparas, birth may be imminent at this time.

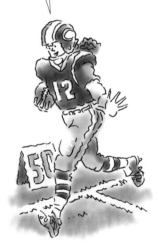

Contractions reach maximum intensity during the transition phase of labour. I'm at maximum intensity ALL the time.

What she's feeling

When in the transition phase, the woman may experience intense pain or discomfort as well as nausea and vomiting. She may also experience intense mood swings and feelings of anxiety, panic, irritability and loss of control because of the intensity and duration of contractions.

What you're doing

Midwifery care during the transition phase includes monitoring vital signs and FHR and encouraging proper breathing techniques. The midwife should be with the woman at all times because there's a possibility that birth is imminent. Make sure to provide emotional support to the woman and her partner or support person during this time.

Second stage

The second stage of labour starts with full dilation and effacement of the cervix and ends with the delivery of the baby. It lasts about 1–2 hours for the primipara and 30–60 minutes for the multipara. During the second stage, the frequency of the contractions slows to about one every 3–4 minutes; however, they continue to last 60–90 seconds and are accompanied by the uncontrollable urge to push or bear down. The decreased frequency of the contractions gives the woman a chance to rest.

Vigilance!

During the second stage of labour (including pushing), auscultate FHR in between contractions.

Movin' out

Whereas the previous stage of labour primarily involved thinning and opening of the cervix, the second stage involves moving the fetus through the birth canal and out of the body.

As the uterine contractions work to accomplish this movement, the fetus pushes on the internal side of the perineum, causing the perineum to bulge and become tense. When the widest part of the fetal scalp becomes visible at the opening to the vagina (called *crowning*). The vaginal opening changes from a slit to an oval and then to a circle. The circular opening then gradually increases in size to allow the baby's head to emerge. The combination of involuntary uterine contractions and the mother pushing with her abdominal muscles helps the fetus proceed through the mechanisms of labour and expel from the body.

The physiological changes that began in the first stage of labour continue throughout the second stage. In addition, the mother's oxytocin level increases, which helps to intensify the contractions.

> All the world's a stage, and although the second stage of labour ends with delivery of the baby, there are still two stages yet to go!

Mechanisms of labour

The mechanisms of labour are fetal position changes that occur during the second stage of labour. They help the fetus pass through the birth canal. These movements are necessary because of the size of the fetal head in relation to the irregularly shaped pelvis. Specific, deliberate and precise, the various movements allow the smallest diameter of the fetus to pass through the corresponding diameter of the woman's pelvis. (See *Mechanisms of labour*, page 281.)

Descent

Descent, the first of the mechanisms, is the downward movement of the fetus. It's determined when the biparietal diameter of the head passes the ischial spines and moves into the pelvic inlet.

May the forces be with you

Descent progresses intermittently with contractions and occurs because of several forces:
- direct pressure on the fetus by the contracting uterine fundus
- pressure of the amniotic fluid

Mechanisms of labour

These illustrations show the fetal movements that occur during the mechanisms of labour.

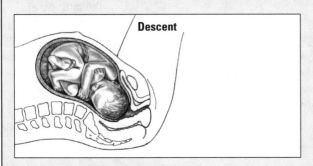
Descent

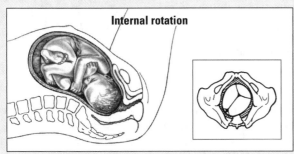
Internal rotation

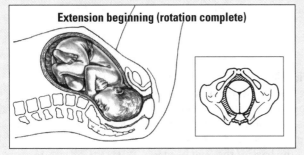
Extension beginning (rotation complete)

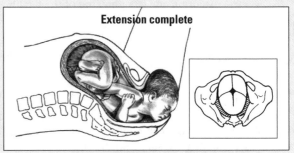
Extension complete

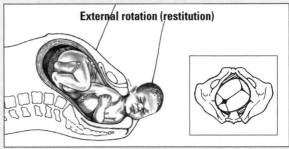
External rotation (restitution)

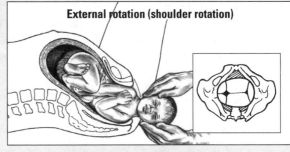
External rotation (shoulder rotation)

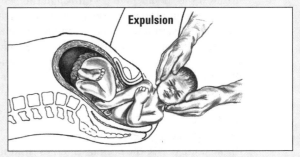
Expulsion

- contraction of the abdominal muscles (fetal pressure on the mother's sacral nerves causes her to experience an uncontrollable need to push)
- extension and straightening of the fetal body.

Making contact

Full descent is accomplished when the fetal head passes beyond the dilated cervix and contacts the posterior vaginal floor.

Flexion
Flexion, the second of the mechanisms, occurs during descent. It's caused by the resistance of the fetal head against the pelvic floor. The combined pressure from this resistance and uterine and abdominal muscle contractions forces the head of the fetus to bend forward so that the chin is pressed to the chest. This allows the smallest diameter of the fetal head to descend through the pelvis.

A different angle

Flexion causes the presenting diameter to change from occipitofrontal (nasal bridge to the posterior fontanelle) to suboccipitobregmatic (posterior fontanelle to subocciput) in an occiput anterior position. If the fetus is in an occiput posterior position, flexion is incomplete and the fetus has a larger presenting diameter, which can prolong labour.

Internal rotation
The fetal head typically enters the pelvis with its anteroposterior head diameter in a transverse (right to left) position. This position is beneficial when entering the pelvis because the diameter at the pelvic inlet is widest from right to left. However, if the head remains in the transverse position, the shoulders are in a position where they're too wide to pass through the pelvic inlet.

Shifting towards the same plane

To allow the shoulders to pass through the pelvic inlet, the fetal head rotates about 45° as it meets the resistance of the pelvic floor. With the head rotated, the anteroposterior diameter of the head is in the anteroposterior plane of the pelvis (front to back), which places the widest part of the shoulders in line with the widest part of the pelvic inlet and outlet. At this point, the face of the fetus is usually against the mother's back and the back of the fetal head is against the front of the mother's pelvis.

Extension
Extension occurs after the internal rotation is complete. As the head passes through the pelvis, the occiput emerges from the vagina and the back of the neck stops under the symphysis pubis (pubic arch). Further descent is temporarily halted because the fetus's shoulders are too wide to pass through the pelvis or under the pubic arch.

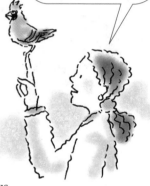

Mechanisms of labour are the fetal position changes that occur during the second stage of labour and help the fetus pass through the birth canal.

Pivotal movements

With the back of the fetal neck resting against the pubic arch, the arch acts as a pivot. The upward resistance from the pelvic floor causes the head to extend. As this occurs, the brow, nose, mouth and chin are born.

External rotation

External rotation (also called *restitution*) is necessary because the shoulders, which previously turned to fit through the pelvic inlet, must now turn again to fit through the pelvic outlet and under the pubic arch.

Return the fetus to the transverse position . . .

After the head is born, the face, which is facing down after the completion of extension, is turned to face one of the mother's inner thighs. The head rotates about 45°, returning the anteroposterior head diameter to the transverse (right to left) position assumed during descent.

. . . and prepare for shoulder delivery

The anterior shoulder (closest to the mother's pubic bone) is delivered first with the possible assistance of downward flexion on the head. After the anterior shoulder is delivered, a slight upward flexion may be necessary to deliver the posterior shoulder.

Weighing in

During external rotation, a baby who weighs more than 4.5 kg (9.9 lb) has a greater likelihood of experiencing shoulder dystocia than one who weighs less. Shoulder dystocia occurs when lack of room for passage causes the shoulders to stop at the pelvic outlet. Commonly, shoulder dystocia is resolved by sharply flexing the maternal thighs against the maternal abdomen. This movement reduces the angle between the sacrum and the spine and allows the shoulders to pass through; however, the baby may sustain some injury to the brachial plexus.

Expulsion

After delivery of the shoulders, the remainder of the body is delivered quickly and easily. Termed *expulsion*, this step signifies the end of the second stage of labour.

Third stage

The third stage of labour, also called the *placental stage*, occurs after delivery of the baby and ends with the delivery of the placenta. It consists of two phases: placental separation and placental expulsion. This stage of labour is important because a placenta that remains in place may cause haemorrhage, shock, infection or even death.

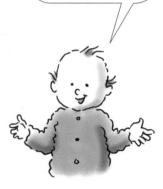

I turned out all right. I turned to fit through the pelvic inlet, then turned again to fit through the pelvic outlet and under the pubic arch.

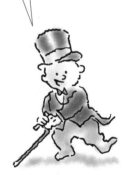

Look Ma! I've been expulsed! Aren't I wonderful?!

From round to discoid

After the baby has been delivered, uterine contractions commonly stop for several minutes. During this time, the uterus is a round mass located below the level of the umbilicus that feels firm to the touch. When contractions resume, the uterus takes on a discoid shape until the placenta has separated from the uterus.

The duration of the third stage varies widely. It may last from several minutes to up to 60 minutes.

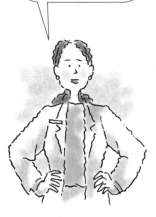

The placenta may cause haemorrhage, shock, infection or death if it isn't delivered.

Placental separation

Separation of the placenta from the uterus occurs after the uterus resumes contractions. Uterine contractions continue to occur in the wavelike pattern that they assumed throughout the other stages of labour; however, in the other stages, the fetus exerted pressure on the placenta during contractions, which prevented the placenta from separating prematurely. When the fetus is no longer in the uterus, the uterine walls contract on an almost empty space. Nothing exerts reverse pressure on the placenta. As a result, the placenta folds and begins to separate from the uterine wall. This separation causes bleeding that further pushes the placenta away from the uterine wall, ultimately causing the placenta to fall to the upper vagina or lower uterine segment.

Ready to roll

Signs that the placenta has separated and is ready to be delivered include:
- absence of cord pulse
- lengthening of the umbilical cord
- sudden gush of vaginal blood
- change in the shape of the uterus.

Separating from the centre…

Approximately 80% of all separated placentas are Schultze's placentas. A Schultze's placenta starts to separate at the centre and folds onto itself. It delivers with the fetal surface exposed and appears shiny and glistening from the fetal membranes.

…or the edge

A Duncan placenta separates at the edges, then slides down the surface of the uterus and delivers with the maternal surface exposed. It appears red, raw and irregular because of the ridges that separate the blood collection spaces.

Placental expulsion

Natural bearing down by the mother aids in the delivery of the placenta. To avoid possible eversion (turning inside out) of the uterus, which can result in gross haemorrhage, never exert pressure on the uterus when it isn't contracted. Manual removal of the placenta may be indicated if it doesn't deliver spontaneously.

Memory jogger

To help remember which type of placenta is which, think 'Shiny Schultze's' and 'Dirty Duncan'. The Schultze's placenta is shiny from the fetal membrane. The Duncan placenta exposes the maternal side and appears red and dirty with an irregular surface.

Active or expectant?

In the UK, mothers are offered the choice of managing the third stage of labour in two ways:

- **Active management**   An oxytocic drug is administered I.M. with the birth of the baby's anterior shoulder – this may be Syntometrine 1 amp (contains 5 IU of Syntocinon + 0.5 mg Ergometrine) or Syntocinon 10 IU.

  When the signs of separation are confirmed, the placenta and membranes are delivered by controlled cord traction. This means that the midwife must 'guard' the uterus above the symphysis pubis as she applies a downward traction on the cord. If any resistance is felt, the midwife should stop. Once the placenta is visible, it should be cupped in both hands and eased out of the vagina, into a receiver along with blood loss and clots. The mother's uterus is checked for consistency – it should feel hard and contracted and blood loss should be minimal.

- **Physiological management**   No oxytocic agents are given. The cord is left unclamped to allow drainage of blood from the placenta and contraction/retraction of the uterus to occur naturally. Delayed clamping is not advised in Rh-negative women because of the danger of maternal-fetal transfusion.

  Often the baby is put to the breast and this releases oxytocin which assists separation of the placenta. The abdomen should not be handled excessively as it may interfere with the natural process – the mother's bladder should be empty as well.

  The mother can assume the squatting position and when she feels a contraction, she may push involuntarily. Once the cord lengthens further, it is a sign the placenta is in the vagina and the mother can be encouraged to push gently. This will probably expel the placenta and membranes with ease. The whole process may take a lot longer than in active management – up to an hour or more.

Check it out

After delivery, keep your gloves on and examine the placenta to make sure it's intact and normal in appearance. This helps determine whether any has been retained in the uterus. Hold the placenta and membranes by the cord and let the membranes hang down – check them for completeness – are there any blood vessels running out into the membranes? If there are, this could be an indication that there was a succenturate lobe (an extra lobe) which was situated away from the main placenta. If this lobe is not attached to the membranes, then it is likely it could still be inside the woman's uterus – this could cause further bleeding and eventually, infection.

Fetal surface

This surface is bluish-grey and contains some major blood vessels. You should check where the cord is inserted – some insertions are abnormal and should be documented in the mother's notes.

Umbilical cord

Check that the cord has three vessels – two arteries and a vein. Absence of one vessel has been associated with possible renal disease. Note the thickness of the cord and the approximate length – purely out of interest!

Maternal surface

Run your hands over the maternal surface of the placenta. There are 18–20 lobes and you should look to make sure they are all present – if there are any gaps in the surface, it may be the woman has retained products.

Check for calcification – this looks like greyish, gritty areas and is often seen when a placenta is postdates.

Also look for creamy/whitish areas that are likely to be infarcted areas. These can be caused by a reduced blood supply to that area or it can be where the placenta has separated during pregnancy. Look at the placenta to see if it looks normal – if it has any unusual features such as colour or smell – it would be wise to send it to pathology laboratory for further investigations. This can be very useful if infection is suspected in the baby. Placentas are sometimes kept in delivery suite for a short period after delivery – some are used for research purposes.

Additional layers

An outer area of decidua (the lining of the uterus) is expelled at the same time as the placenta. The remainder of the decidua separates into two layers:

1. Superficial layer that's shed in the lochia during the postpartum period.
2. Basal layer that remains in the uterus to regenerate new endothelium.

Blood volume matters

Normal bleeding occurs until the uterus contracts with enough force to seal the blood collection spaces. A blood loss of 300–500 ml should be expected. Blood loss exceeding 500 ml from the genital tract in the first 24 hours following birth is classed as a primary postpartum haemorrhage (PPH) and may indicate a cervical tear or a problem at the episiotomy site. Life-threatening haemorrhage occurs in approx. 1 per 1,000 births. It may also indicate that the uterus isn't contracting properly because of retained placenta or a full bladder.

Commonly, after the placenta is delivered, the mother is given I.M. Syntometrine to increase uterine contractions and minimise bleeding; however, this drug shouldn't be given if the mother's blood pressure is increased because it can cause vasoconstriction and hypertension. Syntometrine can also cause nausea and vomiting.

Reestablishing homeostasis (controlling blood loss)

This period of time usually lasts for about 1–4 hours, and it initiates the postpartum period. During this stage, the woman should be monitored closely because her body has just undergone many changes.

Risks associated with this stage include haemorrhage, bladder distention and venous thrombosis. Oxygen, O-negative blood (or blood tested for compatibility) and I.V. fluids must be readily available for 4 hours after delivery.

Inspect and repair

Initially, the labia and vagina are inspected to check for and repair lacerations that may have occurred during birth. If an episiotomy was performed, the incision is sutured with the woman in the lithotomy position (legs in stirrups). Keep in mind that a woman who delivered without the aid of an anaesthetic requires a local anaesthetic for this procedure; a woman who received regional or local anaesthesia during the birth probably won't need additional medication. When suturing is complete, the woman's legs should be lowered from the stirrups. Make sure the legs are lowered simultaneously to prevent back injury.

> After delivery, the woman's pulse, respirations and blood pressure will be slightly increased.

Monitoring mum

Monitor the woman's vital signs for a minimum of 1 hour, then as ordered. Expect the woman's pulse, respirations and blood pressure to be slightly increased at this time because of the birth process, excitement and oxytocin administration. In addition, the woman may experience a normal chill and shaking sensation shortly after the birth. This is common and may be caused by excess epinephrine production during labour or the sudden release of pressure on the pelvic nerves.

The incredible shrinking uterus

After delivery, the uterus gradually decreases in size and descends into its pre-pregnancy position in the pelvis – a process known as *involution*. To evaluate this process, palpate the uterine fundus and determine uterine size, degree of firmness and rate of descent (which is measured in fingerbreadths above or below the umbilicus). Involution normally begins immediately after delivery, when the firmly contracted uterus lies almost at the umbilicus. If the woman is breastfeeding, the release of natural oxytocics should help to maintain or stimulate contraction of the uterus. If it doesn't remain contracted, gently massage the uterus or administer medications as ordered.

Void to avoid interference

Encourage the woman to void because a full bladder interferes with uterine contractions that work to compress the open blood vessels at the placental site. If these blood vessels are allowed to bleed freely, haemorrhage may occur. Observe the amount (measure first one to two volumes passed), colour and consistency of the lochia and watch for its absence, which may indicate that a clot is blocking the cervical os. Sudden heavy bleeding could result if a change of position dislodges the clot.

Clot watch

Pregnant and postpartum women have higher fibrinogen levels, which increase the possibility of clot formation. A woman has an additional risk of clot formation if she has varicose veins or a history of thrombophlebitis or if she had a caesarean delivery. Monitor closely for signs of venous thrombosis, especially if the duration of labour was abnormally long or if the woman was confined to bed for an extended period, for example due to epidural anaesthesia.

Ongoing support

Be sure to take the following steps as well:
• Offer emotional support as needed to the mother and her partner or labour support person.
• Perform perineal care, and apply a clean perineal pad as needed.
• Offer a regular diet as soon as the woman requests food (sometimes this request is made shortly after delivery – tea and toast are always appreciated).
• Encourage full ambulation as soon as possible.
• Provide comfort measures, such as a bath/shower, clean clothes and a warmed blanket.

Midwifery procedures

Midwifery procedures performed during labour and delivery include uterine contraction palpation, intermittent FHR monitoring, continuous external electronic monitoring and vaginal examination.

Uterine contraction palpation

External uterine palpation can tell you the frequency, duration and intensity of contractions and the relaxation time between them. The character of contractions varies with the stage of labour and the body's response to labour-inducing drugs, if administered. As labour advances, contractions become more intense, occur more often and last longer. In some women, labour progresses rapidly, preventing her from travelling to hospital.

Take the following steps to palpate uterine contractions:
• Review the mother's admission history to determine the onset, frequency, duration and intensity of contractions. Also, note where contractions feel strongest or exert the most pressure.
• Describe the procedure to the mother.
• Assist her into a comfortable side-lying position.
• Cover the mother with a sheet.
• Place the palmar surface of your fingers on the uterine fundus, and palpate lightly to assess contractions. Each contraction has three phases: increment (rising), acme (peak) and decrement (letting down or ebbing).

How fast?

• To assess frequency, time the interval between the beginning of one contraction and the beginning of the next.

How long?

- To assess duration, time the period from when the uterus begins tightening until it begins relaxing.

How hard?

- To assess intensity, press your fingertips into the uterine fundus when the uterus tightens. During mild contractions, the fundus indents easily; during moderate contractions, the fundus indents less easily; during strong contractions, the fundus resists indenting.
- Determine how the woman copes with discomfort by assessing her breathing and relaxation techniques.
- Assess contractions in low-risk women every 30 minutes in the latent and active phases, and every 15 minutes in the transition phase. More frequent assessments are required for high-risk women. High-risk fetal status assessments should also occur every 30 minutes during the latent phase, every 15–30 minutes during the active phase and every 5 minutes in the second stage. (See *Contraction without relaxation*.)

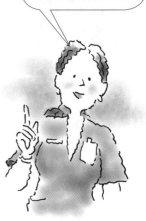

Continuous external fetal monitoring is a noninvasive way to assess contractions and fetal heart rate.

Continuous external electronic monitoring

Continuous external electronic monitoring is an indirect, noninvasive procedure. Two devices, an ultrasound transducer and a tocotransducer, are placed on the mother's abdomen to evaluate fetal well-being and uterine contractions during labour. These devices are held in place with an elastic stockinette or by using plastic or soft straps.

Advice from the experts

Contraction without relaxation

If any contraction lasts longer than 90 seconds and isn't followed by uterine muscle relaxation, or if the relaxation period is less than 1 minute between contractions, notify the doctor. This may indicate hyperstimulation of the uterus or tetanic contractions. When the uterus doesn't relax, or the relaxation period is less than 1 minute, uteroplacental blood flow is interrupted, which can lead to fetal hypoxia and fetal distress.

If you determine that the mother's contractions last longer than 90 seconds or if the relaxation period is less than 1 minute, follow these steps:

- Discontinue the oxytocin infusion to stop uterine stimulations (if the mother is receiving oxytocin).
- Make sure that the mother is lying on her left side; this increases uteroplacental perfusion.
- Administer oxygen via face mask to increase fetal oxygenation.
- Notify the doctor or senior midwife immediately.

Advice from the experts

Applying continuous external monitoring devices

To ensure clear tracings that define fetal status and labour progress, be sure to precisely position continuous external monitoring devices. These devices include an ultrasound transducer and a tocotransducer.

Fetal heart monitor

Palpate the uterus to locate the fetus's back, and place the ultrasound transducer, which reads the fetal heart rate, over the site where the fetal heartbeat sounds the loudest. Then tighten the belt. Use the fetal heart tracing on the monitor strip to confirm the transducer's position.

Tocotransducer

A tocotransducer records uterine motion during contractions. Place the tocotransducer over the uterine fundus where it contracts, either midline or slightly to one side. Place your hand on the fundus, and palpate a contraction to verify proper placement. Secure the tocotransducer's belt, and then adjust the pen set so that the baseline values read between 5 and 15 mmHg on the monitor strip.

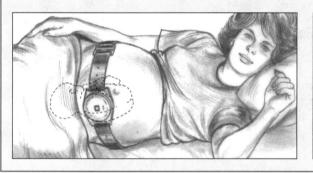
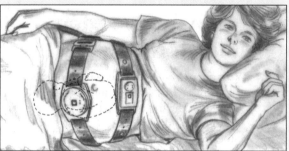

Two readings, one printout

The ultrasound transducer transmits high-frequency sound waves aimed at the fetal heart. The tocotransducer, in turn, responds to the pressure exerted by uterine contractions and simultaneously records the duration and frequency of the contractions. (See *Applying continuous external monitoring devices*.) The monitoring apparatus traces FHR and uterine contraction data onto the same printout paper.

Continuous external fetal monitoring is used for women with a high-risk pregnancy or oxytocin-induced labour.

Monitoring FHR and uterine contractions

Here are the steps you should take when monitoring FHR and uterine contractions:
- Explain the procedure to the woman and ensure she is comfortable before you start.
- Label the monitoring strip with, or enter into the computer, the woman's hospital number, birth date, her name, the date and time – some units require recording observations on the mother's temperature and pulse.

- Assist the mother to a comfortable lying position with her abdomen exposed, and palpate the abdomen to locate the fundus – the area of greatest muscle density in the uterus.

Buckle up and get tracing

- Using transducer straps or a stockinette binder, secure the tocotransducer over the fundus.
- Adjust the pen set tracer controls so that the baseline values read between 5 and 15 mmHg on the monitor strip or as indicated by the model.

Goo for good contact

- Apply conduction gel to the ultrasound transducer, and perform an abdominal palpation to locate the fetal back, through which fetal heart tones resound most audibly.
- Start the monitor, and apply the ultrasound transducer directly over the site having the strongest heart tones.
- Activate the control that begins the printout.
- Observe the tracings to identify the frequency and duration of uterine contractions, but palpate the uterus to determine the intensity of the contractions.

Compare and contract

- Note the baseline FHR, and assess periodic accelerations or decelerations from the baseline. Compare the FHR patterns with those of the uterine contractions.
- Move the tocotransducer and the ultrasound transducer to accommodate changes in maternal or fetal position. Readjust both transducers every hour, and assess the mother's skin for reddened areas caused by the pressure of the monitoring device.
- Clean the ultrasound transducer periodically with a damp cloth to remove dried conduction gel, and apply fresh gel as necessary.
- If the mother reports discomfort in the position that provides the clearest signal, try to obtain a satisfactory 5- or 10-minute tracing with the woman in this position before assisting her to a more comfortable position.
- Make a note of any interventions during the recording, e.g. using a bedpan, on the paper trace and sign it.

Internal electronic monitoring

Internal fetal monitoring, also called *direct monitoring*, is an invasive procedure that uses a spiral fetal scalp electrode (FSE) attached to the presenting fetal part (usually the scalp). This electrode detects the fetal heartbeat and transmits it to the monitor, which converts the signals into a fetal electrocardiogram (ECG) waveform. This helps assess fetal response to uterine contractions, measures intrauterine pressure, tracks labour progress and allows evaluation of short- and long-term FHR variability. Internal monitoring is indicated for high-risk pregnancies. However, it can be performed only if the amniotic sac has ruptured, the cervix is dilated at least 3 cm and the presenting part of the fetal head is at at least the –1 station. Maternal complications of internal fetal monitoring may include uterine perforation and intrauterine infections. Fetal complications may include abscess, haematoma, skin abrasions and infection.

Monitoring FHR with an FSE

Follow these steps when monitoring FHR:
- Help the woman into a comfortable position so the midwife/doctor can perform a vaginal examination.
- After identifying the presenting fetal part and level of descent, the midwife applies a scalp electrode to the fetal scalp.
- Attach the internal FSE to a cable from the monitor. Then secure the electrode to the mother's body.
- Finally, observe the FHR. (See *Reading a fetal monitor strip*, page 293.)

Check and compare

- Check the baseline FHR, and assess periodic accelerations or decelerations from the baseline. Compare the FHR pattern with the uterine contraction pattern. Note the interval between the onset of deceleration and uterine contractions, the interval between the lowest level of an FHR deceleration and the peak of a uterine contraction and the range of FHR deceleration.
- Check for FHR variability, which is a measure of fetal oxygen reserve and neurological integrity and stability. (See *Understanding fetal heart rate variability*, page 293.)

The recent NICE guidelines categorised FHR patterns into normal, suspicious and pathological.

The four key features in CTG are:
- baseline (bpm)
- variability (bpm)
- decelerations
- accelerations.

Decisions, decisions . . .

When interpreting the CTG trace the midwife has to look at the overall pattern and decide if it looks normal, suspicious or pathological. The decision is made by using the following categories.
- Normal – all four features are reassuring.
- Suspicious – one feature is classified as non-reassuring and the remaining features are reassuring.
- Pathological – an FHR trace with two or more features is classified as non-reassuring, and with one or more features is classified as abnormal.

Access the NICE guidelines for Intrapartum Care (2008) where there is a full discussion on monitoring women in normal and high-risk labour (http://www.nice.org.uk/nicemedia/pdf/CG55FullGuideline.pdf).

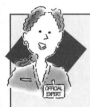

Advice from the experts

Reading a fetal monitor strip (cardiotocograph [CTG] trace)

Presented in two parallel recordings, the CTG trace records the fetal heart rate (FHR) in beats per minute in the top recording and uterine activity (UA) in millimetres of mercury (mmHg) in the bottom recording. You can obtain information on fetal status and labour progress by reading the strips horizontally and vertically.

Reading horizontally on the FHR or the UA trace, each small block represents 10 seconds. Six consecutive small blocks, separated by a dark vertical line, represent 1 minute. Reading vertically on the CTG trace, each block represents an amplitude of 10 beats/minute. Reading vertically on the UA trace, each block represents 5 mmHg of pressure.

Assess the baseline FHR (the 'resting' heart rate) between uterine contractions when fetal movement diminishes. This baseline FHR (normal range: 110–160 beats/minute) pattern serves as a reference for subsequent FHR tracings produced during contractions.

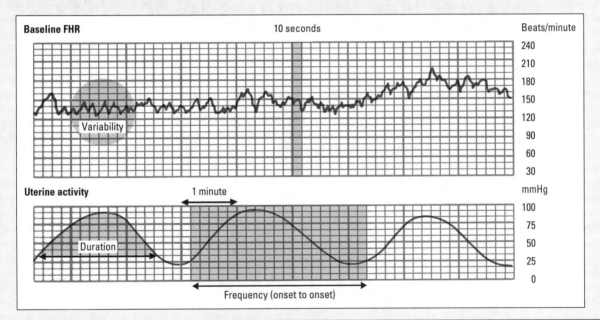

Understanding fetal heart rate variability

Fetal heart rate (FHR) is the fluctuation of the baseline FHR of at least two cycles per minute. This fluctuation represents the interaction between the sympathetic and parasympathetic nervous systems of the fetus. The constant interactions between these systems result in a moment-to-moment change in the FHR. It signals that both nervous systems are working. This interaction can be termed as *absent, minimal, moderate* or *marked* and is determined by the beats per minute (bpm).

Variability	Amplitude range
Absent	Undetectable
Minimal	> undetectable < 5 bpm
Moderate	6–25 bpm
Marked	> 25 bpm

- Until recently, the DRCBRAVADO mnemonic was used for assessing or scoring the trace – some midwives still like this method but be careful to use the chosen method in your unit, as per policy.

  DR – document risks
  C – contractions
  BR – baseline rate
  A – accelerations
  VA – variability
  D – decelerations
  O – overall plan
- High-risk mothers need continuous FHR monitoring, whereas low-risk mothers should have FHR auscultated every 15–30 minutes after a contraction during the first stage of labour and between contractions during the second stage. First, determine the baseline FHR within 10 beats/minute, and then assess the degree of baseline variability. Identify changes such as decelerations (early late, variable or mixed) and nonperiodic changes such as a sinusoidal pattern. (See *Identifying baseline FHR irregularities*, pages 295, 296 and 297.) If vaginal delivery isn't imminent (within 30 minutes) and fetal distress patterns are identified, a fetal scalp pH may be done before proceeding to a caesarean birth.

Intermittent fetal heart rate monitoring

Intermittent FHR monitoring is the periodic auscultation of FHR by either Pinard's stethoscope or a handheld sonicaid device. Because the sonicaid is more sensitive to fluctuations in FHR, it's more commonly used. However, the midwife should always 'listen in' using a Pinard when possible – it is an acquired, invaluable skill and is readily available when modern technology may not be!

Up and about

Intermittent FHR monitoring allows the mother to ambulate during the first stage of labour. Because auscultation isn't done until after a contraction, this type of monitoring doesn't document how the fetus is responding to the stress of labour as well as continuous FHR monitoring does.

Limited

Intermittent FHR monitoring can detect FHR baseline and rhythm as well as changes from the baseline; however, it can't detect variability in FHR as documented by electronic fetal monitoring.

Baseline

To establish the baseline FHR, auscultate FHR for a full minute after a contraction has ended. This type of auscultation can be done until a change in the mother's condition occurs, such as the onset of bleeding or rupture of

amniotic fluid membranes. Assess FHR after vaginal examination, or after
pain medication administration.

Vaginal examination

During first-stage labour, a vaginal examination may be done to assess cervical
dilation and effacement; membrane status and fetal presentation, position and

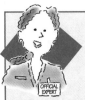

Advice from the experts

Identifying baseline FHR irregularities

When monitoring fetal heart rate (FHR), you need to be familiar with irregularities that may occur, their possible
causes and midwifery interventions to take. Here's a guide to these irregularities.

Irregularity	Possible causes	Clinical significance	Midwifery interventions
Baseline tachycardia FHR > 160 beats/minute *(chart: 240, 210, 180, 150, 120, 90, 60, 30)*	• Early fetal hypoxia • Maternal fever • Parasympathetic agents, such as atropine and scopolamine • Beta-adrenergics, such as ritodrine and terbutaline • Amnionitis (inflammation of inner layer of fetal membrane, or amnion) • Maternal hyperthyroidism • Fetal anaemia • Fetal heart failure • Fetal arrhythmias	Persistent tachycardia without periodic changes doesn't usually adversely affect fetal well-being, especially when associated with maternal fever. However, tachycardia is an ominous sign when associated with late decelerations, severe variable decelerations or lack of variability.	• Intervene to alleviate the cause of fetal distress, and provide supplemental oxygen as ordered. Also administer I.V. fluids as prescribed. • Discontinue oxytocin infusion to reduce uterine activity. • Turn the mother onto her left side. • Continue to observe FHR. • Document interventions and outcomes. • Notify the practitioner; further medical intervention may be necessary.
Baseline bradycardia FHR < 160 beats/minute *(chart: 240, 210, 180, 150, 120, 90, 60, 30)*	• Late fetal hypoxia • Beta-adrenergic blockers, such as propranolol, and anaesthetics • Maternal hypotension • Prolonged umbilical cord compression • Fetal congenital heart block	Bradycardia with good variability and no periodic changes doesn't signal fetal distress if FHR remains higher than 80 beats/minute. However, bradycardia caused by hypoxia and acidosis is an ominous sign when associated with loss of variability and late decelerations.	• Intervene to correct the cause of fetal distress. Administer supplemental oxygen as ordered. Start an I.V. line and administer fluids as prescribed. • Discontinue oxytocin infusion to reduce uterine activity. • Turn the mother onto her left side. • Continue observing FHR. • Document interventions and outcomes. • Notify the obstetric registrar; further medical intervention may be necessary.

(continued)

Identifying baseline FHR irregularities (continued)

Irregularity	Possible causes	Clinical significance	Midwifery interventions
Early decelerations beats/minute mmHg 	Fetal head compression	Early decelerations are benign, indicating fetal head compression at cervical dilation of 4–7 cm.	• Reassure the mother that the fetus isn't at risk. • Observe FHR. • Document the frequency of decelerations.
Late decelerations beats/minute mmHg 	• Uteroplacental circulatory insufficiency (placental hypoperfusion) caused by decreased intervillous blood flow during contractions or a structural placental defect such as placental abruption • Uterine hyperactivity caused by excessive oxytocin infusion • Maternal hypotension • Maternal supine hypotension	Late decelerations indicate uteroplacental circulatory insufficiency and may lead to fetal hypoxia and acidosis if the underlying cause isn't corrected.	• Turn the mother onto her left side to increase placental perfusion and decrease contraction frequency. • Increase the I.V. fluid rate to boost intravascular volume and placental perfusion, as prescribed. • Administer oxygen by mask to increase fetal oxygenation as ordered. • Assess for signs of the underlying cause, such as hypotension or uterine tachysystole. • Take other appropriate measures such as discontinuing oxytocin as prescribed. • Document interventions and outcomes. • Notify the obstetric registrar; further medical intervention may be necessary.

engagement. If the woman has excessive vaginal bleeding, which may signal placenta praevia, vaginal examination is contraindicated.

Obstetricians and midwives can perform vaginal examinations. In early labour, perform the vaginal examination between contractions, focusing on the extent of cervical dilation and effacement. At the end of first-stage labour, perform the examination during a contraction to focus on assessing fetal descent.

Identifying baseline FHR irregularities *(continued)*

Irregularity	Possible causes	Clinical significance	Midwifery interventions
Variable decelerations beats/minute mmHg	Umbilical cord compression causing decreased fetal oxygen perfusion	Variable decelerations are the most common deceleration pattern in labour because of contractions and fetal movement.	• Help the mother change position. No other intervention is necessary unless you detect fetal distress. • Assure the mother that the fetus tolerates cord compression well. Explain that cord compression affects the fetus the same way that breath-holding affects her. • Assess the deceleration pattern for reassuring signs: a baseline FHR that isn't increasing, short-term variability that isn't decreasing, abruptly beginning and ending decelerations and decelerations lasting less than 50 seconds. If assessment doesn't reveal reassuring signs, notify the practitioner. • Start I.V. fluids and administer oxygen by mask at 10–12 L/minute, as prescribed. • Document interventions and outcomes. • Discontinue oxytocin infusion to decrease uterine activity.

Get into position

Follow these steps during vaginal examination:
• Explain the procedure to the mother.
• Ask her to empty her bladder.
• Use abdominal palpation to identify the fetal presenting part and position.
• Help the mother into a comfortable position. Get her to make two fists and place them under her buttocks – this will tilt her pelvis and make the examination easier on her – and you!
• Place a waterproof pad under her bottom.
• Put on sterile gloves, and lubricate the index and middle fingers of your examining hand with a sterile water-soluble lubricant.

Breathe and release

• Ask the woman to relax by taking several deep breaths and slowly releasing the air.
• Insert your lubricated fingers (palmar surface down) into the vagina. Keep your uninserted fingers flexed to avoid the rectum. You should take note of the vaginal walls – temperature, muscle tone and moistness.

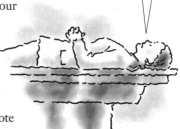

A vaginal examination works best when the woman is relaxed. Take a moment to help her breathe deeply.

Cervical effacement and dilation

As labour advances, so do cervical effacement and dilation, promoting delivery. During effacement, the cervix shortens and its walls become thin, progressing from 0% effacement (palpable and thick) to 100% effacement (fully indistinct, or effaced, and paper thin). Full effacement obliterates the constrictive uterine neck to create a smooth, unobstructed passageway for the fetus.

At the same time, dilation occurs. This progressive widening of the cervical canal – from the upper internal cervical os to the lower external cervical os – advances from 0 to 10 cm. As the cervical canal opens, resistance decreases. This further eases fetal descent.

No effacement or dilation

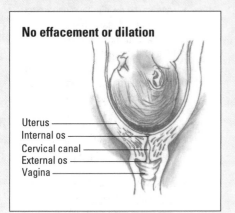

Uterus
Internal os
Cervical canal
External os
Vagina

Full effacement and dilation

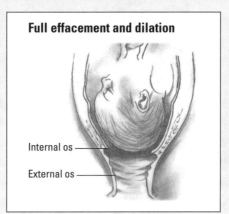

Internal os

External os

- Locate the cervix, noting its consistency. The cervix gradually softens throughout pregnancy, reaching a buttery consistency before labour begins. (See *Cervical effacement and dilation*.)
- After identifying the presenting fetal part and position and evaluating cervical dilation, effacement, engagement, station and membrane status, gently withdraw your fingers.
- Help the woman clean her perineum, and change the sanitary pad, as necessary.

Flood zone

If the amniotic membrane ruptures during the examination, record FHR and time and describe the colour, odour and approximate amount of fluid. If FHR becomes unstable, determine fetal station and check for umbilical cord prolapse. After the membranes rupture, perform vaginal examinations only when labour changes significantly, minimising the risk of introducing intrauterine infection.

Comfort and support issues

Labour and birth usually involve a significant amount of discomfort and can be emotionally draining for the woman. Comfort and support measures, such as antenatal education, a birth plan and the presence of a birthing partner or coach, can promote relaxation and decrease or eliminate the need for analgesia or anaesthesia during labour and birth.

Expect the unexpected

Although it's helpful for the woman to make decisions about the issue of pain relief during labour before the actual event, advise the woman to keep an open mind. She should be aware of the other acceptable pain relief options available in case the situation changes during labour and birth. No matter what method of pain relief is used, the woman should feel comfortable with it and it should be medically safe.

To provide comfort and support to the woman during labour and birth, you must understand sources of pain, pain perception and how it affects the woman's response to relief measures, cultural and familial influences on responses to pain and different approaches to relieving pain.

Sources of pain

The pain experienced during labour and birth comes from several sources.

Uterine contractions

The contraction of the uterine muscles is a prominent source of pain during labour and birth. Like the heart, stomach and intestine, the uterus is part of an involuntary muscle group. Although most muscles of this type don't cause pain when they contract, uterine contractions do. During a contraction, the blood vessels constrict, which reduces the blood supply to the uterine and cervical cells, causing temporary hypoxia or anoxia and pain. As labour progresses and contractions increase in intensity and duration, the blood supply to the cells decreases further, thus increasing the pain.

Dilation

Dilation and stretching of the cervix and lower uterine segment also cause pain during labour. Similar to the intestinal pain caused by accumulated gas in the bowel, this pain increases as the dilation increases.

Distention

Distention of the vagina and perineum to accommodate passage of the fetal head also causes pain during labour. As the fetal head is delivered, an episiotomy or possible tearing of the perineum intensifies this pain.

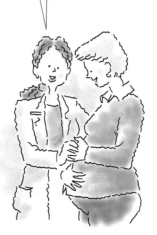

To decrease the need for analgesia or anaesthesia during labour and birth, try using appropriate comfort and support measures.

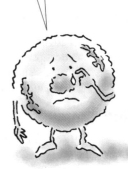

Hey! Where'd everybody go? When contractions increase in intensity and duration, the blood supply to cells decreases.

Pressure on adjacent organs

Another source of pain during labour is the pressure of the presenting part on the adjacent organs, such as the bladder, urethra or lower colon. This varies depending on the position of the fetus.

Tension

Tension also contributes to pain during labour and birth. The woman's anticipation of pain and her inability to relax commonly cause tension or constriction of the voluntary muscles, including the muscles of the abdominal wall. Tense abdominal muscles increase the pressure on the uterus by preventing the uterus from rising with the contractions.

Pain perception

Pain is a subjective symptom that's unique to each individual who experiences it. What may be slight discomfort to one person may be intense, unbearable pain to another. Only the woman who's experiencing the pain can describe it or know its extent. When assessing the woman in labour, watch for signs of pain, such as increased respiratory and pulse rates, clenched fists, facial tenseness and flushed or pale areas of the skin.

Under the influence of endorphins

Many factors influence how pain is perceived. A woman's pain threshold (the amount of pain perceived at a given time) may be influenced by her level of endorphins, the opiate-like substances that are produced by the body in response to pain.

If you expect it, pain will come

Expectations of pain can also affect how pain is perceived. A woman who expects the pain of labour to be the most horrible pain she has ever experienced commonly becomes increasingly tense with each contraction and episode of pain, which can intensify her overall perception of the pain.

Too tired and weak for distractions

Fatigue, nutritional status and sleep deprivation can also affect pain perception. A tired or malnourished individual has less energy than a rested one and can't focus on distraction strategies.

Mind games

Psychological factors, including fear, anxiety, body image, self-concept and feelings of having no control over the situation, also affect a woman's pain perception. In addition, memories of previous childbirth experiences affect how the labour pains of the current pregnancy are perceived.

Ouch! Pain is subjective. Each woman's experience during labour and birth will be unique, just like her!

More pieces to the pain puzzle

Other factors that influence pain perception during labour include the intensity of labour, pelvic size and shape and the interventions of caregivers (which can be a positive or negative influence on pain perception).

Cultural influences on pain

Individuals tend to react to pain in ways that are acceptable to their culture and family. Commonly learned through previous experience and conditioning, some women react to pain by becoming silent and avoiding interaction with other individuals; others may scream, verbalise their feelings of distress or become verbally abusive to other individuals. Make sure that you determine the level of comfort each woman desires to receive and the manner in which she chooses to express her discomfort.

Nonpharmacological pain relief

Most nonpharmacological pain relief methods are based on the gate control theory of pain, which poses that local physical stimulation can interfere with pain stimuli by closing a hypothetical gate in the spinal cord, thus blocking pain signals from reaching the brain. Nonpharmacological pain relief methods may be used as the only method of pain management during labour and delivery, or they may be used in conjunction with pharmacological interventions. Be flexible when a woman chooses an alternative method of pain relief, and provide support and reassurance if she finds that the method she has chosen isn't working effectively.

Nonpharmacological pain relief methods include various relaxation techniques, breathing techniques, heat and cold application, counterpressure, transcutaneous electrical nerve stimulation (TENS), hypnosis, acupuncture and acupressure and yoga.

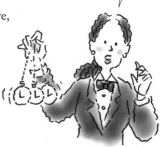

You're getting sleepy. Relaxation techniques take focus away from the pain.

Relaxation techniques

Most childbirth education classes teach relaxation techniques to their students. Relaxation turns the woman's focus away from the pain, which reduces tension. The reduced tension leads to a perceived decrease in pain, which then further reduces tension, thus breaking the pain cycle.

Let the sound take you away . . .

Relaxation techniques include positioning, focusing and imagery, therapeutic touch and massage, music therapy and the support of a birthing partner or coach. Many women find these techniques helpful in the early stages of labour, even if they later decide that they need supplemental analgesia or anaesthesia. Usually, the amount of pharmacological assistance that's needed is reduced when used in conjunction with relaxation techniques.

Positioning

Part of the relaxation process involves positioning. The woman should be taught to shift her position during labour until she finds the one that's most comfortable for her. Commonly, the position of the fetus and its presenting part determines the most comfortable position for the mother. For example, a woman with the fetus in an occipitoposterior position usually experiences intense back pain during labour. The woman should be encouraged to move about as much as possible – in and out of the bed. Sitting in the squatting position, either on a mat or a chair – or birthing stool, can be very comfortable for many women. Birthing balls are very effective at easing pelvic pain and can encourage descent of the fetal head, particularly if the woman rocks from side to side.

A change from a back or side-lying position to one on her hands and knees with her head lower than her hips usually helps to ease this pain. Left side-lying position provides the greatest perfusion of blood to the mother's organs and to the placenta, so it's the position of choice no matter what the fetal position is.

Focusing and imagery

Focusing is a relaxation technique that's used to keep the sensory input perceived during the contraction from reaching the pain centre in the cortex of the brain. During contractions, the woman concentrates intently on an object that has special meaning or appeal to her, such as a photograph.

> When using imagery, the woman mentally places herself in a relaxing environment.

Picture this

In imagery (also known as *visualisation*), the woman concentrates on a mental image of a person, place or thing. The woman may picture herself on a beach with the waves crashing on shore, in a forest or meadow with the sound of rustling leaves or singing birds or near a stream or river with the sound of the water flowing by.

Stop, hey, what's that sound?

The sounds the woman hears during this process are an important part of effective imagery because they help her stay concentrated on the image. She may want to use an item such as a music box playing her favourite tune to help her visualise her image. If a person participating in the delivery is included in the woman's visualisation, the individual should speak softly and offer words of comfort. The person could also sing or read a favourite poem to the woman.

Zip the lip

You shouldn't talk to the woman or ask her questions when she's using focusing or imagery techniques because the dialogue could break her

Education edge

Using imagery during contractions

Teach the mother about using imaging techniques by telling her to follow these steps:

- Begin with a deep cleansing breath.
- Close your eyes.
- Relax every part of your body: head and neck, shoulders, arms, hands, fingers, chest, back, stomach, hips, bottom, legs, feet and toes.
- Picture a place in your mind where you feel warm and safe. The place could be your home, a place you remember from your childhood or a place that reminds you of peacefulness, such as a warm sandy beach or a quiet meadow. Keep these details in your mind so that when a contraction gets closer, you can focus on this image and have all the details in place.
- Slowly breathe with the contraction.
- When the contraction ends, take a deep cleansing breath and return to reality.
- Open your eyes.

concentration and allow the painful stimuli to cross into the brain. An exception should be made if a coach or other support person is assisting her in maintaining her concentration by providing verbal cues. (See *Using imagery during contractions*.)

Therapeutic touch and massage

Therapeutic touch is based on the premises that the body contains energy fields that lead to either good or ill health and that the hands can be used to redirect the energy fields that lead to pain. Touching and massage actually offer a distraction that directs the woman's focus from the pain to the action of the hands. Although not well documented, it's also believed that touch and massage cause the release of endorphins that block the perception of pain. Having her back massaged or stroked, can be very soothing to the mother – and a great way of involving her partner!

Music therapy

As an adjunct to relaxation, focusing and imagery, it's usually helpful for the woman to have her favourite music available during labour and delivery. Listening to her favourite tunes usually helps the woman throughout the focusing or imagery process. It also acts as a form of diversion. Although it's recommended that the music be soft and soothing, many women find greater distraction from dance or rock 'n' roll rhythms. It may also be used in conjunction with breathing exercises; however, depending on the rhythm, music may serve to disrupt an established breathing pattern, rather than support it.

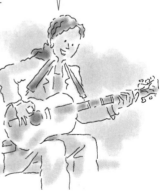

You won't strike a wrong chord when playing music to divert attention from the pain of labour and delivery.

Birthing partner

Having a capable birthing partner to provide support during labour and delivery is one of the most important factors in making the birth experience a positive one. The presence of a birthing partner can alleviate the woman's anxiety and increase her self-esteem and feelings of control over the experience, which can effectively reduce the pain or at least increase her ability to deal with it. The birthing partner may be the woman's husband, partner, parent, sibling or friend. The most important factor in choosing a support person is determining who will provide the most effective support without being influenced on an emotional level.

Doula on duty

Sometimes, a woman doesn't have someone close to her who can take on birthing partner responsibilities. In such cases, the woman may use a doula, an independent contractor with or without formal medical training who provides support during labour and delivery. However, it is important that the doula recognises and acknowledges the role of the midwife when accompanying a mother to the delivery suite of the hospital.

Breathing techniques

Breathing techniques are an important part of nonpharmacological pain relief and are taught in most childbirth preparation classes. They distract the woman from the pain of the contractions and also help to relax the abdominal muscles. When a woman is focusing on slow-paced, rhythmic breathing, she's less likely to concentrate on the pain she's experiencing.

Easing pain one breath at a time

The most common breathing technique used is the Lamaze method. Originally developed in Russia and based on Pavlov's conditioning studies, the Lamaze method was popularised by Ferdinand Lamaze, a French physician. The method incorporates the theory that women can learn to use controlled breathing to reduce the pain felt during labour through the use of stimulus-response conditioning.

In Lamaze, the woman is encouraged to direct her attention to a focal point, such as a spot on the wall, at the first sign of a contraction. This focus creates a visual stimulus that goes directly to the woman's brain. The woman then takes a deep cleansing breath, which is followed by rhythmic breathing. During the contraction, the woman's partner provides a series of commands or verbal encouragements to provide an auditory stimulus to her brain.

Relief at your fingertips

The rhythmic breathing is followed by effleurage (a light fingertip massage) that the woman or her partner performs on the abdomen or thighs. The massage introduces a tactile stimulus that goes directly to her brain, calming

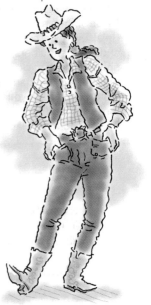

Howdy pardner! A birthing partner helps alleviate anxiety during labour and delivery.

Effective effleurage patterns

Effleurage is a light fingertip massage that the woman or her partner performs on her abdomen or thighs during contractions. This illustration shows the tracing patterns used for effleurage.

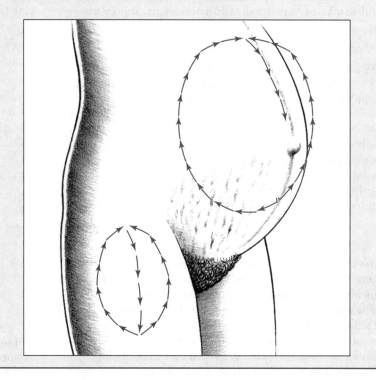

the nerves and promoting relaxation. The rate of effleurage is slow and remains constant, even though the rate of breathing may change. (See *Effective effleurage patterns*.)

It isn't too late to educate

If a woman hasn't attended childbirth preparation classes and hasn't received instruction in breathing and relaxation techniques, the techniques can be taught to her while she's in the early stages of labour. Although techniques learned under these circumstances usually aren't as effective, they may at least help to delay the use of analgesics.

Breathing on so many levels

Different levels of breathing are used depending on the intensity of the contractions. The woman's birthing partner/midwife assists in determining the level of breathing by resting a hand on her abdomen. As the strength of the contraction changes, the partner/midwife calls out the key words that act as commands to the woman.

At the start and finish of each breathing exercise, the woman takes a cleansing breath – she breathes in slowly and deeply and then exhales in the same manner. This decreases the chance of hyperventilation during rapid breathing and also helps to maintain adequate oxygen supply for the fetus.

First level

At the first level, the woman uses slow chest breathing. These full respirations should be done at a rate of 6–12 breaths/minute. The woman is instructed to use this level of breathing for early contractions.

Second level

At the second level, breathing should be heavy enough so that the rib cage expands but light enough so that the diaphragm barely moves. The rate of respirations is up to 40 breaths/minute. The second level of breathing is recommended when cervical dilation is 4–6 cm.

Third level

The third level involves shallow, sternal breathing at a rate of 50–70 breaths/minute. As the respirations become faster, the exhalation must be a little stronger than the inhalation to promote good air exchange and prevent hyperventilation. The woman can achieve a stronger exhalation than inhalation if she practises saying 'out' with each exhalation. The woman should use this level of breathing for contractions that occur during the transition phase of labour. To help prevent the oral mucosa from drying out during such rapid breathing, instruct the woman to keep the tip of her tongue against the roof of her mouth.

Fourth level

At the fourth level, the woman should use a 'pant-blow' pattern of breathing by taking three or four quick breaths in and out and then forcefully exhaling. The breathing pattern is 'hee-hee-hee-hoo' (shallow breath, shallow breath, shallow breath, long exhalation). This type of breathing is often referred to as 'choo-choo' breathing because it sounds like a train.

Fifth level

At the fifth level, the woman should perform continuous chest panting. Breaths are shallow and occur at about 60 breaths/minute. This type of breathing can be used during strong contractions or during the second stage of labour to prevent the woman from pushing before full cervical dilation. It might be useful to apply vaseline to the mother's lips to maintain moisture levels.

> Ahhh! A cleansing breath decreases the chance of hyperventilation and helps maintain the fetus's oxygen supply.

> 'Choo-choo' breathing can engineer some relief from labour pain.

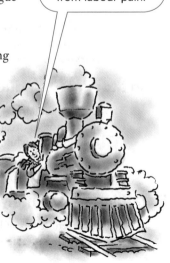

Heat and cold application

Heat application to the lower back is considered effective in reducing labour pain. A heating pad, moist compress, warm shower or bath can significantly aid relaxation if the membranes are still intact. Many women now use water immersion as an effective means of reducing pain and anxiety during labour – some enjoy it so much, they stay in the bath to have their baby!

Applying a cool cloth to the mother's forehead and providing ice chips to relieve dry mouth are other measures that can increase her comfort level. An electric fan may help to reduce her temperature but should be turned off just before the baby is born to avoid hypothermia.

Counterpressure

Counterpressure is the application of firm or forceful pressure, using the heel of the hand or fist, to the woman's lower back or sacrum during a contraction. It relieves back pain during labour by countering the pressure of the fetus against the mother's back.

The amount of force applied varies, depending on the woman. Some women prefer considerable force during a contraction, whereas others prefer firm support on the back. The exact spot for applying pressure also varies from woman to woman and may change throughout the labour. If the partner is using considerable force on the back, suggest that he hold the front of the woman's hipbone to help maintain his balance.

Transcutaneous electrical nerve stimulation (TENS)

TENS is the stimulation of large-diameter neural fibres via electric currents to alter pain perception. Although not documented as being a significant factor in reducing the pain caused by uterine contractions, TENS may be effective in reducing the extreme back pain that some women have during contractions.

Hypnosis

Hypnosis, though used infrequently, can provide a satisfactory method of pain relief for the woman who follows hypnotic suggestions. The woman must meet with the hypnotherapist several times during her pregnancy for evaluation and conditioning. If it's determined that she's a good candidate for this method of pain relief, she's given a posthypnotic suggestion that she'll experience either reduced pain during labour or no pain at all.

Acupuncture and acupressure

Acupuncture and acupressure are also methods of pain relief that are sometimes used during labour. Acupuncture is the stimulation of key trigger points with needles. It isn't necessary for the trigger points to be near the affected organ because their activation causes the release of endorphins, which reduce the perception of pain. Acupressure is finger pressure or massage at the same trigger points. Holding and squeezing the hand of a woman in labour may trigger the point most commonly used for acupuncture and acupressure during labour.

Reflexology and Aromatherapy

Many midwives now provide these services to mothers, during pregnancy, labour and postnatally.

The midwife will know which treatments are effective for the mother and will employ all her skills in making the mother more comfortable and relaxed.

Yoga

Yoga uses a series of deep breathing exercises, body stretching postures and meditation to promote relaxation, slow the respiratory rate, lower blood pressure, improve physical fitness, reduce stress and ease anxiety. It may help reduce the pain of labour through the ability to relax the body and possibly through the release of endorphins that may occur.

Pharmacological pain relief

Pharmacological pain relief during labour includes analgesia and regional or local anaesthesia. These approaches differ in the degree to which pain sensation is decreased. The main goal of using medication during labour is to relax the woman and relieve her discomfort without having a significant effect on her contractions, her pushing efforts or the fetus.

The right amount at the right time

Almost all medications given during labour have an effect on the fetus because they cross the placental barrier, so it's important to give as little medication as possible. It's also important that medications be given at the proper time. When given after cervical dilation of 5 cm in a primipara or after 3 cm dilation in a multipara, medications may, in some cases, speed the progress of labour because the woman can relax and focus on working with the contractions rather than against them. If given too early in labour, medications may slow or stop the contractions. If given within 1 hour of birth, the neonate is likely to experience neuromuscular, respiratory and cardiac depression after delivery.

Know your drugs

The midwife must be familiar enough with anaesthetic and analgesic agents to answer a woman's questions, assist the anaesthetist and obstetrician and identify adverse maternal, fetal and neonatal effects quickly.

Inhalational analgesic – Entonox

Ideal for use by the woman who does not want injections or epidurals and wants to be in control of her analgesia. It is available to all midwives and can be easily used. It may come in cylinder form or it may be piped directly into the wall of delivery suite. Entonox is composed of 50% nitrous oxide and 50% oxygen and can be administered through a mask or mouthpiece, depending on what the mother feels more comfortable with. The gas works quickly – about 20–30 seconds after she first starts to inhale it – the midwife must instruct the mother to breathe it in as soon as she feels a contraction coming so that she gets the full effect of the Entonox as her contraction reaches its peak. The important thing is that the mother administers the Entonox herself – you must never hold a mask over her face – she will lose consciousness when she has had enough and recover again quickly. There are no harmful effects from this gas – it wears off very quickly.

Some women dislike the odour from the mask, some complain of feeling dizzy and nauseous.

Entonox is ideal for procedures like suturing, or vaginal examinations which can be distressing and uncomfortable for the mother, or just to keep her pain free if it is too late for systemic analgesia to be given.

See Midwives Rules and Standards (2008) for administration of Entonox and other analgesics by accessing the Nursing & Midwifery website (www.nmc-uk.org).

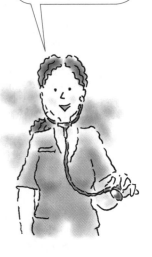

Now hear this. Opioids may cause respiratory depression in the fetus.

Opioids

Opioids are commonly used during labour because they significantly reduce pain. Some opioids have additional effects that are beneficial during labour, such as relaxing the cervix, which facilitates dilation. However, opioids depress the central nervous system of the fetus, which may lead to respiratory depression. In a preterm neonate or one who's already compromised in some way, this could be fatal.

Pethidine

Pethidine is commonly used to relieve labour pains because of its sedative and antispasmodic actions. It also gives the mother feelings of well-being and allows her to sleep, while helping to relax the cervix. Pethidine is given when the mother is more than 3 hours from birth so that there's less risk of respiratory depression in the fetus. Pethidine 100 mg/150 mg is given I.M. When given I.M., Pethidine usually begins to act within 30 minutes and its effects last approximately 3–4 hours. The possible maternal adverse effects from Pethidine are nausea, reduced gastric motility, vomiting and hypotension.

Neonatal adverse effects are depression of the central nervous system, mainly the respiratory centre, leading to reduced respiratory effort at birth – the antidote to this would be Naxalone 100 µg/kg body weight I.M.

Remifentanil

Remifentanil is an ultra short-acting opiate related to fentanyl (q.v.) that can be used to provide pain relief during labour. The mother is given the drug via a cannula in her arm or hand – she is taught how to administer the drug by pressing a button and her clinical condition is monitored closely by the midwife during labour – it is one form of patient-controlled analgesia (PCA)

How does it work?

Remifentanil hydrochloride is a short-acting, µ-receptor opioid agonist that achieves its peak analgesic effect within a minute of administration (much faster than morphine). Unlike the other opioid drugs currently in use, it's rapidly absorbed, but 95% of the metabolite is then excreted in the urine. The half life, both in infancy and in later life, is just 5 minutes. A single I.V. dose provides pain relief within 1 minute that normally only lasts for 5–10 minutes irrespective of the magnitude of the dose given. As a result, sustained analgesia for labour, or longer operative procedures requires the administration of a continuous infusion.

Is there a 'down' side?

Its commonest side effects are nausea, vomiting and headache. Not a lot is known about the potential effect on the baby due to maternal use during pregnancy or lactation but, given the drug's short biological half life, adverse effects seem unlikely. There is evidence, however, that use during operative delivery could cause brief respiratory depression in the newborn baby.

How much do I need?

Sustained use: Start by giving 1 µg/kg per minute I.V., and adjust as necessary to give 'real time' control over pain of variable intensity. Any dose high enough to provide pain relief tends to depress respiration in the newborn infant, so it should only be used as one component of a full anaesthetic strategy, and by a clinician prepared to take control of the airway if necessary (if that has not been done already).

Remifentanil has been used successfully in mothers who like being in control of their pain relief because it wears off quickly and allows them to mobilise quickly after giving birth.

Regional anaesthesia

Regional anaesthesia is used to block specific nerve pathways that pass from the uterus to the spinal cord. It relieves pain by making the nerve unable to conduct pain sensations. This form of anaesthesia allows the woman to be completely awake, aware of what's happening, and – depending on the region anaesthetised – aware of contractions, which gives her the opportunity to push at the appropriate time.

Regional results

Although regional anaesthetics aren't injected into the maternal circulatory system, they still can produce adverse effects in the neonate, such as flaccidity, bradycardia, hypotension and convulsions; however, these effects aren't as common or severe as with systemic anaesthetics.

Other side effects are sleepiness which delays or inhibits breastfeeding.

Lumbar epidural anaesthesia is the method of regional anaesthesia which is frequently used for labour and delivery. Another commonly used method is spinal anaesthesia, often used primarily for caesarean deliveries and in emergency situations.

Lumbar epidural anaesthesia

Lumbar epidural anaesthesia (also known as an epidural block) is the injection of an opioid medication, such as fentanyl (Sublimaze), bupivacaine (Marcaine) or a lidocaine-like drug (along with an opioid, such as fentanyl or morphine,

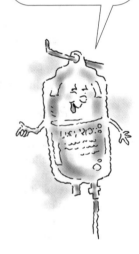

I'm just hanging around looking for some action – like taking care of labour pains.

A closer look at epidural anaesthesia

This illustration shows the placement of the epidural catheter used for injecting pain-relieving medication into the epidural space. This process anaesthetises the nerves that carry pain signals from the uterus and perineum to the brain.

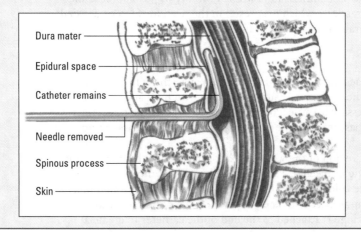

Dura mater

Epidural space

Catheter remains

Needle removed

Spinous process

Skin

to decrease the amount of motor blockage incurred). The medication is injected through a needle or catheter into the epidural space (the vacant space just outside the membrane in the lumbar region containing the cerebrospinal fluid that bathes the spinal column and brain). When the drug is administered into this space, it anaesthetises the nerves that carry pain signals from the uterus and perineum to the brain, thus dulling or eliminating the perception of pain for the woman. Women with preexisting medical conditions, such as heart disease, diabetes and gestational hypertension, tend to choose this method because it makes labour almost pain-free, which can reduce physical and emotional stress. (See *A closer look at epidural anaesthesia*.)

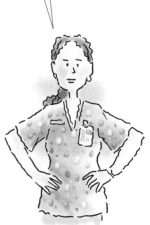

Regional anaesthesia makes the nerves unable to conduct pain sensations.

The down side, part one

Lumbar epidural anaesthesia is relatively safe, but it can lower the woman's blood pressure, which can decrease the flow of blood to the uterus and the placenta. Before receiving lumbar epidural anaesthesia, the woman should be cannulated so that in the event of sudden or severe hypotension, she can be given I.V. fluids or drugs.

Jacking up the pressure

If the woman does become hypotensive, treatment may include placement in the left side-lying position, oxygen administration, increased I.V. fluids and administration of a medication, such as ephedrine, to elevate blood pressure. Monitor FHR closely (CTG trace) during and after the epidural and especially during periods of maternal hypotension. Fetal distress can occur as a result of reduced blood flow to the placenta from hypotension.

The down side, part two

Lumbar epidural anaesthesia can also slow labour if it's given before the cervix is 5 cm dilated. It may also diminish the woman's ability to push because she's unaware of the contractions, which may result in the need for forceps-assisted delivery, vacuum extraction or caesarean birth.

How it's done

Lumbar epidural anaesthesia is administered by an anaesthesiologist. The woman is placed on her side or in a sitting position with her back straight. This position is necessary because a back in flexion increases the possibility that the needle will pass through the epidural space into the subarachnoid space.

After the lumbar region of the woman's back is cleaned with an antiseptic and a local anaesthetic is injected, a special needle is passed through the L3–L4 space into the epidural space. A catheter is then passed through the needle into the epidural space and taped in place on the skin. The needle is withdrawn, and a syringe is attached to the end of the catheter to create a closed system.

Test the waters

A small dose of the anaesthetic is injected through the catheter, and the woman is observed to make sure that the catheter is in the proper position and the desired effect is obtained. When this is ascertained, the initial dose of the anaesthetic is given. The anaesthetic takes effect within 10–15 minutes and lasts from 40 minutes to 2 hours. An infusion pump is used and the anaesthetic is infused at a slow, continuous rate. Close observation of the woman is necessary to avoid a toxic reaction from too much anaesthetic.

Step up to the baseline

Here's what you should do during the procedure:
• Perform baseline vital signs and assess FHR before the epidural is initiated.
• Monitor the woman for signs of adverse reactions to the narcotic, such as a change in sedation level, respiratory depression or itching. Also monitor the woman for adverse effects of the local anaesthetic, which may include numbness in the arms, hands or around mouth; ringing in the ears; seizure activity; nausea and vomiting and metallic taste.
• Once you've determined that the woman isn't experiencing adverse reactions to the test, monitor maternal vital signs every 5 minutes for 15 minutes, then every 15 minutes for 45 minutes and then every 30 minutes for the duration of the epidural and labour, or according to your unit's protocol.

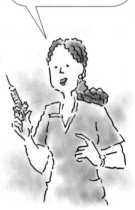

A small dose of anaesthetic is injected through the catheter before the initial dose. This verifies catheter placement and patient response.

Ins and outs

- Monitor the woman's intake and output because the woman can't feel the sensations associated with a full bladder. Encourage the woman to void at least once every 2 hours, and regularly palpate for bladder distention. In most cases the woman is usually catheterised.
- Monitor FHR and observe for fetal distress, which can result from maternal hypotension.

Continuous lumbar epidural infusion

Once the epidural block is established, 10–15 mg/hour of 0.1 or 0.125% Marcaine solution is administered via an infusion pump attached to the epidural cannula. This can be combined with a patient-controlled device which allows the woman to control how much of the drug she gets (with a strict limit). Midwives are specially trained to carry out 'top-ups' of this type of epidural infusion.

Spinal anaesthesia

With spinal anaesthesia, a local anaesthetic is injected into the cerebrospinal fluid in the subarachnoid space at the third or fourth lumbar interspace. Recently, the use of spinal anaesthesia has significantly declined, having been replaced by lumbar epidural anaesthesia. Currently, spinal anaesthesia is used more widely for caesarean birth.

For spinal anaesthesia administration, place the woman in a side-lying or sitting position with her head bent forward and her back flexed as much as possible. If she's lying down, make sure that her head and upper body are higher than her abdomen and legs so that the anaesthetic doesn't rise too high in the spinal canal.

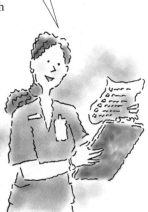

Local anaesthesia is used only for pain relief during the actual birth of the fetus because it doesn't provide relief from the pain of contractions.

The down side

As with epidural anaesthesia, hypotension is a possible adverse effect of spinal anaesthesia. Preventive measures should be taken before injecting anaesthetic, and the woman should be closely monitored afterward.

Other disadvantages of spinal anaesthesia include the possibility of a spinal headache, the risk of transient complete motor paralysis, increased incidence and degree of hypotension and urine retention.

Local anaesthesia

Local anaesthesia is used only for pain relief during the actual birth of the fetus because it doesn't provide relief from the pain of contractions.

For when labour keeps going and going and going

In most cases, the pressure of the fetal head on the perineum causes a natural anaesthesia, making local anaesthesia administration unnecessary. However, after hours of exhaustive labour, many women need this relief, especially if an episiotomy is to be performed.

Local infiltration location

Local infiltration is the injection of a local anaesthetic (usually lidocaine [Xylocaine]) into the superficial perineal nerves. This illustration shows the location of the injection.

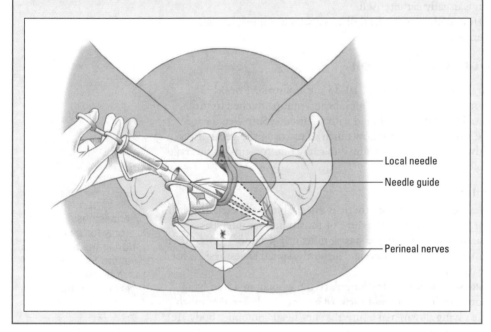

Local needle

Needle guide

Perineal nerves

Local infiltration

Local infiltration is the injection of a local anaesthetic (usually lidocaine) into the superficial perineal nerves. It's commonly used by the midwife or doctor in preparation for or before suturing an episiotomy; however, anaesthesia with this method isn't as effective as a pudendal block. (See *Local infiltration location*.)

There are no significant risks to local infiltration except rare allergic reactions and inadvertent intravascular injections. However, some practitioners believe that injection may weaken the perineal tissue and increase the likelihood of tearing.

Midwifery interventions

Midwifery interventions during labour and delivery focus on providing the woman comfort and support. Here's what you should do:

• To promote the woman's comfort and general body cleanliness, advise her to take a warm shower or, if her membranes haven't ruptured, a warm bath. If she can't walk, perform a sponge or bed bath with meticulous perineal care.

• To increase the woman's comfort and reduce the risk of infection, change her nightie and sheets whenever they become soiled. Also be sure to change the disposable underpad, especially after a vaginal examination.

- Wipe the woman's face and neck with a cool, clean washcloth, especially during the transition phase of labour.
- Psychological care is vital in labour and one of the most important aspects is support and encouragement for the mother – never leave her alone when she is frightened and give her information that allows her to make informed choices – she will feel more in control of her labour.

Comforts of home

- To increase the woman's feelings of comfort and well-being, advise her to use her own toiletries, if available.
- To maintain throat and mouth moisture, offer the woman frequent sips of water or allow her to suck on some ice, boiled sweets or a washcloth saturated with ice water. Provide mouth care during labour, and encourage the woman to brush her teeth or use mouthwash to freshen her breath.
- To moisturise and heal dry, cracked lips, help the woman to apply lip balm or petroleum jelly to her lips.
- To give the woman a sense of control over her pain, advise her about the possible causes of back pain during labour and the coping strategies that she can use.
- To help the woman relax during labour, teach her to use relaxation techniques and slow, paced breathing (not less than one-half the normal respiratory rate) between contractions.
- To help maintain relaxation during the later part of labour and to prevent hyperventilation, advise her to increase her respiratory rate (not more than twice the normal rate) and to modify her breathing pattern during contractions.
- Encourage her to listen to her favourite music as she moves about – she may want to watch TV.

Under pressure

- To reduce the woman's pain and promote her comfort, show her partner how to apply firm counterpressure with the heel of one hand to the sacral area.
- To prevent feelings of helplessness during a difficult labour, encourage the woman to let her partner know the amount and location of counterpressure that relieves the most pain. Feedback allows the partner to relieve pain most effectively.
- To allow the pressure of the fetus to fall away from the mother's back, help her to assume a side-lying, upright forward-leaning, or hands-and-knees position.
- To promote the woman's comfort and further anterior rotation of the fetus (if the fetus is in the occipitoposterior position), help her to change positions at least every 30 minutes – from side-lying to hands-and-knees to the opposite side-lying positions.
- To reduce back discomfort, apply a warm, moist towel, an ice bag or a covered rubber glove filled with ice chips to the woman's lower back.

Documentation

Ensure that all clinical observations, care discussed and given, drugs administered and staff involved in any interventions, have all been documented clearly and concisely in the mother's notes. This should be done as close to the time as possible and records should be updated as and when necessary. Verbal reports should also be given at intervals to the midwife in charge and also to any staff taking over the care of the mother.

Quick quiz

1. Which option isn't a primary factor in determining the presentation of the fetus during birth?
   A. Fetal attitude
   B. Fetal heart rate
   C. Fetal lie
   D. Fetal position

Answer: B. The primary factors that determine fetal presentation are fetal attitude, lie and position.

2. In the LOA and ROA fetal positions, the presenting part is the:
   A. olecranon.
   B. chin.
   C. occiput.
   D. buttocks.

Answer: C. The occiput is the presenting part in the LOA and ROA fetal positions.

3. Transition is part of which stage of labour?
   A. First stage
   B. Second stage
   C. Third stage
   D. Fourth stage

Answer: A. The first stage of labour is divided into three phases: latent, active, and transition.

4. In which order do the mechanisms of labour occur?
   A. Flexion, extension, internal rotation, external rotation, descent, expulsion
   B. Descent, flexion, internal rotation, extension, external rotation, and expulsion
   C. Descent, internal rotation, flexion, external rotation, extension, expulsion
   D. Descent, extension, internal rotation, flexion, external rotation, expulsion

Answer: B. The mechanisms of labour occur in this order: descent, flexion, internal rotation, extension, external rotation, and expulsion.

5. Which sign isn't a sign of true labour?
   A. Bloody show
   B. Painful uterine contractions
   C. Lightening
   D. Rupture of the membranes

Answer: C. Lightening is a preliminary sign of labour – not a sign of true labour.

6. Which uncommon fetal attitude results in a brow presentation?
    A. Partial extension
    B. Complete extension
    C. Moderate flexion
    D. Complete flexion

Answer: A. Partial extension is an uncommon fetal attitude that results in a brow presentation through the birth canal.

Scoring

☆☆☆   If you answered all six questions correctly, terrific! You certainly delivered the goods on that challenge.

☆☆   If you answered four or five questions correctly, great! Your labouring paid off.

☆   If you answered fewer than four questions correctly, keep your head up. You'll present well in the next quiz.

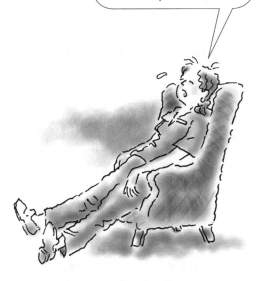

Exhausted after labouring through Labour and birth? Take a breather, and then let's move on to the next exciting chapter, Labour and birth complications.

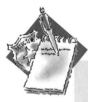

8 Complications of labour and birth

Just the facts

In this chapter, you'll learn:

♦ various complications that can occur with labour and birth
♦ ways to assess and detect problems occurring with labour and birth
♦ treatment and management of various complications.

A look at complications

Although labour usually proceeds without problems, about 8% of births involve complications. A problem can arise at any point in the labour process and can involve uterine contractions, the fetus or the birth canal.

Stress stinks, honesty works

Emotional support is essential for the mother and her birthing partner during labour and birth. Even when labour and birth progress normally, the process is stressful and usually lengthy. It's important to periodically assure the labouring woman that everything is going well and that she and the fetus are fine, as appropriate. When a complication arises, stress increases and honesty and sincerity remain just as important.

The importance of being careful

Because complications can occur at any point in the process, the mother and fetus need to be carefully monitored, this is important for several reasons. A malpositioned fetus is a major factor in birth complications. Midwives can be instrumental in identifying malposition by carrying out regular abdominal palpations to avoid complications. Early detection of signs and symptoms of uterine rupture can help reduce maternal morbidity during labour. When

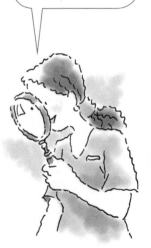

Identifying a malpositioned fetus by performing an abdominal examination is one thing a midwife can do to help avoid complications.

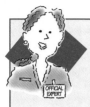

Advice from the experts

Tips for continuous electronic monitoring

When applying an external electronic fetal and uterine monitoring device, remember to explain monitoring and why it must be used to the woman in labour to ensure compliance with the technology. Also, to avoid causing the mother distraction and stress, explain in advance that the alarms may sound even when everything is going smoothly.

Don't forget

When reading the monitor pattern, remember:

- to assess the mother and fetus to verify what the various patterns suggest
- that the woman may move as a result of pain or a desire to adjust her position
- that movement may result in artefacts on the tracings that require monitor adjustment.

working with a monitoring device, be sure to explain its importance to the woman and her partner. (See *Tips for continuous electronic monitoring*.)

C is for 'complication'

In addition to problems arising from the condition of the mother or fetus, medical interventions to prevent or manage complications can cause other problems. One of the most invasive of these interventions is caesarean birth, in which a surgical incision is made in the abdominal and uterine walls for delivery of the baby. Because this procedure is commonly performed, many times as a result of other complications, it's listed below with other birth complications.

Amniotic fluid embolism

Amniotic fluid embolism occurs as rarely as 1 in 8,000 births. Occurring during labour or during the postpartum period, amniotic fluid embolism happens when amniotic fluid is forced into an open maternal uterine blood sinus due to some defect in the membranes themselves or after membrane rupture or partial premature separation of the placenta. Solid particles then enter the maternal circulation and travel to the lungs, causing pulmonary embolism. Amniotic fluid embolism isn't preventable and requires prompt intervention and lifesaving treatment.

What causes it

The exact cause of amniotic fluid embolism is unknown, but possible risk factors include:
• oxytocin administration
• placental abruption
• polyhydramnios.

How it's detected

Signs of amniotic fluid embolism are dramatic. The woman, who's commonly in strong labour when the problem occurs, may sit up suddenly and grasp her chest. She may also complain of a sharp pain in her chest and an inability to breathe. In assessment, her colour markedly pales and then turns the typical bluish grey associated with pulmonary embolism and lack of blood flow to the lungs.

What to do

Prognosis of the mother and fetus depends on the size of the emboli and the skill and speed of the emergency interventions. Immediate management of this complication includes oxygen administration by face mask or nasal cannula. Because vital organs are deprived of oxygen supply due to the emboli, within minutes the woman develops cardiopulmonary arrest, necessitating cardiopulmonary resuscitation (CPR). Even so, CPR may be ineffective because, despite providing oxygen transport to organs, it does nothing to remove the emboli. If the emboli aren't removed, blood can't circulate to the lungs. Death may occur within minutes.

Here are some other facts you should consider:
• Even if the initial insult (the emboli) is resolved, disseminated intravascular coagulation (DIC) is highly likely from the presence of particles in the bloodstream, further complicating the woman's condition.
• If the woman survives initial emergency procedures, she'll need continued management (such as endotracheal intubation) to maintain pulmonary function and therapy with fibrinogen to counteract DIC.
• Prompt transfer to the intensive care unit (ICU) is necessary.
• The prognosis for the fetus is guarded because reduced placental perfusion results from the severe drop in maternal blood pressure.
• The fetus may be delivered immediately by caesarean birth or vaginally using forceps if she is in the second stage of labour.

Cephalopelvic disproportion

A narrowing, or *contraction*, of the birth canal, which can occur at the inlet, mid-pelvis or outlet, causes a disproportion between the size of the fetal head and the pelvic diameters, or cephalopelvic disproportion (CPD). CPD results in failure of labour to progress.

Primary problems

Malpositioning can occur because the fetus's head isn't engaged in the pelvis. Malpositioning can lead to further complications. For example, if membranes rupture, the risk of cord prolapse increases significantly.

What causes it

A small pelvis is a major contributing factor in CPD. The small size of the pelvis may be the result of rickets in the early life of the mother, a genetic predisposition, or a pelvis that isn't fully matured in a young adolescent.

A perfect fit

In primigravidas, the fetal head normally engages with the pelvic brim at 36–38 weeks gestation. When this event occurs before labour begins, it's assumed that the pelvic inlet is adequate. Engagement of the head proves that the head fits into the pelvic brim and indicates that the head will probably also be able to pass through the mid-pelvis and through the outlet. In CPD, the fetal head may be too large to fit or the overall fetal size may be prohibitively large (known as *macrosomia*, or a birthweight of more than 4,000 g [8.8 lb]).

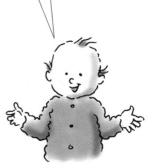

CPD means the fetal head can't fit through the mum's pelvis. It's like trying to fit a square peg through a round hole.

Inlets and outlets

Inlet contraction occurs when the narrowing of the anteroposterior diameter (from the symphysis pubis to the sacral prominence) is less than 11 cm or a maximum transverse diameter (between the ischial spines) is less than 12 cm. In outlet contraction, the transverse diameter narrows at the outlet to less than 11 cm. The outlet measurement is the distance between the ischial tuberosities.

Positional faux pas

Abnormal positions of the fetus can also cause CPD. Posterior, transverse, face, brow or breech presentations can make it difficult or impossible for the fetal presenting part to fit through the pelvis.

Fetal faux pas

Fetal anomalies such as hydrocephalus, hydrops fetalis and tumours of the fetal head can also result in CPD.

How it's detected

When engagement doesn't occur in a primigravida, a problem exists. This problem may be a fetal abnormality, such as a larger-than-usual head, or a pelvic abnormality, as in a smaller-than-usual pelvis. It's important to note that engagement doesn't usually occur in multigravidas until labour begins. In this situation, a previous delivery of a full-term infant vaginally without problems is substantial proof that the birth canal is considered adequate.

What to do

If the mother appears to have a small pelvis, or the fetus is large, the obstetrician and midwife should assess the possible risks of allowing this woman to labour for a long period of time. A decision must be made as to whether a 'trial of labour' will be allowed to assess the suitability of the pelvis for vaginal delivery. A trial labour may be allowed to continue if descent of the presenting part and dilation of the cervix are occurring. In other words, normal labour and delivery are occurring and no complications have been detected.

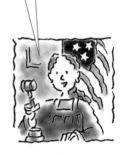

Trial labour failed! The verdict is clear: Caesarean birth is the best way to deliver a healthy baby.

Giving it a try

If a trial labour is anticipated, the following midwifery care issues are important:
• Monitor fetal heart sounds and uterine contractions continuously if possible to detect abnormalities promptly.
• Make sure that the woman's bladder is kept as empty as possible, such as by urging her to void every 2 hours, to allow the fetal head to use all the space available, making delivery possible.
• After rupture of the membranes, assess fetal heart rate (FHR) carefully. Alterations in FHR may indicate an increased danger of prolapsed cord and fetal anoxia. If the fetal head is still high, this might be an indication that the pelvic diameters are indeed reduced.
• Monitor progress of labour. After 6–12 hours, if fetal descent and cervical dilation isn't documented or fetal distress occurs at any time, the woman should be scheduled for a caesarean birth.
• Keep in mind that a woman undertaking a trial of labour may feel she'll be unable to complete the process, which may lead her to feel she's being needlessly subjected to pain. Emphasise that it's best for the baby to be born vaginally, if possible.
• If the trial of labour fails and caesarean birth is scheduled, explain why the procedure is necessary and why it's a better alternative for the baby at that point. At this point, it is vital that the woman is given as much information about the situation as possible so that she is able to give informed consent for the procedure.
• Make sure that clinical observations are recorded and all care, medications given and personnel involved are carefully documented in the mother's records.

Support

• A woman having a trial labour may feel as if she's on trial herself. She may feel she's being judged and may be self-conscious if labour doesn't go well as hoped.
• When cervical dilation doesn't occur, the woman may feel discouraged and inadequate, as if she's somehow at fault. A woman may not be aware how much she wanted the trial labour to work until she's told that it isn't working.
• Remember to support the support person. He or she may also be frightened and feel helpless when a problem occurs.

- Assure the parents that a caesarean birth isn't an inferior method of birth. Remind them that it's an alternative method. In this instance, it's the method of choice, allowing them to achieve their goal of a healthy mother and a healthy child.

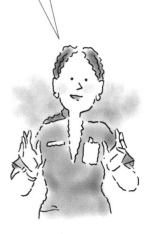

When vaginal birth isn't possible, all roads lead to caesarean birth.

Caesarean birth

Also known as *caesarean section (C/S)* or *caesarean delivery*, caesarean birth is one of the oldest surgical procedures known. It may be performed as a planned surgery (elective), or an emergency procedure when vaginal birth isn't possible. (See *Caesarean factors.*)

Follow the plan

A caesarean birth is sometimes planned when the mother has had a previous caesarean birth and for specific reasons, a vaginal birth (VBAC) isn't recommended this time. It's considered elective because the woman and her obstetrician choose the date that the caesarean birth will be performed based on her expected date of delivery and the maturity of the fetus.

VBACS

Vaginal birth after caesarean section (VBACS) is quite controversial in some regions of the UK. Some obstetricians still believe that after a mother has had a C/S, she is at high risk of uterine rupture and other complications associated with labour. For this reason, not all women will be encouraged to try for a normal birth after C/S. Some obstetricians will be very supportive of mothers who wish to try for a normal birth but will ensure that they are

---

Caesarean factors

Caesarean birth may be a planned or an emergency procedure. Factors that lead to caesarean birth may be maternal, placental or fetal in nature.

Maternal

- Cephalopelvic disproportion
- Active genital herpes or papilloma
- Previous caesarean birth by classic incision
- Disabling conditions, such as severe gestational hypertension and heart disease, that prevent pushing to accomplish the pelvic division of labour

Placental

- Placenta praevia
- Premature separation of the placenta

Fetal

- Transverse fetal lie
- Extremely low fetal size
- Fetal distress
- Compound conditions, such as macrosomic fetus in a breech lie

closely observed for potential complications and they will not be encouraged to labour for long periods where no progress is taking place.

Still dangerous

Because it's an invasive surgical procedure, caesarean birth is considered more hazardous than vaginal birth. Thus, it's usually only performed when the health and safety of the mother or fetus are in jeopardy. In addition, caesarean birth is generally contraindicated when there's a documented dead fetus. In this situation, labour can be induced to avoid an unnecessary surgical procedure.

On the rise

The incidence of caesarean birth is on the rise. In the United Kingdom, around 25% of pregnancies end in caesarean birth. In regional maternity units that care for mothers with high-risk deliveries, the rate has risen to as high as 35%. Some theories have attributed this rise to recent medical and technological advances in fetal and placental surveillance and care. However, midwifery-led units have a lower incidence of caesarean birth than more mainstream hospital services. Some suggest that the midwifery model of continuous support during labour may be a reason for the difference. A few maternity units, whose midwives and obstetricians support the promotion of normal labours and births, have caesarian section rates as low as 12%. You can access the most recent statistics on the NHS statistics website, available on http://www.ic.nhs.uk/statistics-and-data-collections/hospital-care/maternity/nhs-maternity-statistics-2006-07

Other possible influences on the rising rate of caesarean birth include:
• combination of the increasing safety of caesarean birth and the use of fetal monitors, which provide for early detection of fetal problems that would necessitate caesarean birth.
• doctors becoming increasingly skilled in the procedure while not acquiring comparable experience in alternative methods, such as external cephalic version (ECV) and exercises to encourage a breech presentation to move into a vertex presentation – or assisting in a normal, vaginal delivery.
• doctors' fears of malpractice allegations, which may result when a fetus is allowed to be delivered vaginally and then discovered to have suffered anoxia.

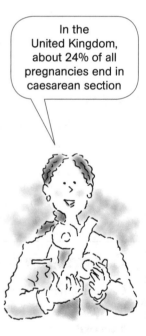

In the United Kingdom, about 24% of all pregnancies end in caesarean section

Double trouble

Occasionally, a woman may refuse to submit to a caesarean birth. Because women have a right to decide if they'll undergo surgery, the right to refuse the procedure is respected. In some instances, however, a court order to go ahead with the procedure may be obtained when caesarean birth is seen as necessary to save the life of the fetus as well as the mother. Midwives working in delivery units should be aware of the opinion of their Trust's ethics committee on this issue and should also be aware of the proper channels to take should this situation arise. Another issue which often arises is that of women requesting C/S early (<37 weeks) for no good reason, other than social. This can lead to a premature baby being admitted to the neonatal unit (NNU) requiring special/intensive care. Some midwives believe this to be wrong and potentially dangerous to the newborn infant.

Body system effects

Because caesarean birth requires a surgical procedure, it can result in systemic effects, including thrombophlebitis from interference in the body's natural stress response as well as alterations in body defences, circulatory function, organ function, self-image and self-esteem.

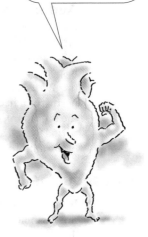

The stress response ensures that the body is ready for action with increased heart rate, lung function and glucose for energy.

Stress response

Whenever the body is subjected to stress, either physical or psychological, it responds by trying to preserve function of all major body systems. This response includes the release of epinephrine and norepinephrine from the adrenal medulla. Norepinephrine release leads to peripheral vasoconstriction, which forces blood to the central circulation and increases blood pressure. Epinephrine causes changes resulting in:

- increased heart rate
- bronchial dilation
- elevation of blood glucose levels.

These responses are considered normal and are elicited when the woman is tensed. The body is then ready for action with an increased heart rate and lung function as well as glucose for energy.

Antagonise, not minimise

However, these responses may antagonise anaesthetic action aimed at minimising body activity in the mother undergoing a caesarean birth. In addition, the stress response may result in reduced blood supply to the woman's lower extremities. The pregnant woman is prone to thrombophlebitis due to the stasis of blood flow; the stress response compounds this potential, greatly increasing the risk. Combined with other effects of stress on major body systems, the stress response can significantly increase the risks associated with surgery.

Altered body defences

The skin is the first line of defence against bacterial invasion. When the skin is incised for a surgical procedure, as in caesarean birth, this important line of defence is automatically lost. In addition, if caesarean birth is performed after membranes have been ruptured for hours, the woman's risk of infection doubles. Of course, precautions should be taken to minimise the risk to the mother through strict adherence to sterile technique during surgery and the days following the procedure.

Altered circulatory function

During caesarean birth, blood vessels are incised, a consequence of even the simplest surgical procedure. A surgical wound results in blood loss that, if extensive, can lead to hypovolaemia and decreased blood pressure. When blood pressure decreases, inadequate perfusion of body tissues results, especially if the problem isn't recognised and corrected quickly. The amount of blood lost in caesarean birth can be relatively high compared with vaginal birth. Pelvic vessels are usually congested with blood needed to supply the placenta. When pressure is placed on these vessels, blood loss occurs freely. During a vaginal birth, a woman may loose up to 500 ml of blood. This loss increases dramatically to a potential 1,000 ml with a caesarean birth.

Altered organ function

Like any body organ, the uterus may respond to being manipulated, cut or repaired with a temporary disruption in function. Pressure from oedema or inflammation can occur as fluid moves into the injured area. This normal response can further impair function of the uterus. In addition, handling of the uterus may result in a decrease in its ability to contract, which can lead to postpartum haemorrhage. Because complications may not be evident during the procedure, close assessment of the uterus is required in the postoperative period as well as an assessment of total body function to determine the degree of disruption.

What about the others?

In addition to effects on the uterus, other organs may be directly affected. For example, to reach the uterus, the bladder must be displaced anteriorly. To perform the caesarean birth, pressure must be exerted on the intestine, possibly leading to paralytic ileus or halting of intestinal function. Because of these manipulating events, uterine, bladder, intestine and lower circulatory function must be carefully assessed after a caesarean birth to detect complications early and avert potential problems.

Altered self-image or self-esteem

Surgical procedures almost always leave incisional scars that are noticeable to some extent afterwards. In some situations, the resulting scar from a caesarean birth may be quite noticeable, such as when a horizontal incision is performed across the lower abdomen. The appearance of this scar may cause the woman to feel self-conscious later. She may also experience decreased self-esteem. This decrease may stem from a belief that she's marked as someone who can't give birth vaginally.

Incision types

Depending on the type of caesarean incision, a woman may be able to deliver vaginally after previously delivering by caesarean birth. VBAC is becoming an increasingly successful alternative to elective caesarean birth. The type of incision chosen depends on the presentation of the fetus and the speed with which the procedure can be performed. In general, there are two types of caesarean incisions: classic and lower uterine segment.

Decreased blood pressure results in inadequate perfusion – especially in caesarean birth, in which blood loss is greater than in other procedures.

Classic caesarean incision

In a classic caesarean incision, the incision is made vertically through the abdominal skin and the uterus. It's made high on the uterus, for example in the case of a placenta praevia, to avoid cutting the placenta. The result of this incision type is a wide skin scar that runs through the active contractile portion of the uterus. This scarring pattern carries an additional risk of complication in future pregnancies. Because this type of scar could cause uterine rupture during labour, the woman will need very close monitoring during her next labour – the plan will include a trial of labour to assess progress within a limited time period – if she doesn't make adequate progress within this time, she will need a caesarean section. Induction would not be advised in such a mother.

Low-segment incision

Low-segment incision is the most common type of caesarean incision. Unlike the classic incision, a low-segment incision is made horizontally across the lower abdomen just over the symphysis pubis and occurs horizontally across the uterus just over the cervix. This incision type is also referred to as *Pfannenstiel's incision* or a *bikini incision* because even a low-cut bathing suit should cover it. Because it's made through the nonactive portion of the uterus, or the part of the uterus that contracts minimally, it's less likely to cause rupture in subsequent labours. Thus, the low-segment incision makes it possible for a woman to attempt VBAC. Other advantages of this incision type include:
* decreased blood loss
* ease of suturing
* minimal postpartum uterine infection risk
* decreased risk of postpartum gastrointestinal (GI) complications.

The downside

The major disadvantage of this incision is that it takes longer to perform. So if the caesarean must be done in a hurry, such as in an emergency, low-segment incision may become impractical because of time constraints.

No assumptions, please

Sometimes a skin incision is made horizontally and the uterine incision is made vertically, or vice versa. Thus, during a future pregnancy, don't assume that a small skin incision indicates a small uterine incision.

When is it necessary?

Caesarean birth is indicated when labour or vaginal birth carries an unacceptable risk for the mother or fetus, such as in CPD and transverse lie or other malpresentations. It may also be necessary if induction is contraindicated or difficult, or if advanced labour increases the risk of morbidity and mortality.

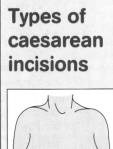

Types of caesarean incisions

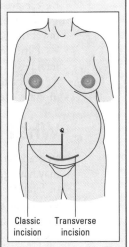

Classic incision   Transverse incision

The most common reasons for caesarean birth are:
- malpresentation of the fetus (such as shoulder or face presentation)
- evidence of fetal intolerance of labour stress
- CPD in which the pelvis is too small to accommodate the fetal head
- certain cases of pre-eclampsia
- previous caesarean birth, especially with a classic incision
- inadequate progress in labour (failure of induction).

Fetus in distress

Conditions causing fetal distress can also indicate a need for caesarean birth. These conditions include:
- living fetus with prolapsed cord
- fetal hypoxia
- abnormal FHR patterns
- unfavourable intrauterine environment, such as from infection
- moderate to severe rhesus factor (Rh) isoimmunisation.

Mum needs help

Less commonly, maternal conditions may necessitate caesarean birth. These conditions include:
- complete placenta praevia
- placental abruption
- placenta accreta
- malignant tumours
- chronic diseases in the mother in which delivery is indicated before term.

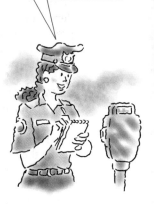

When labour or vaginal birth carries an unacceptable risk for the mother or fetus, caesarean birth is just the ticket.

How it's detected

Special tests and monitoring procedures provide early indications of the need for caesarean birth:
- X-ray or magnetic resonance imaging (MRI) pelvimetry may be carried out if the pelvis is thought to be contracted (after delivery).
- Ultrasonography shows pelvic masses that interfere with vaginal birth and fetal position.
- Auscultation of FHR (by foetoscope, Doppler unit or electronic fetal monitor) determines acute fetal intolerance of labour.

What to do

In preparation for caesarean birth, an anaesthetic is administered. Mothers may have general or regional anaesthetic, depending on the extent of maternal or fetal distress. The woman is then positioned on the operating table. A towel may be placed under her left hip to help relocate abdominal contents so that they're up and away from the surgical field. This can also assist in lifting the uterus off the vena cava, promoting better circulation to the fetus as well as maternal blood return.

Blocking bacteria as well as the view

A screen or some other type of shielding may be placed at the mother's shoulder level and covered with a sterile drape. This not only serves as a courtesy to help obstruct her view of the necessary surgical incision, but also helps to block the flow of bacteria from the woman's respiratory tract to the incision site. Placement of the drape also blocks the support person's line of vision, preventing additional anxiety and fear that may arise from the sight of blood.

Support for the support

The support person is usually positioned at the mother's head as long as the mother is conscious – if the mother has been intubated and is unconscious, the support person waits outside theatre. The incision area on the woman's abdomen is then scrubbed, and drapes are placed around the area of incision so that only a small area of skin is left exposed. In many cases, watching a caesarean birth is the first surgery the father or support person has witnessed. Thus, the person may be too overwhelmed by the whole event or too interested in the procedure to be of optimum support. He or she may become concerned about the amount of manipulation and cutting that occurs before the uterus itself is cut, assuming fetal distress isn't extreme. Remember to prepare the mother and support person for what they might see. This can help avert too much shock or surprise as well as promote open discussion about how much they would like to see or not see.

Remember to prepare the mother and support person for what they might see in the operating room.

The down side

Possible maternal complications of caesarean birth include:
- respiratory tract infection
- wound infection or haematoma
- thromboembolism
- paralytic ileus
- haemorrhage
- genito-urinary tract infection
- bowel, bladder or uterine injury.

Before surgery

Preoperative care measures involve both the mother and fetus. Here are some measures you should take:
- Assess maternal and fetal status frequently until delivery – document all observations.
- If ordered, make sure that an ultrasound has been obtained. The doctor may have ordered the test to determine a definite fetal position.
- Explain caesarean birth to the mother and her partner, and answer any questions they may have.
- Provide reassurance and emotional support to help improve the self-esteem and self-concept of the mother and her partner. Remember that a

caesarean birth is commonly performed after hours of labour, resulting in an exhausted woman and partner. Be brief but clear and stress the essential points about the procedure.

• For an elective, planned caesarean birth, discuss the procedure with both parents and provide preoperative information.

• Observe the mother for signs of imminent delivery.

• Restrict food and fluids after midnight if a general anaesthetic is ordered to prevent aspiration of vomitus.

• Prepare the woman by shaving the pubic region from about 2 cm above the pubic hairline.

• Make sure the woman's bladder is empty, use an indwelling urinary catheter as ordered, and check for flow and patency – this could be done when she has been given her anaesthetic. Tell the mother that the catheter may remain in place for 24 hours or longer.

• Administer ordered preoperative medication and record it in the mother's medicine kardex.

• Give the mother an antacid to help neutralise stomach acid.

• The mother will have an I.V. infusion for fluid replacement therapy using her nondominant hand if required. Use an 18 G or larger catheter to allow blood administration through the I.V. if needed.

• Make sure that grouping and crossmatching of the mother's blood has been carried out and that two units of blood are available.

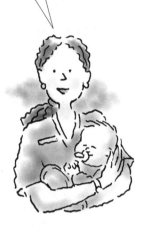

As soon as possible after delivery, encourage 'skin-to-skin' with mother and baby to promote bonding.

After surgery

Postoperative care measures of the mother and infant include:

• As soon as possible, encourage the mother to see, touch and hold her baby, either in the delivery room or after she recovers from the general anaesthetic. Contact with the baby promotes bonding.

• Check the perineal pad and abdominal dressing on the incision every 15 minutes for 1 hour, then every half-hour for 4 hours, every hour for 4 hours and finally every 4 hours for 24 hours.

• Check the dressing frequently for bleeding, and report it immediately. Be sure to keep the incision clean and dry.

• Monitor vital signs every 5–10 minutes until stable. Then check vital signs when you evaluate perineal and abdominal drainage.

• The doctor may order Syntocinon mixed with the first 1 L of I.V. fluids infused, to promote uterine contraction and decrease the risk of haemorrhage. Make sure the I.V. is patent and monitor the woman carefully for effects of the medication.

• Monitor intake and output as ordered. Expect the mother to receive I.V. fluids for 12–24 hours.

• Make sure the catheter is patent and urine flow is adequate. Observe the colour of the urine – it is possible, in emergency cases, that the bladder may have been touched by the scalpel during surgery leading to haematuria. When the catheter is removed, make sure that the woman can void without difficulty and that urine colour and amount are adequate.

- Maintain a patent airway for the mother and the baby.
- Encourage the mother to cough and deep-breathe to encourage respiratory recovery.
- If a general anaesthetic was used, remain with the woman until she's responsive.
- If regional anaesthetic was used, monitor the return of sensation to the legs.
- Help the mother to turn from side to side every 1–2 hours.
- If prescribed, show the woman how to administer patient-controlled analgesia (PCA)
- Administer pain medication as ordered and note the effect.
- If the mother wants to breastfeed, offer encouragement and help.
- Recognise 'afterpains' in multiparas and monitor the effects of pain medication. Timing of administration of pain medication and breastfeeding may need to be coordinated; this is so that the baby won't receive as much of the sedating effect, but the mother is as pain free as possible.
- Document all care given, medication administered and complete care plans as per unit policy.
- Promote early ambulation to prevent cardiovascular and pulmonary complications. Remember to assist the mother initially and make sure she doesn't suffer from orthostatic hypotension. Warn her that lochia may flow freely when she moves from a supine to an upright position.

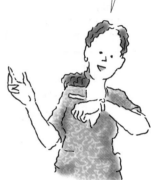

After caesarean birth, check the perineal pad and abdominal dressing frequently for the first 24 hours.

Going home

Home care instructions should also be provided to a woman who has had a caesarean birth, including:
- Encourage the mother to get as much rest as possible to promote healing and recovery.
- Discourage her from heavy household duties or lifting heavy weights as this could induce strain injury or bleeding from her genital tract.
- Instruct the woman to immediately report haemorrhage, chest or leg pain (possible thrombosis), dyspnoea or separation of the wound's edges.
- Tell her to also report signs and symptoms of infection, such as fever, lower abdominal pain, difficulty urinating and flank pain.
- Remind the woman that her community midwife will be visiting her for up to 10 days and she will give her support and advice during that time – and for longer if necessary.
- Remind the woman to keep her follow-up appointment. At that time, she can talk to the doctor about using contraception and resuming intercourse.

Fetal presentation or position

Problems can occur with the fetus's presentation or position during labour and delivery. Although most fetuses move into the proper birthing position, alternative positions and presentations can occur, making vaginal delivery difficult and, in some situations, impossible.

A briefing on brow presentation

A brow presentation (the rarest of the presentations) may occur with a multipara or in an individual with relaxed abdominal muscles. Here are some key points about this type of presentation.

- It almost invariably results in obstructed labour because the head becomes jammed in the brim of the pelvis as the occipitomental diameter presents.
- Unless the presentation spontaneously corrects, caesarean birth is necessary to safely deliver the baby.
- Because brow presentation leaves extreme bruising on the baby's face and head, his parents may need additional reassurance that he's healthy.

Problematic presentations and positions

Some presentations and positions that can be problematic include occipitoposterior position, breech presentation, face presentation and transverse lie. A fifth type of presentation, called *brow presentation*, is rarely seen. (See *A briefing on brow presentation*.)

Occipitoposterior position

In about one-tenth of labours, the fetal position may be posterior rather than the traditional anterior position. When this occurs, the occiput, assuming the presentation is vertex, is directed diagonally and posteriorly, right occipitoposterior or left occipitoposterior. In these positions, during internal rotation, the fetal head must rotate through an arc of approximately 135°, rather than the normal 90° arc.

This rotation through the 135° arc may not be possible if the fetus is above average in size or isn't in a well flexed position, or if contractions are ineffective. Ineffective contractions may occur in:
- uterine dysfunction from maternal exhaustion
- fetal head arrested in the transverse position (transverse arrest).

1-2-3 rotate!

If rotation through the 135° arc doesn't occur but the fetus has reached the mid-portion of the pelvis, he may be rotated manually to an anterior position with forceps and then delivered. As an alternative, caesarean delivery may be preferred because the risk of a mid-forceps manoeuvre exceeds the risk of caesarean delivery. If mid-forceps are used for birth, the woman is at risk for reproductive tract lacerations, haemorrhage and infection in the postpartum period.

Breech presentation

Most fetuses are in a breech presentation early in pregnancy. However, in many pregnancies, the fetus turns to a cephalic presentation by week 38, only 3–4% of fetuses will stay in breech presentation. Although the fetal head is the widest single diameter, the fetus's buttocks (breech), plus the lower extremities, takes up more space. The fundus, being the largest part of the uterus, promotes fetal turning so that the buttocks and lower extremities are within it. Additionally, some evidence suggests that a breech presentation is less likely to occur if a woman assumes a knee–chest position for approximately 15 minutes three times per day during pregnancy.

Styles of breech from frank to complete

There are several types of breech presentations:
- frank breech – in which the buttocks are the presenting part and the legs are extended and rest on the fetal chest
- footling breech – which can be either one foot (single-footling breech) or both feet (double-footling breech) and the thighs or lower legs aren't flexed
- complete breech – in which the fetal thighs are flexed on the abdomen and both the buttocks and the tightly flexed feet are against the cervix.

Danger, danger!!

Breech presentation is more hazardous than a cephalic presentation because there's a greater risk of:
- anoxia from a prolapsed cord
- traumatic injury to the aftercoming head, which can result in intracranial haemorrhage or anoxia
- fracture of the spine or arm
- dysfunctional labour
- early rupture of the membranes because of the poor fit of the presenting part
- meconium aspiration (the inevitable contraction of the fetal buttocks from cervical pressure commonly causes meconium to be extruded into the amniotic fluid before birth).

Same stages

In a breech birth, the same stages of flexion, descent, internal rotation expulsion and external rotation occur as in a cephalic birth. (See *A look at breech birth*, page 334.)

Turn, turn, turn

An alternative to vaginal or caesarean birth of a fetus in breech presentation is a method called *external cephalic version*. In this method, the fetus is manually turned from a breech to a cephalic position before birth. Use of external version can decrease the number of caesarean births due to breech presentations if done by a skilled practitioner. To turn the fetus:

The breech and vertex of the fetus are located and grasped transabdominally by an examiner's hands on the woman's abdomen.

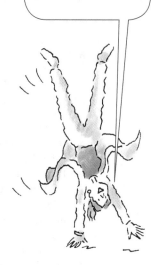

To put a different spin on things, in external cephalic version, the fetus is manually turned from a breech presentation to a cephalic position before birth.

A look at breech birth

A breech presentation follows the same stages of descent, flexion and rotation as a cephalic presentation.

As the breech fetus enters the birth canal, descent and external rotation occur, as shown below.

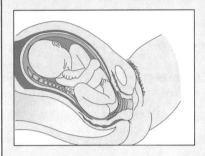

If the presenting part is the buttocks, the doctor/midwife reaches up into the birth canal and pulls the legs down and out, as shown below. The breech delivery continues as the shoulders turn and present in the anteroposterior diameter of the mother's pelvis. Hands off the Breech!!

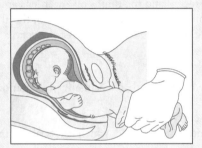

The head is then delivered by laying the baby across the doctor/midwife's left hand while the index and 3rd finger are placed on the baby's cheekbones, the other hand is placed on the back of the neck to apply gentle pressure to flex the head fully, as shown below. At the same time, gentle upward and outward traction is applied to the shoulders. An assistant may need to gently apply external abdominal wall pressure to ensure that head flexion occurs.

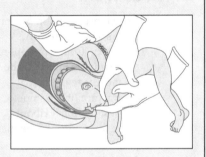

Gentle pressure is then exerted to rotate the fetus. The fetus must be moved in a forward direction to a cephalic lie. (See *A look at external cephalic version*, page 335.)

However, this procedure is not without risks to the mother and the fetus:
- It can be painful.
- It has been known to cause placental abruption.
- It has been known to cause uterine rupture.
- It causes foetomaternal haemorrhage.

ECV is contraindicated when:
- C/S is required
- mother has had an Antepartum Haemorrhage (APH) within the previous 7 days
- abnormal cardiotocograph (CTG)
- major uterine anomaly
- ruptured membranes
- multiple pregnancy (except for 2nd twin)

Let's face this head on. A face presentation results from some abnormality in the fetus or mother.

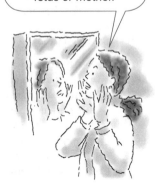

A look at external cephalic version

In external cephalic version, the practitioner manually rotates the fetus. The fetus is rotated by external pressure to a longitudinal lie, with cephalic presentation, aiding the possibility of a normal vaginal delivery.

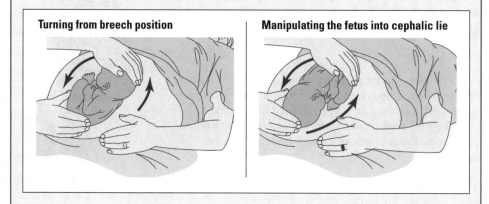

Turning from breech position | **Manipulating the fetus into cephalic lie**

- unstable lie
- pre-eclamptic mother

Remember the anti-D!

All mothers who are Rh-negative must be given anti-D following ECV and this should be prescribed by the obstetrician, administered by the midwife and documented in the mother's records.

Occipitoposterior position

Posterior positions tend to occur in women with these pelvic structures:
- android pelvis
- anthropoid pelvis
- contracted pelvis.

On assessment, a posteriorly presenting head will be found to not fit the cervix as snugly as one occurring in an anterior position. Because this increases the risk of prolapse of the umbilical cord, the position of the fetus should be confirmed by abdominal palpation and vaginal examination (some doctors may use ultrasound scan). On abdominal examination, a 'saucer' shaped dip might be observed around the umbilical area of the woman's abdomen, indicating that the fetal spine is lying parallel to the mother's. On palpation, it is difficult to feel a back to either side of the abdomen, and the head may be well above the brim.

A posterior position may also be suspected when dysfunctional labour patterns occur, such as:
- prolonged active phase
- arrested descent
- fetal heart is heard best at the lateral sides of the abdomen.

Oops! Am I early? Gestational age less than 40 weeks can contribute to breech presentation.

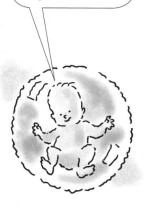

Getting into position

Most fetuses presenting in posterior positions rotate during labour, and birth can proceed normally. This scenario is most common when the fetus is of average size and in good flexion. This rotation is also aided by forceful uterine contractions causing the fetus to rotate through the large arc. The fetus arrives at a good birth position for the pelvic outlet in these situations and can be delivered satisfactorily. The fetus may experience slightly increased moulding and caput formation.

Drawing it out

One of the drawbacks to the posterior position is the duration of the labour process. Because the arc of rotation is greater, it's common for the labour to be somewhat prolonged. Labour pain is also different in this type of positioning. Because the fetal head rotates against the sacrum, the woman may experience pressure and pain in her lower back from sacral nerve compression during labour.

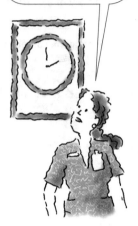

Posterior position may be suggested by a prolonged active phase.

Breech presentation

Breech presentation may occur for various reasons, including:
• gestational age less than 40 weeks
• fetal abnormality from anencephaly, hydrocephalus or meningocele
• hydramnios, which allows free fetal movement so the fetus doesn't have to engage for comfort
• congenital anomaly of the uterus, such as a mid-septum, that traps the fetus in a breech position
• space-occupying mass in the pelvis that doesn't allow engagement, such as a fibroid tumour of the uterus and placenta praevia
• pendulous abdomen in the mother that occurs when the abdominal muscles are lax, which may cause the uterus to fall so far forward that the head comes to lie outside the pelvic brim, causing breech presentation
• multiple gestation in which the presenting fetus can't turn to a vertex position.

Breech presentation is detected by these findings:
• Fetal heart is commonly heard high in the abdomen.
• Abdominal palpation will identify the fetal head in the uterine fundus.
• Vaginal examination reveals the presence of the buttocks or the foot (or both) as the presenting part, although, if the breech is complete and firmly engaged, the tightly stretched gluteal muscles may be mistaken on vaginal examination for a head and the cleft between the buttocks may be mistaken for the sagittal suture line.
• Ultrasound reveals the position of the fetus and provides information on pelvic diameter, fetal skull diameter and the existence of placenta praevia.

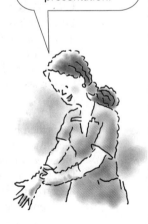

Be careful! Tightly stretched gluteal muscles can be mistaken for a head during vaginal examination for breech presentation.

Face presentation

In a face presentation, the chin, or mentum, is the presenting part. Although this presentation is rare, when it does occur, birth usually can't proceed because the diameter of the presenting part is too large for the maternal pelvis. A fetus in a posterior position, instead of flexing the head as labour proceeds, may extend the head, resulting in a face presentation. The situations in which this occurs include:

- a woman with a contracted pelvis
- placenta praevia
- relaxed uterus of a multipara
- prematurity
- hydramnios
- fetal malformation.

When a face presentation is suspected, an ultrasonography can be performed to confirm the position of the fetus. If indicated, measurements of the pelvic diameters are made. Other signs of face presentation include:

- fetus's head that feels more prominent than normal with no engagement apparent on abdominal palpation
- fetus's head and back that are both felt on the same side of the uterus on palpation
- difficulty outlining the fetus's back (because it's concave)
- fetal heart is heard on the side of the fetus where feet and arms can be palpated (in extremely concave back, which causes transmission of fetal heart to the forward-thrust chest)
- vaginal examination that reveals the nose, mouth or chin as the presenting part.

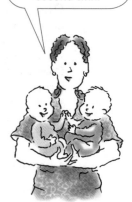

Seeing double? Multiple gestation can cause transverse lie, especially in a second twin.

Transverse lie

Transverse lie occurs in these conditions:

- a woman with a pendulous abdomen
- a uterine mass, such as fibroid tumour, that obstructs the lower uterine segment
- contraction of the pelvic brim
- congenital uterine abnormalities
- hydramnios
- hydrocephalus or other gross abnormalities that prevent the head from engaging
- prematurity
- room for free fetal movement in the uterus
- multiple gestation (particularly in a second twin)
- short umbilical cord
- placenta praevia
- fetal abnormalities.

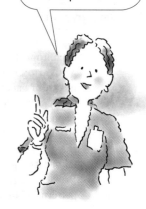

Intervention depends on the specific presentation and position.

How it's detected

Detection of abnormalities also depends on the specific fetal position or presentation abnormality.

A transverse lie is usually obvious on inspection, when the ovoid of the uterus is found to be more horizontal than vertical. Other detection methods include:
• abdominal palpation when the midwife may discover the fetus in a transverse lie position
• ultrasonography, which confirms transverse lie and provides other information (such as placenta praevia).

What to do

Management of fetal position or presentation abnormalities depends on the specific type of abnormality.

Occipitoposterior position

Because labour pain may be intense when a fetus is in the occipitoposterior position, management can be a challenge. Commonly, the labouring woman asks for medication for relief of the intense pressure on and pain in her back. Consider alternative methods to help relieve back pressure, such as those mentioned here:
• Place pressure on the sacrum, such as with a back rub, or suggest a position change to relieve some of the pain.
• Apply heat or cold, depending on which is more successful in obtaining relief.
• Ask the woman to lie on the side opposite the fetal back or maintain a hands-and-knees position to help the fetus rotate. Sitting on the birthing ball is great for encouraging fetal rotation and descent.
• Encourage the woman to void approximately every 2 hours to keep the bladder empty to avoid impeding the descent of the fetus and additional discomfort.
• Because of the commonly lengthy labour, be aware of how long it has been since the woman last ate. During a long labour, she may need I.V. glucose solutions to replace glucose stores used for energy.

I.V. glucose may be necessary for energy in a prolonged labour when the woman hasn't eaten in a long time.

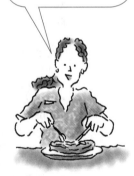

Something else to consider

Here are some other considerations for the woman delivering a baby in the occipitoposterior position:
• During labour, the woman needs a great deal of support to prevent her from becoming panicked over the length of the labour. In addition, you should provide practical, step-by-step explanations of what's happening.
• Be aware that the woman who's best prepared for labour is commonly the most frightened when deviations occur because she realises that her labour isn't going 'by the book', or as described by the doctors and midwives. Provide frequent reassurance to her that, although the labour is long, her pattern of labour is still within safe, controlled limits.

Breech presentation

If the fetus in a breech presentation can be born vaginally, when full cervical dilation is reached, the woman is allowed to push and the breech, trunk and shoulders are delivered. Here's what else you can expect:
• As the breech spontaneously emerges from the birth canal, it's steadied and supported by a sterile towel held against the baby's inferior surface.
• The shoulders present towards the outlet, with their widest diameter anteroposterior. If the shoulders don't deliver readily, the arm of the posterior shoulder may be drawn down by passing two fingers over the baby's shoulder and down the arm to the elbow and then sweeping the flexed arm across the baby's face and chest and out.
• The other arm is then delivered in the same way. External rotation is allowed to occur to bring the head into the best outlet diameter.
• Hands off the breech! – It is vital that at this point, the baby's lower abdominal area is not grabbed or squeezed unduly as this can result in rupture of his liver, spleen or kidneys.

Everything comes to a head

Birth of an aftercoming head involves a great deal of judgment and skill. Here's how it's done:
• To aid delivery of the head, the trunk of the baby is usually straddled over the doctor's right forearm.
• He places one finger of his right hand on each of the baby's cheekbones.
• The doctor slides his left hand into the mother's vagina, palm down, along the baby's back.
• Pressure is applied to the occiput to flex the head fully.
• Gentle traction applied to the shoulders (upward and outward) delivers the head.

Pied Piper

An aftercoming head may also be delivered using Barnes Neville forceps to control the flexion and rate of descent. (See *Using Barnes Neville forceps*.)

Using Barnes Neville forceps

Occasionally, the fetal head can't be easily delivered in a breech presentation. Barnes Neville forceps may be used to apply traction directly to the head, preventing damage to the fetal neck.

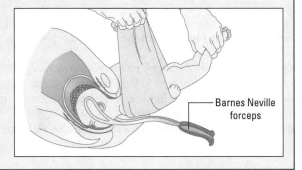

Barnes Neville forceps

Head hazards

Birth of the head is the most hazardous part of a breech birth. Here are some complications to consider:
- Because the umbilicus comes before the head, a loop of cord passes down alongside the head and automatically becomes compressed. This compression is due to the pressure of the head against the pelvic brim.
- With a cephalic presentation, moulding to the confines of the birth canal occurs over hours. With a breech birth, this pressure change occurs instantaneously. Tentorial tears can occur as a result of this pressure change. These tears may cause gross motor malfunction, mental problems or lethal damage to the fetus.
- The baby may be delivered suddenly to decrease the duration of cord compression. Doing so, however, may result in an intracranial haemorrhage.
- A baby delivered gradually in order to reduce the possibility of intracranial injury may suffer hypoxia.

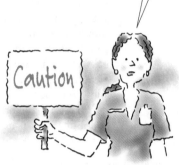

Here's a heads up. The most hazardous part of a breech birth is the birth of the head.

What happened?

Parents and health care providers usually inspect a breech newborn baby a little more closely than a baby from a normal delivery for many reasons:
- The cause of the breech birth may be unknown. The parents and the person who makes the initial physical assessment of the infant may look for the reason that made the presentation breech.
- Remember that a baby who was delivered in a frank breech position may resume his fetal position. He may keep his legs extended and at the level of the face for the first 2–3 days of life.
- The baby who presented in a footling breech may keep the legs extended in a footling position for the first few days.
- The baby, who was in breech presentation during a long labour, may have very bruised buttocks, or in the case of the male infant, his scrotum could be very sore for a few days.
- Be sure to point out these possible positions to the parents to avoid undue worry or a misinterpretation of the baby's unusual posture.

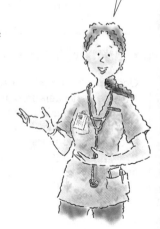

Be sure to point out these possible positions to the parents to avoid undue worry or a misrepresentation of the baby's unusual posture.

Alternate version

If ECV is performed before the birth to turn the fetus to a cephalic position, remember the following considerations:
- FHR and, possibly, ultrasound should be recorded continuously.
- A tocolytic agent may be administered to help relax the uterus.
- Provide support to the woman to help her tolerate the discomfort from the pressure experienced during the procedure.
- Women who are Rh-negative should receive anti-D in case minimal bleeding occurs.

Face presentation

If the chin is anterior and the pelvic diameters are within normal limits, the fetus in face presentation may be delivered without difficulty. However, certain complications must be considered:
• There may be a long first stage of labour because the face doesn't mould well to make a snugly engaging part.
• If the chin is posterior, caesarean delivery is the optimal method of birth because a vaginal birth would require posterior-to-anterior rotation, which could take a long time. In addition, such rotation can result in uterine dysfunction or a transverse arrest.

Oedema dilemma

Babies born after a face presentation have a great deal of facial oedema and may be purple from ecchymotic bruising. Additional considerations include:
• Lip oedema may be so severe that the baby can't suck for 1 or 2 days.
• The baby may need gavage feedings to obtain enough fluid until he can suck effectively.
• The baby must be observed closely for a patent airway.
• The baby is usually transferred to a neonatal ICU for the first 24 hours.
• Assure the parents that the oedema will disappear in a few days and usually causes no long-term effects.

Transverse lie

A mature fetus in a transverse lie can't be delivered vaginally. Although the membranes usually rupture at the beginning of labour, there's no firm presenting part. Thus, the cord or arm may prolapse or the shoulder can come down and obstruct the cervix. Caesarean birth is mandatory in this instance. Thus, to manage transverse lie presentation, follow the care measures for caesarean birth.

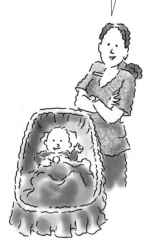

Assure parents that facial oedema will disappear in a few days and usually causes no long-term effects.

Fetal size

The size of the fetus may be an indication of a difficult delivery. In general, a fetus who weighs more than 4,500 g (9.9 lb) may lead to a difficult delivery. An abnormally large fetal size may pose a problem at birth because it can cause fetal pelvic disproportion or uterine rupture from obstruction. The risk of perinatal mortality in larger neonates is substantially higher than in normal-sized neonates. The large baby born vaginally also has a higher-than-normal risk of:
• cervical nerve palsy
• diaphragmatic nerve injury
• fractured clavicle because of shoulder dystocia.

Mum, too

During the postpartum period, the mother has an increased risk of haemorrhage because an overdistended uterus may not contract as readily.

Shoulder dystocia

Shoulder dystocia is increasing in incidence along with the increasing average weight of neonates. The problem occurs at the second stage of labour when the fetal head is born but the shoulders are too broad to enter the pelvic outlet. This situation can cause vaginal or cervical tears in the mother or cord compression leading to a fractured clavicle or brachial plexus injury in the fetus.

What causes it

Large fetuses are most common in women who are diabetic. Large babies are also associated with multiparity, because each baby born to a diabetic woman tends to be slightly heavier and larger than the one born just before. Shoulder dystocia is most apt to occur in babies of women with diabetes, multiparas and in postterm pregnancies.

How it's detected

Although fetal size can usually be detected using palpation, it may be missed in an obese woman because the fetal contours are difficult to palpate. Also, just because she's obese doesn't mean the woman has a larger-than-usual pelvis; in fact, her pelvis may be small. Pelvimetry or sonography is the best way to compare fetal size with the woman's pelvic capacity.

Head and . . . shoulders?

Shoulder dystocia, however, commonly isn't identified until the head has been born. The wide anterior shoulder then seems to lock beneath the symphysis pubis. Shoulder dystocia may be suspected earlier if:
• second stage of labour is prolonged
• arrest of descent occurs
• the head, when it appears on the perineum (crowning), retracts instead of protruding with each contraction (turtle sign).

What to do

If the fetus is so large that he can't be delivered vaginally, caesarean delivery becomes the method of choice. Shoulder dystocia is a major obstetrical emergency and needs urgent, efficient management by a well-trained, efficient team. The emergency should be managed by instigating the following steps in the HELPERR mnemonic:

1. H – HELP. Call appropriate staff for help: sister in charge, 2nd midwife, senior obstetrician, anaesthetist and paediatrician – explain to the family what is happening.
2. E – Evaluate. Is this a real shoulder dystocia, or is it caused by maternal posture, with sacrum pushed up, leaving not enough room at the outlet? In this case, consider left lateral position, or (in the absence of an epidural), squatting or kneeling (all fours).

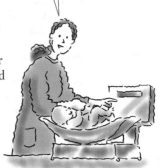

The incidence of shoulder dystocia is increasing along with the increasing average weight of newborn babies.

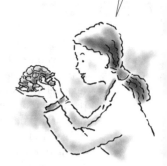

When the head of the fetus appears on the perineum and then retracts with each contraction, it's known as the 'turtle' sign.

3. L – Legs into McRoberts position. Hips are abducted, rotated outwards and flexed, so that thighs touch the mother's abdomen, with the aid of two assistants. The buttocks need to come over the edge of the bed, allowing the sacrum to rotate backwards.

4. P – Pubic bone. Apply suprapubic pressure: another assistant puts hand laterally and pushes in direction that the baby is facing and posteriorly to try and disimpact the anterior shoulder. This is done at the same time as moderate traction of head; 91% of cases will be delivered by this stage. It is vital that the fetal position was established before so that the midwife is pushing in the right direction.

5. E – Enter/evaluation. Evaluate for episiotomy, make or enlarge episiotomy; this enables access to the vagina for step 6 or 7. Internal rotation can be attempted here.

   There is *NO* place for fundal pressure or undue traction on the head. The brachial plexus is already under stretch and further traction results in neurological damage. Fundal pressure can only increase impaction of the shoulder under the symphysis pubis.

6. Woodscrew manoeuvre. Rotation of the posterior shoulder by 180° to deliver the anterior shoulder from under the symphysis pubis. Rubin's manoeuvre is turning the baby in the opposite direction (reverse Woods manoeuvre). This has the advantage of abducting the shoulders, thereby decreasing the diameter.

OR

7. R – Remove the posterior arm. To deliver the posterior arm, insert hand into sacral hollow to identify the posterior shoulder, arm down to the wrist. Sweep this across the fetal chest, flexing the elbow, to deliver the arm posteriorly.

8. R – Roll the woman over onto all fours.

9. Zavanelli manoeuvre (cepahalic replacement). This manoeuvre can be attempted, whereby there is manual return of the partially born, but undeliverable fetus, to the vagina for extraction by caesarian section. This is done by rotating the head back to the anterior occipital position, flexing the head with pressure on the occiput whilst using the other hand to replace the chin back into the vagina. Tocolytics can help the procedure.

OR

Symphysiotomy. This is the division of the fibrocartilagenous symphysis pubis. Using local anaesthetic, infiltrate the joint with the woman in the lithotomy position, (thighs supported at no more than 90°, so as not to put too great a strain on the sacroiliac joints). Use the index and middle fingers of the left hand on the posterior aspect of the symphysis. Push the indwelling catheter aside with the index finger and use the middle finger to monitor the action of the scalpel. The latter is used like a pencil, keeping it vertical and using the entry point as a fulcrum, to bring the blade down towards the operator. Remove, turn 180° and in original point to divide the upper half of the symphysis. If completed, the middle finger can fit into the space created by the separation.

Step 9 is only resorted to if all the other manoeuvres have failed. The CEMACH recommendations state that clinicians should be aware of these if desperate measures are sought. There needs to be regular audit of shoulder dystocia cases, irrespective of the outcome and CEMACH ensure that all cases where there is an unfavourable outcome are recorded so that clinicians might examine current practices and improve management of emergency cases such as these. (See *The HELPERR mnemonic for management of shoulder dystocia*.)

Accurate record keeping:
- time head delivered
- time each manoeuvre was performed
- time body delivered
- staff present
- times at which others were summoned
- medications given
- resuscitation of infant
- observations throughout.

Emergency drills

There is a real need for regular scenario training and ward drills in all maternity settings so that if an emergency such as this arises, all staff have an in-depth knowledge of the actions that should be taken and the possible consequences of each. The advanced life support in obstetrics (ALSO) course is a vital tool in ensuring that midwives, doctors, anaesthetists and paediatricians train together in managing emergencies like shoulder dystocia and that they achieve a good outcome for all. Find out more about this course on their website: http://www.also.org.uk/providercourses.asp

More information on the management of shoulder dystocia and training tools can be accessed on the following websites:
http://www.perinatal.nhs.uk/reviews/oe/oe_shoulder_dystocia.htm
http://www.rcog.org.uk/index.asp?PageID=1317
http://www.cemach.org.uk/

The HELPERR mnemonic for management of shoulder dystocia
H Call for help
E Evaluate for episiotomy
L Legs (the McRobert's manoeuvre)
P Suprapubic pressure
E Enter manoeuvres (internal rotation)
R Remove the posterior arm
R Roll the woman

Ineffective uterine contractions

Uterine contractions force the moving fetus through the birth canal. Usually, contractions are initiated at one pacemaker point in the uterus. When a contraction occurs, it sweeps down over the uterus, encircling it. Repolarisation then occurs, a low resting tone is achieved, and another pacemaker-activated contraction begins. This process is aided by:
- hormones – adenosine triphosphate, oestrogen and progesterone
- electrolytes – calcium, sodium and potassium
- proteins – actin and myosin
- epinephrine and norepinephrine
- oxytocin
- prostaglandins.

Ineffective = increased mortality

Most labours are completed with contractions following a predictable, normal course; however, in some cases, ineffective labour can occur. The incidence of maternal puerperal infection and haemorrhage and infant mortality is higher in women who have a prolonged labour than in those who don't. Therefore, it's vital to recognise and prevent ineffective labour.

Although effective labour can become ineffective at any time, there are two general types:

 primary (at beginning of labour)

secondary (later in labour).

Be productive

Abnormal labour can produce anxiety, fear or discouragement in the woman as well as her partner. You should provide continuous explanations of what's happening to the woman and her support person. (See *Helping to reduce stress in the mother*.) In addition, there are some measures you can employ to try to promote a more productive labour. (See *Promoting productive labour*, page 346.)

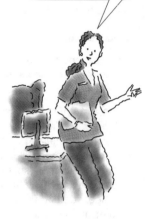

Infant mortality is higher in women who have a prolonged labour than in those who don't.

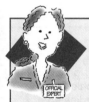

Advice from the experts

Helping to reduce stress in the mother

Stress results from and can lead to, or increase, dysfunctional labour. If a woman is tense or frightened during labour, her cervix won't dilate as rapidly, making labour prolonged.

Employ these management techniques to help the mother and her partner reduce stress:

- Ask directly if the woman has concerns.
- Offer explanations of all procedures.
- Make the support person just as welcome and comfortable as the woman herself.
- Pose questions such as 'Is labour what you thought it would be?' to both the woman and her support person to help them express concerns.
- Remember that pain is exhausting and rest promotes adequate cervical dilation. Encourage the mother to rest or sleep (if possible) in between contractions.

- Encourage the use of nonpharmacological comfort measures.
- Employ comfort measures, such as breathing with the woman, giving back rubs, changing sheets and using cool washcloths. If breathing exercises are effective, the need for analgesia (which can lead to hypotonic contractions) can be reduced.
- Urge the mother to lie on her side so the uterus is lifted off the vena cava to promote comfort, increase blood supply to the uterus and prevent hypotension.
- If a mother is more comfortable lying supine, place a hip roll under one buttock to tip her pelvis and move the uterus to the side.
- Play music in the room that the mother likes.
- Encourage her to mobilise so that she feels in control of what's happening.

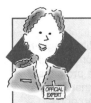

Advice from the experts

Promoting productive labour

Some measures used to promote productive labour can help avoid serious complications from ineffective labour. Consider the following measures for a woman suffering from abnormal labour.

Glucose stores

Because labour is work, it can cause a woman to deplete her glucose stores. To investigate this possibility:

- On a mother's admission to a birthing room, ask the time of her last meal to help determine if she's at risk for depleting her glucose stores.
- If the mother is still in early labour, she may be able to eat small snacks or drink some high-carbohydrate fluid such as an orange drink (Lucozade). I.V. fluid therapy may also be necessary later on to provide glucose for energy.
- Most obstetricians/midwives also encourage women to have lollipops or boiled sweets to suck on during labour to supply additional glucose.

Fluid replacement

Many women don't want to receive I.V. fluid therapy during labour. Some perceive it as losing control over their bodies or having the naturalness of labour and birth taken away.

Take these measures to allay the mother's concerns:

- Explain the purpose of I.V. fluid therapy before arriving with the bag of fluid and tubing.
- When inserting the I.V. catheter device, try to use an insertion site in the woman's nondominant hand.
- Assure the woman that she can be out of bed and walking as well as turn freely or move about during labour as desired because none of these acts should interfere with the infusion.

When the force isn't with you

Complications due to ineffective uterine force can impede the natural course of labour. These complications include:
- hypertonic contractions
- hypotonic contractions
- incoordinate contractions. (See *Comparing and contrasting contractions*, page 347.)

Hypertonic contractions

Hypertonic uterine contractions are marked by an increased resting tone to more than 15 mmHg. Even so, the intensity of contractions may be no stronger than with hypotonic contractions. Hypertonic contractions tend to occur frequently. They're most commonly seen in the latent phase of labour, and may result in precipitous labour. (See *Precipitous labour*, page 348.)

Hypotonic contractions

Contractions are termed *hypotonic* when the number or frequency of contractions is low. For example, they might not increase beyond two or three in a 10-minute period. The strength of contractions doesn't rise above 25 mmHg.

> Hypertonic, hypotonic and uncoordinated contractions are three major complications that impede the natural course of labour.

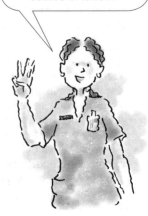

Advice from the experts

Comparing and contrasting contractions

Here are illustrations of the different uterine activity types. Depending on your assessment, you may need to intervene to promote adequate labour contractions.

Typical contractions

Typical uterine contractions occur every 2–5 minutes during active labour and typically last 30–90 seconds.

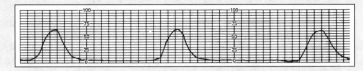

Hypertonic contractions

Hypertonic contractions don't allow the uterus to rest between contractions, as shown by a resting pressure of 40–50 mmHg.

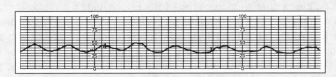

Hypotonic contractions

Hypotonic contractions are evident by a rise in pressure of no more than 10 mmHg during a contraction.

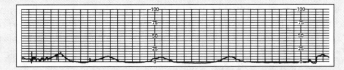

Utter exhaustion

Hypotonic contractions tend to increase the length of labour because so many of them are necessary to achieve cervical dilation. This can result in exhaustion of the mother as well as of the organs involved. This exhaustion can lead to:
• ineffective contraction of the uterus, increasing the woman's chance for postpartum haemorrhage
• risk of infection in the uterus and the fetus because of the extended period of cervical dilation.

Incoordinate contractions

Incoordinate contractions occur erratically, such as one on top of another followed by a long period without any. The lack of a regular pattern to contractions makes it difficult for the woman to rest or to use breathing exercises between contractions. Incoordinate contractions may occur so closely together that they don't allow good filling time.

What causes it

The causes of ineffective uterine force depend on the type of dysfunction.

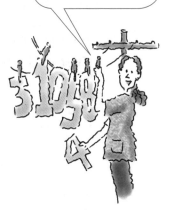

Contractions are termed hypotonic when the number or frequency of contractions is low.

Precipitous labour

Precipitous labour and birth occur when uterine contractions are so strong that the woman delivers with only a few rapidly occurring contractions. It's commonly defined as labour completed within less than 3 hours. Such rapid labour may occur with multiparity. It may also follow induction of labour by oxytocin or when an amniotomy is performed.

Dangerous force

In precipitous labour, contractions may be so forceful that they lead to premature separation of the placenta, placing the mother and fetus at risk for haemorrhage. The woman may also sustain injuries such as lacerations of the birth canal from the forceful delivery. Precipitous labour is also disconcerting and the woman may feel as if she has lost control.

Rapid labour poses an additional risk to the fetus as well. Subdural haemorrhage may result from the sudden release of pressure on the fetal head.

Graphic evidence

A precipitous labour can be detected from a partograph. This can occur during the active phase of dilation, when the rate is greater than 5 cm/hour (1 cm every 12 minutes) in a nullipara and more than 10 cm/hour (1 cm every 6 minutes) in a multipara. If this situation occurs, a tocolytic may be administered to reduce the force and frequency of contractions.

Even shorter next time

Because labours tend to be quicker with subsequent pregnancies, inform the multiparous woman by week 28 of pregnancy that her labour might be shorter than a previous one. She should plan for appropriately timed transportation to the hospital or birthing centre. When labour begins, alert a woman who has had a prior precipitous labour and birth that she may deliver this way again. When preparing for delivery, both grand multiparas and women with histories of precipitous labour should have the birthing room converted to birth readiness before full cervical dilation. Then birth can be accomplished in a controlled surrounding.

Hypertonic contractions

Hypertonic contractions occur because the muscle fibres of the myometrium don't repolarise after a contraction, making it ready to accept a new pacemaker stimulus. They can occur when more than one pacemaker is stimulating the contractions, unlike the normal single stimulus found with normally occurring contractions. Syntocinon administration may also cause hypertonic contractions. (See *Hypertonic contractions and Syntocinon*, page 349.)

Hypotonic contractions

Hypotonic contractions usually occur during the active phase of labour. They may occur when:
- analgesia has been administered too early (before cervical dilation of 3–4 cm)
- bowel or bladder distention is present, preventing descent or firm engagement
- the uterus is overstretched due to multiple gestation, larger-than-normal single fetus, hydramnios or grand multiparity.

Incoordinate contractions

With incoordinate contractions, more than one pacemaker may initiate contractions. In addition, receptor points in the myometrium act independently of the pacemaker.

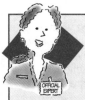

Advice from the experts

Hypertonic contractions and Syntocinon

When assessing the woman receiving Syntocinon, monitor for hypertonic uterine contractions. These contractions can be as high as 100 mmHg in intensity. With these contractions, the fetus may experience late decelerations and FHR increases, as depicted here.

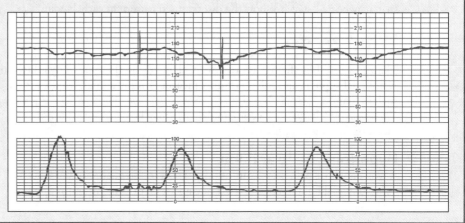

How it's detected

Ineffective uterine force is determined through physical examination and monitoring. Signs and symptoms depend on the type of dysfunction.

Hypertonic contractions

Hypertonic contractions are determined by the presence of painful uterine contractions that are either palpated or observed on an electronic monitor. On the electronic monitor, these uterine contractions show a high resting tone, and a lack of relaxation between contractions is also present. Fetal monitoring may even reveal bradycardia and fetal distress in the form of late decelerations because the absence of uterine relaxation doesn't allow the best possible uterine filling, which results in diminished oxygenation to the fetus. The woman won't be able to relax between contractions and may find it difficult to breathe with her contractions. These contractions are painful because the myometrium becomes tender as a result of inadequate relaxation.

Hypotonic contractions

Hypotonic contractions usually aren't abnormally painful because they aren't intense. However, pain is subjective; one woman's interpretation of uterine contractions may be different from another. Thus, some women may interpret these contractions as very painful.

Lack of progress

Hypotonic contractions are detected by lack of labour progression and cervical dilation. The contractions are insufficient to dilate the cervix and won't register as intense on an electronic uterine contraction monitoring strip.

Hypertonic contractions can occur when more than one pacemaker stimulates contractions. It's like trying to ride two waves at once.

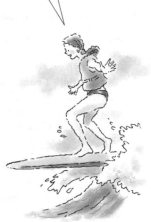

Incoordinate contractions

Incoordinate contraction patterns may be detected with the application of a fetal and uterine external monitor. Monitoring allows assessment of the rate, pattern, resting tone and fetal response to contractions, revealing an abnormal pattern. Usually this pattern may be detected within 15 minutes; however, a longer time span may be necessary to show the disorganised pattern in early labour.

What to do

Management of ineffective uterine force depends on the type of dysfunction. Emotional support and other comfort measures are essential. Medication such as Syntocinon may be required. (See *Syntocinon adverse effects*; *Preventing Syntocinon complications*.) Caesarean delivery may be necessary if other measures are unsuccessful.

Hypertonic contractions

A woman whose pain seems out of proportion to the quality of her contractions should have both a uterine and fetal external monitor applied

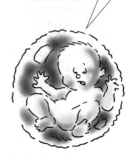

I don't want to sound like a baby, but hypertonic contractions can cause me distress.

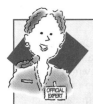

Advice from the experts

Preventing Syntocinon complications

Syntocinon infusion can cause excessive uterine stimulation – leading to hypertonicity, tetany, rupture, cervical or perineal lacerations, premature placental separation, fetal hypoxia or rapid forceful delivery – and fluid overload – leading to seizures and coma. To help prevent these complications, follow these guidelines:

Excessive uterine stimulation

- Administer oxytocin with a volumetric pump/dripcounter and use piggyback infusion so that the drug may be discontinued, if necessary, without interrupting the main I.V. line.
- Every 15 minutes, monitor uterine contractions, intrauterine pressure, FHR and the character of blood loss.
- If contractions occur less than 2 minutes apart, last 90 seconds or longer, or exceed 50 mmHg, stop the infusion, turn the mother onto her side (preferably the left), and notify the obstetrician. Contractions should occur every 2–3 minutes, followed by a period of relaxation.
- Keep magnesium sulphate (20% solution) available to relax the myometrium.
- Utopar, GTC sprays or Terbutaline S.C can also be used effectively

Fluid overload

- To identify fluid overload, monitor the mother's intake and output, especially in prolonged infusion of doses above 20 milliunits/minute.
- The risk of fluid overload also increases when oxytocin is given in hypertonic saline solution after abortion.

Syntocinon adverse effects

When administering Syntocinon, be aware of its possible adverse effects and intervene to avoid complications. Adverse effects include:

- dizziness
- headache
- nausea and vomiting
- tachycardia
- hypotension
- fetal bradycardia or tachycardia
- hypertonic contractions
- decreased urine output.

for at least a 15-minute interval to ensure that the resting phase of the contractions is adequate and to determine that the fetal pattern isn't showing late deceleration. If the woman is having Syntocinon, the rate should be decreased, or stopped, depending on how hypertonic her contractions are and how the fetus is responding.

For good measures

Other management measures include:
• promoting rest
• providing analgesia with a drug such as Pethidine
• possibly inducing sedation so the woman can rest
• comfort measures, such as changing the linen and the woman's clothing, darkening room lights and decreasing noise and stimulation.

If it isn't working

If decelerating FHR, an abnormally long first stage of labour, or lack of progress with pushing (second stage arrest) occurs, caesarean birth may be necessary. The woman and her support person need to understand that, although the contractions are strong, they are, in reality, ineffective and aren't achieving cervical dilation.

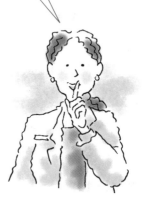

Decreasing noise and stimulation, changing the woman's bedlinen and gown and dimming lights are comfort measures for hypertonic contractions.

Hypotonic contractions

Management of hypotonic contractions includes these considerations:
• If hypotonicity is the only abnormal factor (including ruling out CPD or poor fetal presentation by sonogram), then rest and fluid intake should be encouraged.
• If the membranes haven't ruptured spontaneously, rupturing them at this point may be helpful.
• Syntocinon may be administered I.V. to augment labour by causing the uterus to contract more effectively.
• If hypertension occurs, discontinue Syntocinon and notify the doctor.

Incoordinate contractions

Management includes these considerations:
• Syntocinon administration may be helpful in uncoordinated labour to stimulate a more effective and consistent pattern of contractions with a better, lower resting tone.
• If hypertension occurs, discontinue Syntocinon and notify the doctor.

Discontinue Syntocinon and notify the obstetrician if hypertension occurs.

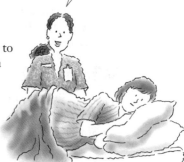

Intrauterine fetal death

Intrauterine fetal death is described as death of the fetus that occurs after a gestation of 24 weeks or longer. It can also be defined as a weight of 500 g (1.1 lb) or more.

What causes it

There are four causes of intrauterine fetal death:

 fetal

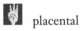 maternal

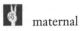 placental

 unknown.

Fetal

Fetal causes include genetic or congenital abnormalities and infection.

Maternal

Maternal causes include advanced maternal age, hypertension, diabetes and pregnancy-related complications, such as pre-eclampsia and eclampsia, uterine rupture, Rh incompatibility and maternal infection.

Placental

Placental causes include placental abruption (most common cause), prolapsed cord or a true knot in the cord, premature rupture of membranes (PROMs) and twin-to-twin transfusion.

No one's fault

Sometimes, there's no clear or accountable cause for the intrauterine death.

What to look for

A pregnant woman reporting that she can no longer feel her baby move is the first sign of possible fetal death. Or, the midwife may not be able to detect a fetal heartbeat.

What tests tell you

The only way to confirm fetal death is through an ultrasound, which can assess the cardiac movement of the fetal heart. Lack of fetal cardiac movement confirms fetal death.

How it's treated

Treatment consists of inducing labour within the next few days after it has been determined that the fetus is dead because the longer the woman carries the fetus, the greater her risk of developing DIC. If the gestation is less than

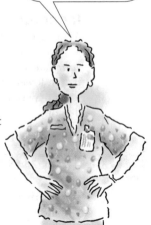

The only way to confirm fetal death is through an ultrasound scan.

28 weeks, the woman's cervix may not be favourable for an induction; she may need to have labour induced with prostaglandin E_2 vaginal suppositories or intravaginal misoprostol (Cytotec).

What to do

Midwifery care for a woman who has experienced an intrauterine fetal death is no different from that for a woman giving birth to a viable fetus; however, the emotional care is certainly more complex.

• Provide sensitive, compassionate care for the woman in a quiet, calm atmosphere.
• Continuity of care is vital – keep staff numbers to a minimum with the same midwife there throughout the labour and birth where possible.
• Try to have the mother in a room that is not too close to other rooms where babys might be heard crying.
• Try to prepare the woman and her partner for what will happen at the birth and afterwards.
• Answer the woman's questions as honestly as possible.
• Remember that each woman goes through the grieving process in different stages.
• Know that the mother and her partner may react to the death of the baby in different ways.
• Offer to call a pastor or a chaplain for the mother, her partner and the family.
• Encourage her to name and hold her baby, if she's able.
• Allow the woman, her partner and the family time to grieve.
• Allow the mother and her partner unhurried private time with the baby to facilitate the grieving process.
• Encourage the mother to assist with bathing and dressing the baby.
• Ask the woman and her partner if there's a particular religious ritual that they may wish to be performed, such as baptism or a blessing.
• According to Trust policy, gather mementos such as a photograph of the baby and distribute them to the family. Some facilities take a photograph of the baby, which is kept on record for a year; if the mother refuses the photograph initially, she may later change her mind.
• Collect footprints, a lock of hair and other reminders of the baby and give to the mother or her partner – with her consent.
• The bereavement midwife or counsellor may be invited to spend time with the parents.

Multiple gestation

A woman with multiple gestation usually causes excitement in the labour suite. Additional personnel are needed for the birth. Midwives are needed to attend to possible preterm babies. Additional paediatricians or advanced neonatal nurse practitioners are required. The mother may get lost in all this activity and may be more frightened than excited.

Twin presentations

There are four types of twin presentations; they are illustrated here.

Vertex

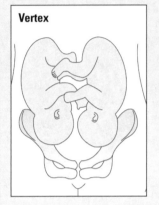

Vertex and breech

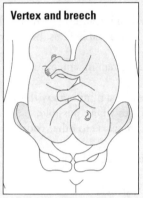

Breech

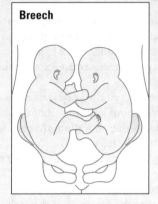

Vertex and transverse lie

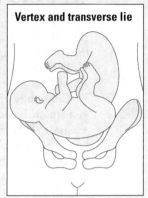

Multiple gestation may be delivered by caesarean birth to decrease the risk of anoxia to the second fetus. This problem is more common in multiple gestation of three or more because of the increased incidence of cord entanglement and premature separation of a placenta.

Twin positions

Most twin pregnancies present with both twins in the vertex position. This is followed in frequency by vertex and breech, breech and vertex and then breech and breech. (See *Twin presentations*.)

What causes it

Multiple gestation may occur spontaneously, especially with a history of twins or multiple births in the family. It may also occur with fertility medications, which cause multiple ova to be released simultaneously, thus increasing the chances of fertilisation of more than one ovum.

How it's detected

Multiple gestation may be suspected when several FHRs are auscultated, the mother is larger than average for gestational age of the fetus or when palpation reveals multiple fetuses. Multiple gestation is confirmed by ultrasound.

Multiple gestation of three or more has extremely varied presentations after the birth of the first child. The lie of the second fetus is usually determined by external abdominal palpation and sonogram.

Multiple gestation may occur spontaneously or with the use of fertility drugs.

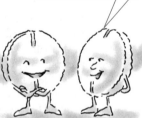

What to do

If a woman with multiple gestation is to deliver vaginally, she's usually instructed to come to the hospital early in labour. Here are some other considerations:
• The first stage of labour won't differ greatly from that of a single-gestation labour, but coming to a hospital early may make labour seem long.
• Urge the woman to spend the early hours of labour engaged in an activity such as playing cards to make the time pass more quickly.
• Analgesia administration is given conservatively so it won't compound respiratory difficulties the babies may have at birth because of their immaturity.
• A Syntocinon infusion may be initiated to assist uterine contractions and shorten the time span between the births. It's usually begun after the first fetus is delivered.
• Support the use of breathing exercises to minimise the need for analgesia or anaesthesia. Remember that multiple pregnancies commonly end before they're full term, so the woman may not yet have practiced breathing exercises. The early hours of labour are an excellent opportunity to practice breathing.
• Having a nice warm bath may relax her – and she could spend a little longer in the water with close monitoring, if it provides pain relief for her.
• Try to monitor each FHR by a separate fetal monitor if possible.

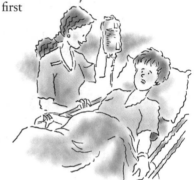

Syntocinon may be initiated to assist uterine contractions and shorten the time span between the births.

Multiple complications

Complications such as these are common in multiple gestation:
• Because the fetuses are usually small, firm head engagement may not occur, which increases the risk of cord prolapse after rupture of the membranes.
• Uterine dysfunction from a long labour may occur.
• An overstretched uterus may result and could cause ineffective labour.
• Premature separation of the placenta after the birth of the first baby is more common in multiple gestation. When separation occurs, there's sudden, profuse bleeding at the vagina, causing a risk of exsanguination for the woman.
• Because of the multiple fetuses, abnormal fetal presentation may occur.
• Anaemia and gestational hypertension occur at higher-than-usual incidences in multiple gestation. Haematocrit and blood pressure should be monitored closely during labour.
• After the birth, the uterus can't contract, placing the woman at risk for haemorrhage from uterine atony.
• Separation of the first placenta may cause loosening of the additional placentas. If a common placenta is involved, the fetal heart sounds of the other fetuses immediately register distress. Careful FHR monitoring is essential. If separation occurs, the fetuses must be delivered immediately to avoid fetal death.

After the event

Keep in mind the following points after the birth of multiple infants:
• The babies need careful assessment to determine their true gestational age and whether twin-to-twin transfusion has occurred.
• Some parents worry that the hospital will confuse their babies through improper identification. Review with them the careful measures that are taken to ensure correct identification.
• Despite preparations for a multiple birth, the woman may have difficulty believing she has given birth to more than one baby. She may find it helpful to discuss her feelings with you as well as view all her babies together to become accustomed to the idea.
• The parents may be unable to inspect the babies thoroughly immediately after the birth because of low birthweight and the danger of hypothermia. Bonding time should be promoted as soon as possible to dispel fears they may have that the babies are less than perfect.

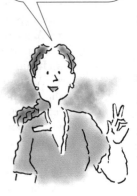

The risk of anaemia and gestational hypertension is greater in multiple gestation.

Preterm labour and delivery

When labour begins earlier in gestation than normal, it's considered preterm. As with normal labour, in preterm labour rhythmic uterine contractions produce cervical change. This change may occur after fetal viability but before fetal maturity. It usually occurs between 20 and 37 weeks' gestation. Premature labour is a major cause of perinatal morbidity and mortality. Neonatal complications may include respiratory distress syndrome, intracranial bleeding and sepsis. Only 5–10% of pregnancies end prematurely, but if the membranes rupture prematurely, then the number rises sharply to 40%.

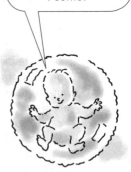

I might be a little early, but here I come!

Weight and length = outcome

The impact on the fetus depends on birthweight and gestation:
• Infants weighing less than 737 g (1 lb, 10 oz) and born at less than 26 weeks' gestation have a survival rate of about 10%.
• Infants weighing 737–992 g (2 lb, 3 oz) and born at 27–28 weeks' gestation have a survival rate of more than 50%.
• Infants weighing 992–1,219 g (2 lb, 11 oz) and born at more than 28 weeks' gestation have a 70–90% survival rate.

What causes it

Causes of preterm labour include:
• PROM
• hydramnios
• fetal death.

When mum is at risk

Numerous maternal risk factors also increase the incidence of preterm labour, including:
- gestational hypertension
- chronic hypertensive vascular disease
- placenta praevia
- placental abruption
- incompetent cervix
- abdominal surgery
- trauma
- structural anomalies of the uterus
- infections (such as group B streptococci)
- genetic defect in the mother.

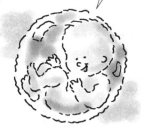

Don't blame me. It could be the genes.

Other contributors

Other factors that may cause preterm labour include:
- stimulation of the fetus via heredity. Genetically imprinted information tells the fetus that nutrition is inadequate and that a change in environment is required for well being, thus provoking the onset of labour.
- sensitivity to the hormone oxytocin. Labour begins because the myometrium becomes hypersensitive to oxytocin, the hormone that usually induces uterine contractions.

How it's detected

As with labour at term, preterm labour produces:
- rhythmic uterine contractions
- cervical dilation and effacement
- possible rupture of the membranes
- expulsion of the cervical mucus plug (operculum)
- bloody discharge.

Combination confirmation

Preterm labour is confirmed by the combined results of:
- antenatal history indicating that the mother is at 20–37 weeks of gestation
- ultrasonography (if available) showing the position of the fetus in relation to the mother's pelvis
- vaginal examination confirming progressive cervical effacement and dilation
- continuous electronic fetal monitoring showing rhythmic uterine contractions
- differential diagnosis excluding Braxton Hicks contractions and urinary tract infection.

What to do

Treatment of premature labour aims to suppress labour when tests show:
- immature fetal pulmonary development
- cervical dilation of less than 4 cm
- absence of factors that contraindicate continuation of pregnancy.

Let's be conservative

Here are some conservative measures to suppress labour:
- A woman in preterm labour requires bed rest, close observation for signs of fetal or maternal distress and comprehensive supportive care.
- During attempts to suppress preterm labour, make sure the woman maintains bed rest and administer medications as ordered.
- Because sedatives and analgesics may be harmful to the fetus, administer them sparingly. Minimise the need for these drugs by providing comfort measures, such as frequent repositioning and good perineal and back care.
- Avoid preterm labour by successfully identifying women at risk and adapting their antenatal visits and screening accordingly.
- Ensure that the woman is taking proper preventive measures, such as good antenatal care, adequate nutrition and proper rest.
- Insertion of a purse-string suture (cerclage) can reinforce an incompetent cervix at 14–18 weeks' gestation to avoid preterm delivery in a woman with a history of this disorder.

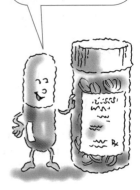

Because sedatives and analgesics may be harmful to the fetus, administer them sparingly.

Drug details

Pharmacological measures to suppress labour include the following:
- Atosiban is recommended by the Royal College of Obstetricians and Gynaecologists (RCOG) for treatment of preterm labour. It is recommended that it is not used for more than 48 hours.
- Ritrodine is also popular, but like all beta-agonists, it has a high frequency of adverse effects.

Monitoring measures

Careful monitoring is essential throughout therapy. The usual monitoring of uterine contractions and fetal heart tones should be conducted. Here are some additional measures:
- During therapy, monitor the woman's haematological status, especially for decreased haematocrit. Report abnormal findings to doctor.
- Monitor the woman's cardiac status continuously and report arrhythmias.
- Check the mother's blood pressure and pulse every 10–15 minutes initially, then every 30 minutes or as ordered.
- Notify the doctor if the woman's pulse rate exceeds 140 beats/minute or if her blood pressure falls 15 mmHg or more.
- If the woman complains of palpitations or chest pain or tightness, decrease the drug dosage and notify the doctor immediately.

- Keep emergency resuscitation equipment nearby.
- Assess pulmonary status every hour during I.V. therapy, and report crackles or increased respirations.
- Monitor intake and output and notify the doctor if urine output drops below 50 ml/hour as pulmonary oedema may result.
- If signs of pulmonary oedema develop, place the woman in high Fowler's position, administer oxygen as ordered and notify the doctor.
- For 1–2 hours after I.V. therapy, monitor the woman's vital signs, intake and output and FHR.
- ECGs may be ordered if any cardiac problems arise during the course of the treatment.
- Immediately report tachycardia, hypotension, decreased urine output or diminished or absent fetal heart sounds.
- Watch for maternal adverse reactions to magnesium sulphate administration, including drowsiness, slurred speech, flushing, decreased reflexes, decreased GI motility and decreased respirations.
- Ensure the mother understands and is compliant with treatment. (See *Informing the woman about preterm labour*.)
- Document all care, drugs administered and evaluate care plans where appropriate.

Preterm delivery

It may be in the best interest of the fetus or the mother and fetus to allow preterm labour to progress and delivery to ensue. Maternal factors

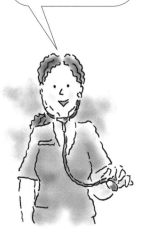

It's important to assess pulmonary status every hour during I.V. therapy, and report crackles or increased respirations.

Education edge

Informing the woman about preterm labour

Here are some guidelines for informing a woman about preterm labour.

- Reassure her that drug effects on her baby should be minimal.
- Tell her to notify the midwife/doctor immediately if she experiences sweating, chest pain or increased pulse rate.
- Her pulse is always checked before oral drug administration. If her pulse exceeds 130 beats/minute, she shouldn't take the drug and the doctor should be notified.
- Emphasise the importance of immediately reporting contractions, lower back pain, cramping or increased vaginal discharge.

- Instruct her to report other adverse reactions requiring a reduction in drug dosage, such as headache, nervousness, tremors, restlessness, nausea and vomiting.
- Her temperature should be checked every day and any fever reported to the doctor because it may be a sign of infection.
- Encourage her to remain in bed as much as possible.
- Tell her to avoid stimulating her breasts in preparation for breastfeeding until about 2 weeks before her due date because this can stimulate the release of oxytocin and initiate contractions.

that jeopardise the mother and fetus, making preterm delivery the lesser risk, include:

- intrauterine infection
- placental abruption
- severe pre-eclampsia.

Factors that jeopardise the fetus can become more significant as pregnancy nears term, and so preterm delivery may be more favourable. These factors include:

- placental insufficiency
- isoimmunisation
- congenital anomalies.

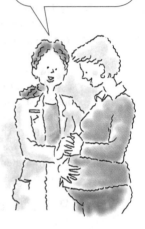

Preterm delivery may be best for mother and fetus when intrauterine infection, placental abruption or severe pre-eclampsia is a factor.

Ideal situation

Ideally, treatment of active preterm labour should take place in a regional maternity unit where there are neonatal ICUs and the staff are specially trained to handle this situation. The infant can also remain close to his parents, promoting bonding. Smaller hospitals often lack the facilities for special neonatal care and have to transfer the infant only to the regional NNU; this can be even more traumatic, for the baby and his parents. Remember, the uterus is the best incubator of all! Better to transfer in utero than out.

Part of a team

Treatment and delivery require an intensive team effort focusing on:

- continuous assessment of fetal health through fetal monitoring
- unless contraindicated, administration of antenatal steroids to assist fetal lung development
- maintenance of adequate hydration through I.V. fluids.

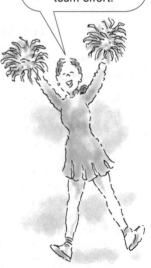

Go, team! Treatment and delivery of a preterm baby require a team effort.

Constant concerns

Also keep in mind:

- Pethidine may cause fetal respiratory depression. They should be administered only when necessary and in the smallest possible dose.
- Amniotomy should be avoided, if possible, to prevent cord prolapse or damage to the fetus's tender skull.
- The preterm newborn baby has a lower tolerance for the stress of labour and is much more likely to become hypoxic than the term infant.
- If necessary, administer oxygen to the mother through a nasal cannula.
- Observe fetal response to labour through continuous monitoring.
- Continually reassure the mother throughout labour to help reduce her anxiety.
- Monitor fetal and maternal response to local and regional anaesthetics.
- Pushing between contractions is ineffective and can damage the premature baby's soft skull.

• Throughout labour, keep the mother informed of her progress and the condition of the fetus.
• Inform the parents of their baby's condition. Describe his appearance and explain the purpose of supportive equipment. It is important to take a photo of their baby before he commences treatment in the NNU.

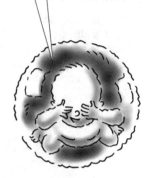

Peek-a-boo. I see you! Remember to keep tabs on my condition throughout labour.

Placental abnormalities

The normal placenta weighs approximately in at approximately 500 g and is 15–20 cm in diameter and 1.5–3 cm thick. Its weight is approximately one-sixth that of the fetus. Problems can occur with the size of the placenta or the blood vessels connected to it. Other abnormalities can involve the placement of the umbilical cord or placental attachment. Types of abnormalities include:
• battledore placenta
• placenta accreta
• placenta circumvallata
• placenta succenturiata
• vasa praevia
• velamentous cord insertion. (See *Abnormal placental formations*, page 362.)

What causes it

Abnormalities may be present for several reasons. For example, a placenta may be unusually enlarged in a woman with diabetes. In certain diseases, such as syphilis or erythroblastosis, the placenta may be so large that it weighs half as much as the fetus. The placenta may be wider in diameter if the uterus has scars or a septum, possibly because it was forced to spread out to find implantation space.

Well, that depends . . .

Other causes of placental abnormalities depend on the type of abnormality:
• Battledore placenta has no known cause.
• Placenta accreta is caused by a defect in decidua formation from implantation over uterine scars or in the lower segment of the uterus.
• Placenta circumvallata has no known cause, although formation of insufficient chorion frondosum, subchorial infarcts and an abnormally implanted blastocyst causes part of the fetal surface to be covered by the decidua.
• Placenta succenturiata is caused when a group of villi distant to the placenta fail to degenerate and implantation is superficial or confined to a specific site so that attachment of the trophoblast also occurs on the opposing wall. This condition can occur in the case of a bicornuate uterus.
• Vasa praevia is caused by rotation of the inner cell mass and body stalk, which aligns in an eccentric insertion.

Abnormal placental formations

Abnormal placental formations occur for various reasons, some of which are unknown. The types of abnormal placental formations and their clinical significance are discussed here.

Battledore placenta

In battledore placenta, the umbilical cord is attached marginally, rather than centrally. It can lead to preterm labour, fetal distress and bleeding from cord compression or vessel rupture.

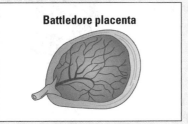

Battledore placenta

Placenta accreta

In placenta accreta, an unusually deep attachment of the placenta to the uterine myometrium doesn't allow the placenta to loosen and deliver as it should. Attempts to remove it manually may lead to extreme haemorrhage. This abnormality is associated with placenta praevia, which can lead to severe maternal haemorrhage, uterine perforation and subsequent hysterectomy.

Placenta circumvallata

In placenta circumvallata, the chorion membrane that usually begins at the edge of the placenta and spreads to envelop the fetus is missing on the fetal side of the placenta. In this condition, the umbilical cord may enter the placenta at the usual midpoint with large vessels spreading out from there. However, the vessels end abruptly at the point where the chorion folds back onto the surface. This abnormality can lead to spontaneous abortion, placental abruption, preterm labour, placental insufficiency and intrapartum and postpartum haemorrhage.

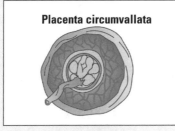

Placenta circumvallata

Placenta succenturiata

In placenta succenturiata, one or more accessory lobes are connected to the main placenta by blood vessels. Identify this abnormality through careful examination of the placenta after birth because the small lobes may be retained in the uterus, leading to severe maternal postpartum haemorrhage.

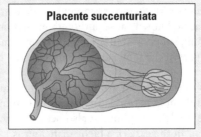

Placente succenturiata

Vasa praevia

In vasa praevia, velamentous insertion of the cord is present and the unprotected and fragile umbilical vessels cross the internal os and lie in front of the presenting fetal head. This abnormal insertion may cause the cord to be delivered before the fetus, possibly causing the vessels to tear with cervical dilation, leading to haemorrhage.

Velamentous cord insertion

Velamentous cord insertion occurs when the cord separates into small vessels that reach the placenta by spreading across a fold of amnion. This form of cord insertion is found most commonly in multiple gestation and may be associated with fetal abnormalities. This condition can lead to vessel tearing and haemorrhage because the vessels are unprotected as they travel through the amnion and chorion before they form the cord.

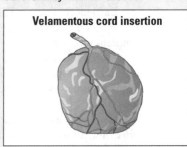

Velamentous cord insertion

- In velamentous cord insertion, the umbilical cord inserts into the membrane, causing the vessles to run between the amnion and chorion before entering the placenta. This condition most likely occurs during implantation.

How it's detected

Placental abnormalities usually aren't detected until after the birth of the placenta. Both the umbilical cord and placenta are examined. However, if sudden painless bleeding occurs with the beginning of cervical dilation, vasa praevia should be suspected. Ultrasound confirms this diagnosis.

What to do

Some placental abnormalities require immediate attention, whereas others may not be significant. For example, if the woman has a placenta succenturiata, the remaining lobes must be removed from the uterus manually. This is done to prevent maternal haemorrhage from poor uterine contraction.

Look before you touch

Some abnormalities must be detected before routine care may be performed. For example, before inserting an instrument (such as an internal fetal monitor), fetal and placental structures must be identified to prevent problems. For example, accidental tearing of a vasa praevia can result in sudden fetal blood loss. If vasa praevia is identified, caesarean delivery of the infant is necessary.

Abnormalities such as placenta accreta require more intense treatment. Placenta accreta requires a hysterectomy or treatment with methotrexate to destroy the still-attached tissue.

Retained placenta

In some instances, the placenta may not separate and remain attached to the uterine wall leading to a retained placenta. In other instances, the cord may snap during cord traction, resulting in a trapped placenta – this is no one's fault – it could be that the cord was very thin and unable to withstand the pressure exerted on it. Once the cervix closes, it may be impossible to deliver the placenta normally and so the mother will need a manual removal performed.

In some cases, it may not be the whole placenta that is left in the uterus but a lobe – this will be picked up when the midwife examines the placenta after 3rd stage is complete. If an ultrasonography reveals that placental tissue has been left behind, the mother will need manual evacuation of her uterus to prevent infection occurring.

What do you do?

- The mother could try breastfeeding her baby in the case of retained placenta – this releases oxytocin and results in uterine contractions which might expel the placenta.

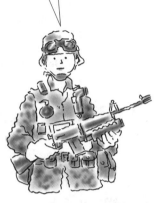

Attention! Battledore placenta has no known cause.

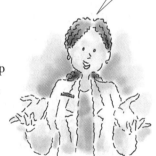

Some placental abnormalities require immediate attention, whereas others may not be significant.

- Monitor her clinical condition carefully and observe for signs of haemorrhage.
- Alert the obstetrician and anaesthetist as the mother will need to go to theatre for a manual removal of her placenta.
- Prepare the mother for theatre – she will need to give consent for the procedure and will require a local anaesthetic prior to the procedure.
- Explain to the mother that afterwards she will have to stay in hospital for at least 48 hours so that she can begin antibiotic therapy and have her condition monitored.
- Document all care given and drugs administered in the mother's records.

Umbilical cord anomalies

Umbilical cord anomalies include absence of an umbilical artery and an unusually long or short umbilical cord.

Absent artery

A normal umbilical cord contains one vein and two arteries. The presence of a single umbilical artery is caused by atrophy of a previously normal artery, presence of the original artery of the body stalk or agenesis of one of the umbilical arteries. The absence of one of the umbilical arteries has been associated with congenital heart and kidney defects because the insult that caused the loss of the vessel probably led to an insult to other mesoderm germ layer structures as well.

The long . . .

An unusually long cord can be compromised more easily because of its greater tendency to twist or knot. When this happens, the natural pulsations of the blood through the vessels and the muscular vessel walls usually keep the blood flow adequate. A long cord that wraps around the fetus's neck is called a *nuchal cord*. If the cord is wrapped tightly enough to restrict blood flow to the fetus, it may cause stillbirth.

. . . and short of it

An unusually short umbilical cord can result in premature separation of the placenta or an abnormal fetal lie. It can also result in fetal asphyxia because of traction on the umbilical cord as the fetus descends.

What causes it

The cause of differences in cord length is unknown. Some researchers suggest that reduced fetal activity, such as in the case of twinning (monoamniotic and conjoined), may be a cause and can be a genetic failure of the cord to elongate.

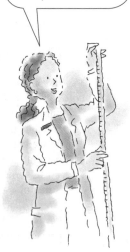

A cord that's either too long or too short can cause problems.

However, the cause of unusual inversions of the cord into the placenta may be a result of rotation of the body stalk (which becomes the cord) as it implants into the placenta. The degree of rotation determines how far the umbilical cord will be from the centre of the placenta.

How it's detected

Cord length abnormalities and abnormal cord insertion can be detected using ultrasound. However, detection of other umbilical cord abnormalities is only possible upon inspection of a cord at birth. Inspection should take place immediately, before the cord begins to dry because drying distorts the appearance.

What to do

Document the number of vessels present. The baby with only two vessels needs to be observed carefully for other defects during the neonatal period.

Calcification and Infarcts

Calcified areas can be found in postterm placentas – they look like little greyish areas and feel gritty to touch.

Infarcts are sometimes found in placentas where the blood supply has been reduced to a particular area making it whitish in colour. This can also happen in areas of the placenta that may have separated during pregnancy.

Umbilical cord prolapse

In umbilical cord prolapse, a loop of the umbilical cord slips down in front of the presenting fetal part. This prolapse may occur at any time after the membranes rupture, especially if the presenting part isn't fitted firmly into the cervix. It happens in 1 out of 200 pregnancies. (See *Prolapse patterns*, page 366.)

What causes it

Prolapse tends to occur more commonly with the following conditions:
- PROMs
- fetal presentation other than cephalic
- placenta praevia
- intrauterine tumours that prevent the presenting part from engaging
- small fetus
- CPD that prevents firm engagement
- hydramnios
- multiple gestation.

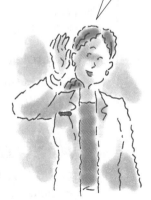

Auscultate heart sounds immediately after rupture of the membranes to rule out cord prolapse.

Prolapse patterns

Prolapse of the umbilical cord may occur in two ways: outwardly prolapsed or hidden. Regardless of the type of prolapse, it means that the fetal nutrient supply is compromised. Both types of prolapse can be detected by fetal monitoring.

Hidden prolapse

The cord still remains within the uterus but is prolapsed.

Outward prolapse

The cord can be seen at the vulva.

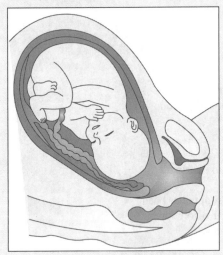

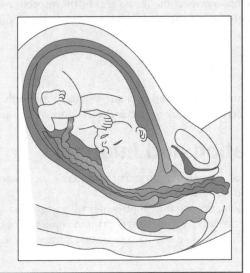

How it's detected

Signs of prolapse include a sudden variable deceleration of FHR pattern with the cord present in the vagina or visible at the vulva. To rule out cord prolapse, auscultate fetal heart immediately after rupture of the membranes (occurring spontaneously or by amniotomy).

Perhaps it's prolapse

Signs of hypoxia and fetal distress suggest prolapse. In rare instances, the cord may be felt as the presenting part on vaginal examination. It can also be identified in this position on scan.

What to do

Cord prolapse leads to immediate cord compression because the fetal presenting part presses against the cord at the pelvic brim. Management is aimed towards relieving pressure on the cord, thereby relieving the compression and avoiding fetal anoxia.

Here are some points that you should consider if this occurs:

• If vaginal examination reveals the cord as the presenting part, caesarean birth is necessary before rupture of the membranes occurs. Otherwise, with rupture, the cord prolapses down into the vagina.

• A gloved hand may be placed in the vagina. This is done to manually elevate the fetal head off the cord.

• The woman may be placed in a knee–chest or Trendelenburg's position, which causes the fetal head to fall back from the cord.

• In some instances, catheterising the woman and filling the bladder with normal saline can distend the bladder, preventing the fetal head from descending.

• Administering oxygen at 10 L/minute by face mask to the mother is also helpful.

• A tocolytic agent may be used to reduce uterine activity and pressure on the fetus.

• If the cord has prolapsed so far that it's exposed to room air, drying begins, leading to atrophy of the umbilical vessels. If this happens, don't attempt to push exposed cord back into the vagina. This may add to the compression and further cause knotting or kinking. Cover the exposed portion with a sterile saline compress to prevent drying.

• If the cervix is fully dilated at the time of the prolapse, the doctor may choose to deliver the baby quickly, possibly with forceps, to prevent a period of anoxia.

• If cervical dilation is incomplete, the birth method of choice is upward pressure on the presenting part by a midwife/doctor's hand in the woman's vagina to keep pressure off the cord until a caesarean delivery can be performed.

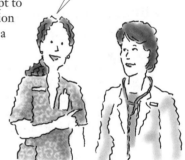

If the cervix is fully dilated at the time of prolapse, the doctor may choose to deliver the baby quickly to prevent a period of anoxia.

Uterine rupture

Rupture of the uterus during labour is a rare occurrence; it happens in about 1 in 1,500 births. A uterus ruptures when it undergoes more strain than it can sustain. If the situation isn't relieved, uterine rupture and death of the fetus may occur. In the placental stage, massive maternal haemorrhage may result because the placenta is loosened but then can't deliver, preventing the uterus from contracting. Uterine rupture accounts for as many as 5% of all maternal deaths. When it occurs, fetal death results 40–50% of the time.

The viability of the fetus depends on the extent of the rupture and the time that elapses between the rupture and abdominal extraction. The woman's prognosis depends on the extent of the rupture and blood loss. It's inadvisable for a woman to conceive again after a rupture of the uterus unless it occurred in the inactive lower segment.

What causes it

The most common cause of uterine rupture is previous caesarean birth, such as when a vertical scar from a previous incision is present. It can also be from hysterotomy repair. Contributing factors include:
- prolonged labour
- faulty presentation
- multiple gestation
- use of Syntocinon
- obstructed labour
- traumatic manoeuvres using forceps or traction.

How it's detected

Strong uterine contractions that occur without cervical dilation are a sign of impending rupture. A more specific sign, called a *pathological retraction ring*, is an indentation that appears across the abdomen over the uterus just before rupture.

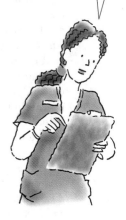

The most common cause of uterine rupture is previous caesarean birth.

The things about rings

Two types of retraction rings can occur in abnormal labour:

Bandl's ring – This sign is evident at the junction of the upper and lower uterine segments. It usually appears during the second stage of labour as a horizontal indentation across the abdomen. It's formed by excessive retraction of the upper uterine segment. The uterine myometrium is much thicker above the ring than below it.

Constriction ring – This sign can occur at any point in the myometrium and at any time during labour. When it occurs in early labour, it's usually the result of incoordinate contractions. Causes may include obstetric manipulation or administration of oxytocin. In a constriction ring, the fetus is gripped by the constriction ring and can't advance beyond that point. The undelivered placenta is also held at that point.

Retraction rings are confirmed by ultrasonography. This finding is extremely serious and should be reported promptly.
- Administration of I.V. morphine or the inhalation of amyl nitrite may relieve the retraction ring.
- A tocolytic may be administered to halt contractions.

Complete rupture

If the rupture is complete, here are some changes you can expect:
- The woman experiences a sudden, severe pain during a strong labour contraction and then contractions stop.
- The woman may report a tearing sensation, and haemorrhaging may occur from the torn uterus into the abdominal cavity and possibly into the vagina. Rupture goes through endometrium, myometrium and peritoneum.

- Signs of shock begin immediately, including rapid, weak pulse; falling blood pressure; cold and clammy skin; and respiratory distress.
- The woman's abdomen changes in contour. Two distinct swellings are visible: the retracted uterus and the extrauterine fetus.
- Fetal heart sounds become absent.

Incomplete rupture

If the rupture is incomplete, the signs are less dramatic:
- The woman may experience only a localised tenderness.
- She may complain of a persistent aching pain over the area of the lower segment.
- FHR falls, there is a lack of contractions and the woman's vital signs deteriorate, revealing fetal and maternal distress. (See *Signs of uterine rupture*.)

What to do

The uterus at the end of pregnancy is a highly vascular organ. This makes uterine rupture an immediate emergency situation. It's comparable to a splenic or hepatic rupture. Most likely, a caesarean delivery is performed to ensure safe birth of the fetus. Manual removal of the placenta under general anaesthesia may be necessary in the event of placental-stage pathological retraction rings. The following measures are also indicated:
- Ensure there is good I.V. access with a wide bore cannula if possible.
- Administer emergency fluid replacement therapy as ordered.
- Anticipate use of I.V. oxytocin to attempt to contract the uterus and minimise bleeding.
- Prepare the woman for a possible laparotomy as an emergency measure to control bleeding and effect a repair.
- The doctor, with consent, may, in some cases, perform a hysterectomy (removal of the damaged uterus) or tubal ligation at the time of the laparotomy. Explain to the woman that these procedures result in loss of childbearing ability.
- The woman may have difficulty giving her consent at this time because it isn't known whether the fetus will live.
- If blood loss is acute, the woman may be unconscious from hypotension. If this is the case, her support person must give consent, relying on the information provided by the operating surgeon to decide whether a functioning uterus can be saved.
- Be prepared to offer information and support and to inform the support person about the fetal outcome, the extent of the surgery and the woman's safety as soon as possible.

Give time for grief

- Expect the parents to go through a grieving process for not only the loss of this child (as applicable) but also the loss of having future children through pregnancies.

Advice from the experts

Signs of uterine rupture

Signs and symptoms of uterine rupture require prompt recognition and intervention. Intervene immediately to save the life of the mother and fetus. Signs and symptoms include:

- severe abdominal pain
- halt in contractions
- absent FHR
- possible vaginal bleeding
- falling blood pressure
- rapid weak pulse.

- Give them time to express these emotions without feeling threatened.
- It is important that they are counselled in relation to the loss of this pregnancy and future pregnancies.

Uterine inversion

Uterine inversion is a rare phenomenon in which the uterus turns inside out. It may occur after the birth of the baby, especially if traction is applied to the uterine fundus when the uterus isn't contracted. It may also occur when there's insertion of the placenta at the fundus, so that during birth, the passage of the fetus pulls the fundus down.

A matter of degrees

Uterine inversion can range from first-degree (incomplete) inversion, in which the corpus extends to the cervix but not beyond the cervical ring, to third-degree (complete) inversion. In complete inversion, the inverted uterus extends into the perineum. An additional condition, called *total uterine inversion*, involves total inversion of the uterus and the vagina.

What causes it

Causes of uterine inversion occur during the third stage of labour and include:
- excessive cord traction
- excessive fundal pressure.

How it's detected

Signs of inversion include:
- a large, sudden gush of blood from the vagina
- inability to palpate the fundus in the abdomen
- signs of blood loss (hypotension, dizziness, paleness, diaphoresis)
- signs of shock (such as increased heart rate and decreased blood pressure) if the loss of blood continues unchecked for more than a few minutes
- inability of the uterus to contract, resulting in continued bleeding (a woman could exsanguinate within a period as short as 10 minutes).

What to do

When exsanguination is imminent, follow these measures:
- Call for help immediately!
- Never attempt to replace the inversion because without good pelvic relaxation this may only increase bleeding.
- Never attempt to remove the placenta if it's still attached because this only creates a larger bleeding area.
- Administering an oxytocic drug only compounds the inversion.

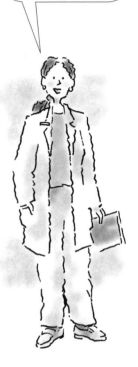

Excessive cord traction or excessive fundal pressure during the third stage of labour can cause uterine inversion.

- Start an I.V. fluid line if one isn't present. Use a large-gauge needle because blood must be replaced. Open an existing fluid line to achieve optimal fluid flow for fluid volume replacement.
- Administer oxygen by mask, and assess vital signs.
- Be prepared to perform CPR if the woman's heart fails from the sudden blood loss.
- The woman should immediately receive general anaesthesia or, possibly, a tocolytic drug I.V.
- The delivering doctor or midwife replaces the fundus manually.
- Syntocinon is administered after manual replacement, which helps the uterus to contract into place.
- Because the uterine endometrium was exposed, the woman requires antibiotic therapy postpartum to prevent infection.
- Document all treatments, drugs given and care provided in the mother's records.

Quick quiz

1. Maternal factors indicating the need for caesarean birth include:
    A. transverse fetal lie.
    B. previous caesarean birth with bikini incision.
    C. active genital herpes.
    D. hypotension.

Answer: C. Maternal factors for caesarean birth include CPD, active genital herpes or papilloma, previous caesarean birth by classic incision and disabling conditions, such as severe hypertension of pregnancy or heart disease, that prevent pushing to accomplish the pelvic division of labour.

2. Contraindications for caesarean birth include:
    A. papilloma.
    B. fetal distress.
    C. transverse fetal lie.
    D. dead fetus.

Answer: D. Caesarean birth is generally contraindicated when there's a documented dead fetus. In this situation, labour can be induced to avoid a surgical procedure.

3. The presence of meconium in the amniotic fluid before birth may indicate:
    A. breech presentation.
    B. transverse lie.
    C. placental abruption
    D. placenta praevia.

Answer: A. In breech presentation, the inevitable contraction of the fetal buttocks from cervical pressure typically causes meconium to be extruded into the amniotic fluid before birth. This, unlike meconium staining that occurs from fetal anoxia, isn't a sign of fetal distress but is expected from the buttock pressure.

4. The child born in breech presentation is at risk for:
    A. hypotension.
    B. hypoxia.
    C. intracranial haemorrhage.
    D. infection.

Answer: C. A danger of breech birth is intracranial haemorrhage. With a cephalic presentation, moulding to the confines of the birth canal occurs over hours. With a breech birth, pressure changes occur instantaneously. The baby who's delivered suddenly to reduce the amount of time of cord compression may, therefore, suffer an intracranial haemorrhage.

5. Administration of Syntocinon should be discontinued when:
    A. contractions are less than 2 minutes apart.
    B. contractions are stronger than 50 mmHg.
    C. contractions are less than 50 seconds long.
    D. contractions are irregular.

Answer: B. General guidelines for Syntocinon use include that contractions should occur no more than every 2 minutes, shouldn't be stronger than 50 mmHg and shouldn't last longer than 70 seconds.

6. Shoulder dystocia should be suspected when:
    A. the baby's head delivers but the neck is not visible – turtle sign.
    B. there is obvious restitution with the shoulders.
    C. there are no signs of restitution.
    D. the head retracts with every contraction.

Answer: A, C and D. In shoulder dystocia, you will not see signs of restitution because the shoulders are impacted and so the head cannot progress forward and cannot restitute with the shoulders because they are stuck.

Scoring

☆☆☆ If you answered all six questions correctly, give yourself a hand! You've got a good grip on a complicated subject.

☆☆ If you answered five questions correctly, capital! You're using your head to grasp these labour complications.

☆ If you answered fewer than five questions correctly, keep your eye on the prize. Going through the chapter again can help you see your way through.

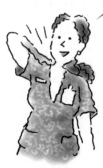

Give yourself a pat on the back for a job well done! Then let's go to the chapter on postpartum care.

9 Postnatal care

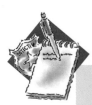

Just the facts

In this chapter, you'll learn:

♦ physiological and psychological changes that occur during the postnatal period

♦ key components of a postnatal assessment

♦ midwifery care measures required during the postnatal period

♦ physiological events that occur during lactation

♦ two feeding methods, including their advantages and disadvantages.

A look at postnatal care

The definition of postnatal is 'the period following the birth'. The *puerperium* refers to the 6–8-week period after delivery during which the mother's body returns to its pre-pregnant state. Some people refer to this period as the *fourth trimester of pregnancy*. Many physiological and psychological changes occur in the mother during this time. Midwifery care should focus on helping the mother and her family adjust to these changes and on easing the transition to the parenting role. The National Institute for Clinical Excellence has produced guidelines for postnatal care which can be accessed from the website: www.nice.org.uk/CG037

Postnatal care in the UK is provided by midwives in the hospital or in the community and many mothers now choose to go home on their second or third postnatal day. Some mothers may go home within 6 hours of delivery, making community care much more important. Care and information should be appropriate and the woman's cultural practices should be taken into account. Each postnatal contact should be provided in accordance with the principles of individualised care. Postnatal services should be planned locally to achieve the most efficient and effective service for women and their babies and this means that the community services, i.e. midwife, general practitioner (GP), health visitor and social worker (if required) all work in a cohesive way to provide seamless care.

Physiological changes

Two types of physiological changes occur during the postnatal period: retrogressive changes and progressive changes.

Getting back to normal

Retrogressive changes involve returning the body to its pre-pregnancy state. These changes include:
- shrinkage and descent of the uterus into its pre-pregnancy position in the pelvis
- sloughing of the uterine lining and development of lochia
- contraction of the cervix and vagina
- recovery of vaginal and pelvic floor muscle tone.

Theory of involution

After delivery, the uterus gradually decreases in size and descends into its pre-pregnancy position in the pelvis – a process known as *involution*. Involution normally begins immediately after delivery, when the firmly contracted uterus lies midway between the umbilicus and symphysis pubis. Soon after, the uterus rises to the umbilicus or slightly above it. After the first postpartum day, the uterus begins its descent into the pelvis at the rate of 1 cm/day (or 1 fingerbreadth/day), or slightly less for the mother who has had a caesarean delivery. Usually by the 10th postpartum day, the uterus lies deep in the pelvis – either at or below the symphysis pubis – and it can't be palpated.

Contraction is key

If the uterus fails to contract or remain firm during involution, uterine bleeding or haemorrhage can result. At delivery, placental separation exposes large uterine blood vessels. Uterine contraction acts as a tourniquet to close these blood vessels at the placental site. Fundal massage, the administration of synthetic oxytocics and the release of natural oxytocics during breastfeeding help to maintain or stimulate contraction.

All systems undergo

Other body systems undergo retrogressive changes as well. These alterations include:
- reduction in pregnancy hormones, such as human chorionic gonadotropin, human placental lactogen, progestin, oestrogen and oestradiol
- extensive diuresis, which rids the body of excess fluid and reduces the added blood volume of pregnancy
- gradual rise in haematocrit, which occurs as excess fluid is excreted

- reactivation of digestion and absorption
- eventual fading of striae gravidarum (stretch marks), chloasma (pigmentation on face and neck) and linea nigra (pigmentation on abdomen)
- gradual return of tone to the abdominal muscles, wall and ligaments
- return of vital signs to normal parameters
- weight loss due to rapid diuresis and lochial flow
- recession of varicosities (although they may never return completely to pre-pregnancy appearance).

In addition, oestrogen and progesterone production drops abruptly after delivery, and follicle-stimulating hormone (FSH) production rises, resulting in the gradual return of ovulation and the menstrual cycle.

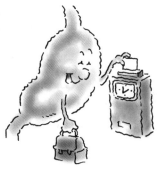

In the postnatal period, I'm working on regaining my muscle tone.

Making progress

Progressive changes involve the building of new tissues, primarily those that occur with lactation and the return of menstrual flow. In the postnatal period, fluid accumulates in the breast tissue in preparation for breastfeeding and breast tissue increases in size as breast milk forms. The changes associated with lactation are discussed in 'Lactation', page 386.

Psychological changes

The postnatal period is a time of transition for the new mother and her family. Even if the family has other children, each family member must adjust to the baby's arrival. The mother, in particular, undergoes many psychological changes during this time in addition to the changes that are occurring in her body.

Don't let the phases faze you

The mother goes through three distinct phases of adjustment in the postnatal period:

 taking in

 taking hold

 letting go.

In the past, each phase of the postnatal period encompassed a specific time span, with women progressing through the phases sequentially. However, with today's shorter hospitalisations for childbirth, women move through the phases more quickly and sometimes even experience more than one phase at a time.

Building relationships

The mother and her family undergo other changes as well. Ideally, these changes lead to the development of parental love for the baby and positive relationships among all family members.

Not all change is good

In some cases, negative psychological reactions may also occur. For example, a mother may feel let down because her baby is now the centre of attention or she may feel disappointed because the baby doesn't meet her preconceived expectations. Tiredness may have a big impact on how well the mother feels – night feeds and recovering from the delivery can all leave her feeling worn out.

A mother may also feel overwhelming sadness for no discernible reason; these feelings are commonly termed '*postnatal blues*' or '*baby blues*'. A mother with postnatal blues may experience emotional lability, a let-down feeling, crying for no apparent reason, headache, insomnia, fatigue, restlessness, depression and anger. These feelings most commonly peak around postnatal day 5 and subside by postnatal day 10. (See *Battling the baby blues*, page 377.)

First contact

Early contact and interaction between the parents, the baby and other siblings – including rooming- in and sibling visitation – encourages bonding and helps integrate the baby into the family.

Postnatal assessment

As with any assessment, a postnatal assessment consists of a maternal history and a physical examination.

Maternal history

Your postnatal maternal history should focus on the woman's pregnancy, labour and birth events. You should be able to find much of this information in the mother's hospital notes. For example, the notes should contain information about:
• problems experienced, such as gestational hypertension or gestational diabetes
• any hospital admissions during the pregnancy prior to onset of labour
• time of labour onset and admission to the hospital
• types of analgesia and anaesthesia used
• length of labour and time of delivery
• type of delivery and any difficulties, e.g. shoulder dystocia
• time of placenta expulsion and appearance of the placenta (completeness)
• sex, weight and condition of the baby.
You'll need this information to plan the mother's care and promote maternal–infant bonding.

Another reliable source

Don't rely on the mother's hospital notes as your sole source of information. Always ask the mother to describe the events and fill in the details in her own

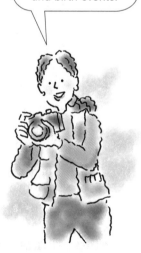

Your postnatal mother's history should focus on her pregnancy, labour and birth events.

Education edge

Battling the baby blues

For most women, having a baby is a joyous experience. However, childbirth leaves some women feeling sad, depressed, angry, anxious and afraid. Commonly called postnatal blues or baby blues, these feelings affect quite a few women after childbirth. In most cases, they occur within the first few days postpartum and then disappear on their own within several days.

Help is on the way

To help the mother with postnatal blues, tell her to:

- get plenty of rest
- ask for help from her family and friends
- take special care of herself
- spend time with her partner
- call her GP if her mood doesn't improve after a few weeks and she has trouble coping (this may be a sign of a more severe depression).

Be sure to explain to the woman that many new mothers feel sadness, fear, anger and anxiety after having a baby. These feelings don't mean that she's a failure as a woman or as a mother. They indicate that she's adjusting to the changes that follow birth.

Blues vs. depression

Unfortunately, about 10% of women experience a more profound problem called postnatal depression. In these cases, maternal feelings of depression and despair last longer than a few weeks and are so intense that they interfere with the woman's daily activities. Postnatal depression can occur after any pregnancy; it isn't specifically associated with first pregnancies. It commonly requires counselling or medication to resolve.

Possible causes of postnatal depression include:

- doubt about the pregnancy
- recent stress, such as loss of a loved one, a family illness or a recent move

- lack of a support system
- unplanned caesarean birth (may leave the woman feeling like a failure)
- breastfeeding problems, especially if a new mother can't breastfeed or decides to stop
- sharp drop in oestrogen and progesterone levels after childbirth, possibly triggering depression in the same way that much smaller changes in hormone levels can trigger mood swings and tension before menstrual periods
- early birth of baby (may cause woman to feel unprepared)
- unresolved issues of not being able to be the 'perfect' mother
- feeling of failure if the mother believes that she should instinctively know how to care for her baby
- disappointment over sex of the baby or other characteristics (baby isn't as mother imagined).

Signs and symptoms that may indicate that postnatal blues are actually postnatal depression include:

- worsening insomnia
- changes in appetite; poor intake
- poor interaction with the baby; views the baby as a burden or problem
- suicidal thoughts or thoughts of harming the baby
- feelings of isolation from social contacts and support systems
- inability to care for self or baby due to lack of energy or desire.

It is vital that the midwife or health visitor in community picks up on potential signs of postnatal depression and supports the woman by referring her to the appropriate services for help.

Women experiencing signs of postnatal depression should seek medical help as soon as possible. (See Chapter 10, *Complications of the postpartum period*.)

words. This is also a good way to find out her emotions and feelings about pregnancy and childbirth.

Also ask the mother about her family and lifestyle, including support systems, other children, other people living in the home, her occupation, her community environment and her socioeconomic level. This information can help you determine whether additional support or follow-up is needed.

> Always ask the mum to describe the events and fill in the details in her own words.

Physical examination

In many cases, you won't need to do a complete physical examination in the postnatal period because the mother already had a complete assessment early in the pregnancy. However, you should complete a review of systems, covering the following areas:
- general appearance – weight, eyes, puffiness – anything unusual
- skin – colour, condition
- energy level, including level of activity and fatigue
- pain, including location, severity and aggravating factors, such as sitting and walking
- GI elimination, including bowel sounds, passage of flatus and haemorrhoids
- fluid intake
- urinary elimination, including the time and amount of first voiding – any pain on micturition
- peripheral circulation.
   In addition, you'll need to assess these five critical areas:
- breasts
- uterus
- lochia
- perineum
- legs.

Clinical observations

It may be necessary to record the mother's temperature, pulse, respiratory rate and blood pressure, depending on her physical condition, for example if she had raised blood pressure before delivery, it should be monitored closely till it settles. Some units routinely record maternal observations on a daily basis and it may be a good way of detecting early problems like infection.

Breasts

It is unnecessary to examine the breasts on the mother's first postnatal day as the changes will be minimal, but thereafter it is wise to check the breasts for redness, trauma (if breastfeeding) and enquire about discomfort or pain. It is important, if the mother doesn't mind, that student midwives have the opportunity to examine 'normal' breasts so that they will be able to recognise deviation from normal.

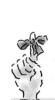

Memory jogger

To help you remember what to evaluate during a postnatal assessment, think of the words BUBBLE.

B – Breasts

U – Uterus

B – Bowel

B – Bladder

L – Lochia

E – Episiotomy

Education edge

Engorgement or something else?

Engorgement, which may result from venous and lymphatic stasis and alveolar milk accumulation, causes the entire breast to appear reddened and to feel warm, firm and tender. The baby will experience difficulty latching onto a severely engorged breast, which further complicates the situation. Encourage the woman to perform frequent and regular breastfeedings to help prevent this problem.

Something else

If the warmth, tenderness and redness are localised to only one portion of the breast and the woman has a fever or flu-like symptoms, suspect mastitis – inflammation of the glands or milk ducts. It usually results from a pathogen that passes from the infant's nose or pharynx into breast tissue through a cracked nipple. Teach the mother about mastitis, and warn her to call the midwife or GP immediately if she has any signs or symptoms.

Inspect and then gently palpate the breasts, noting size and any unusual marks or signs of trauma. At first, the breasts should feel soft and secrete a thin, yellow fluid called *colostrum*. However, as they fill with milk – usually around the third postnatal day – they should begin to feel firm and warm. Between feedings, the entire breast may be tender, hard and tense on palpation. A low-grade temperature (38.3°C) isn't uncommon between days 2 and 5, when the 'milk comes in', but it shouldn't last for more than 24 hours. Engorgement mimics inflammatory response, i.e. redness, heat, pain and swelling. (See *Engorgement or something else?*)

Nodule?

A small, firm nodule in the breast may be caused by a temporarily blocked milk duct or milk that hasn't flowed forward into the nipple. This problem generally corrects itself when the baby breastfeeds – putting a warm compress on the area and gentle massaging might encourage the duct to clear. Be sure to reassess the breast after the baby feeds to determine if the problem has resolved, and report your findings – including the location of the nodule – to the doctor. Inspect the nipples for cracks, fissures or configuration. Cracks or breaks in the skin can provide an entry for organisms and lead to infection. Also look for other problems. Successful breastfeeding can be more challenging if the nipples are flat or inverted. A lactation consultant or a breastfeeding coordinator may be helpful – use of a breast shell or nipple shield may help.

Check that the mother is wearing a good, supportive bra and breast pads to catch any leakage of colostrum or milk.

Uterus

During your examination, gently palpate the uterine fundus to determine uterine size, degree of firmness and rate of descent, which is measured in fingerbreadths above or below the umbilicus. The fundal height and consistency of the uterus should be checked on a frequent basis in the hours immediately following delivery to make sure the uterus is well contracted and that bleeding is controlled. Fundal assessment should be performed more frequently if complications are noted.

Fundal assessment is especially uncomfortable for the woman who has had a caesarean birth and therefore should not be performed. The midwife should assess this mother's condition by checking the blood loss per vaginum and noting amount, colour and smell of the lochia, as well as recording her temperature and pulse rate regularly.

Ready, set, palpate!

Before palpating the uterus, explain the procedure to the woman and provide privacy. Wash your hands and then put on gloves. Also, ask the woman to void. A full bladder makes the uterus 'boggier' and deviates the fundus to the right of the umbilicus or +1 or +2 above the umbilicus. When the bladder is empty, the uterus should be at or slightly above the level of the umbilicus in the first postnatal day.

Next, lower the head of the bed until the woman is lying supine or with her head slightly elevated. Expose the abdomen for palpation and the perineum for inspection, ensuring that you maintain the mother's dignity at all times. Watch for bleeding, clots and tissue expulsion while massaging the uterus.

Performing palpation

To palpate the uterine fundus, follow these steps:
• While supporting the lower segment of the uterus with a hand placed just above the symphysis, gently palpate the fundus with your other hand to evaluate its firmness. (See *Feeling the fundus*.)

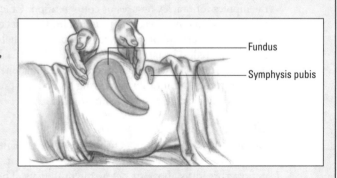

Keep abreast of cracks or breaks in the skin of a breastfeeding mother. They can provide an entry for organisms, leading to infection.

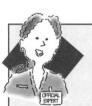

Advice from the experts

Feeling the fundus

A full-term pregnancy stretches the ligaments supporting the uterus, placing it at risk for inversion during palpation and massage. To guard against this, place one hand against the woman's abdomen at the symphysis pubis level, as shown. This steadies the fundus and prevents downward displacement. Then place the other hand at the top of the fundus, cupping it, as shown.

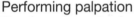

Fundus

Symphysis pubis

Education edge

Complications of fundal palpation

Because the uterus and its supporting ligaments are tender after birth, pain is the most common complication of fundal palpation and massage. Excessive massage can stimulate uterine contractions, causing undue muscle fatigue and leading to uterine atony or inversion. Lack of lochia may signal a clot blocking the cervical os. Heavy bleeding may result if a position change dislodges the clot. Take the woman's vital signs frequently to assess for hypovolaemic shock.

- Note the level of the fundus above or below the umbilicus in centimetres or fingerbreadths.
- If the uterus seems soft and boggy, gently massage the fundus with a circular motion until it becomes firm. Without digging into the abdomen, gently compress and release your fingers, almost cupping the fundus in your hand. Observe the vaginal drainage during massage.
- Massage long enough to produce firmness but not discomfort.
- If the uterus fails to contract and heavy bleeding occurs, take emergency measures to control the bleeding and notify the medical staff. If the fundus becomes firm after massage, keep one hand on the lower uterus and press gently toward the pubis to expel clots. (See *Complications of fundal palpation*.)

Remember the bladder

When assessing the uterine fundus, also assess for bladder distention. A distended bladder can impede the downward descent of the uterus by pushing it upward and, possibly, to the right side. If the bladder is distended and the woman is unable to urinate, you may need to catheterise her.

Lochia

After birth, the outermost layer of the uterus becomes necrotic and is expelled. This vaginal discharge – called *lochia* – is similar to menstrual flow and consists of blood, fragments of the decidua, white blood cells (WBCs), mucus and some bacteria.

Assessing lochia flow

Lochia is commonly assessed in conjunction with fundal assessment. (See *Three types of lochia*.)

Help the woman into a comfortable position – this can be on her side or lying on her back. Be sure to check under her buttocks to make sure that blood isn't pooling there. Then remove the woman's perineal pad and evaluate the amount, colour, odour and consistency (presence of clots) of the discharge.

Three types of lochia

Lochia colour, which typically changes throughout the post-partum period, may be categorised as:

- *lochia rubra* – red vaginal discharge that occurs from approximately day 1 to day 3 postpartum
- *lochia serosa* – pinkish or brownish discharge that occurs from approximately day 4 to day 10 postpartum
- *lochia alba* – creamy white or colourless vaginal discharge that occurs from approximately day 10 to day 14 postpartum (although it may continue for up to 6 weeks).

On the lookout

Here's what to look for when assessing lochia:

- *Amount* – Although it varies, the amount of lochia is typically comparable to the amount during menstrual flow. A woman who's breastfeeding may have less lochia. Also, a woman who has had a caesarean birth may have a scant amount. Lochia may be present for at least 3 weeks postpartum. Lochia flow increases with activity; for example, when the mother gets out of bed the first several times (due to pooled lochia being released) or when she lifts a heavy object or walks up stairs (due to an actual increase in the amount of lochia). If the woman saturates a perineal pad in less than an hour, this is considered excessive flow, and she should notify her midwife.
- *Colour* – Lochia typically is described as lochia rubra, serosa or alba, depending on the colour of the discharge. Lochia colour depends on the postnatal day. A sudden change in colour – for example, from pink back to red – suggests new bleeding or retained placental fragments.
- *Odour* – Lochia should smell similar to menstrual flow. A foul or offensive odour suggests infection.
- *Consistency* – Lochia should have minimal or small clots, if any. Evidence of large or numerous clots indicates poor uterine contraction and requires further assessment – especially if the clots are large (size of a 50p piece or bigger)

Perineum and rectum

The pressure exerted on the perineum and rectum during birth results in oedema and generalised tenderness. Some areas of the perineum may be ecchymotic (bruised), caused by the rupture of surface capillaries. Sutures for an episiotomy or laceration may also be present. Haemorrhoids are also commonly seen.

What's your position?

Assessment of the perineum and rectum mainly involves inspection and is performed at the same time that you assess the lochia. Help the woman into the supine position. This position provides better visibility and causes less discomfort for the woman with a mediolateral episiotomy. A back-lying position can also be used for women with midline episiotomies. Make sure you have adequate light for inspection. Always ensure the woman is covered with a sheet and avoid overexposure.

Checking down under

Observe for intactness of skin, positioning of the episiotomy (if one was performed) or tear and appearance of sutures (from episiotomy or laceration repair) and the surrounding rectal area. Keep in mind that the edges of an episiotomy are usually sealed 24 hours after delivery. Note ecchymosis, haematoma, erythema, oedema, drainage or bleeding from sutures, a foul odour or signs of infection – any of these should be reported to the obstetrician.

Memory jogger

To help you remember what to look for when assessing an episiotomy site or a laceration, think REODA:

R – Redness

E – Erythema and ecchymosis

O – Oedema

D – Drainage or discharge

A – Approximation (of wound edges)

Many women who have a 1° tear may not have been sutured so it is important to look for healing and repair. Also observe for the presence of haemorrhoids as these can cause great discomfort to the mother so she may need cream or suppositories to help ease this. Because the haemorrhoids are often close to the perineal area, she must be careful to keep the area clean – especially after bowel movements. She should be advised to have tepid baths daily and avoid constipation – she might want to shower the area after bowel movements – or use a bidet if she has one.

Perineal care

Perineal assessment also includes perineal care. The goals of postnatal perineal care are to relieve discomfort, promote healing and prevent infection by cleaning the perineal area. Teach the woman how to perform perineal care in conjunction with a perineal assessment. Perineal care should be performed after the woman voids or has a bowel movement.

Two methods of providing perineal care are generally used: vulval toilet if the mother is on bed rest, and the bidet.

Vulval toilet, follow these steps:
- Fill a jug with cleaning solution (usually warm water).
- Help the mother sit on a warmed bedpan.
- Pour the solution over her perineal area.
- After completion, help the woman off the bedpan and remove it.
- Pat the perineal area dry, and help the woman apply a new perineal pad.

Hot and cold comfort

During perineal care, note if the woman complains of pain or tenderness. If she does, you may need to apply cold packs to the area for the first 12 hours after birth. This helps reduce perineal oedema and prevent haematoma formation, thereby reducing pain and promoting healing.

Cold therapy isn't effective after the first 24 hours. Instead, heat is recommended because it increases circulation to the area. Forms of heat include a perineal warm pack (dry heat) or a warm bath (moist heat).

For extensive lacerations, such as third or fourth degree lacerations, frequent warm baths may aid perineal healing, provide comfort and reduce oedema. Because of shortened hospitalisation time, the mother should be advised about perineal hygiene at home, the importance of wearing loose cotton underwear and avoiding talcum, sprays or perfumed bath products until healing is complete.

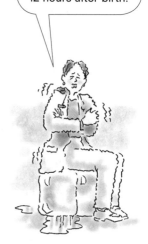

If the woman complains of pain or tenderness, you may need to apply cool packs to the perineal area for the first 12 hours after birth.

Legs

Make the mother comfortable on the bed and expose her legs, examining one at a time. It's a good idea to check with the mother if she has varicose veins and how badly they were affected by her pregnancy. Ask the mother to bend one leg at a time and check carefully for:
- Colour – any reddened areas or discolouration.
- Check the circulation in both her feet – do they both feel warm?
- Look at the legs – are they the same size – deep vein thrombosis (DVT) can cause swelling of the affected leg.

- If the mother has varicose veins make sure they are not inflamed and that there is no signs of thrombophlebitis in any of the veins – this looks like a red track that follows the route of the vein up the leg.
- With the flat of your hand, gently feel, in a continuous movement up the back of the mother's leg – do not grasp or grip parts of her leg – if there was a clot, you could dislodge it. Also look for any reddened areas, swelling, or complaints of pain in the calf when the mother walks.
- Routine use of Homans sign as a tool for evaluation of thromboembolism is not recommended.

High-risk mothers, i.e. obese, smokers, history of DVT, operative delivery, postepidural, are all at potential risk of developing DVT and so they will need anticoagulant therapy postnatally.

In caring for their legs, women should:
- be encouraged to mobilise as soon as appropriate following the birth.
- be discouraged from crossing their legs or putting undue pressure on the calves of their legs
- be evaluated for deep venous thrombosis (emergency action) in case of unilateral calf pain, redness or swelling.

Women experiencing shortness of breath or chest pain should be evaluated for pulmonary thromboembolism (emergency action). Obese women are at higher risk of thromboembolism and should receive individualised care. Any high-risk mother should wear thromboembolic stockings (TED stockings).

Postnatal care measures

Ongoing assessment is crucial during the postnatal period and it is the midwife's duty to examine the postnatal mother on a daily basis and record her findings – usually from day 1 to day 10. Although the midwife can discharge the woman after this period, she is still obliged to care for her up to 28 days postnatally and after, if the mother has problems. The main responsibilities the midwife has to the mother and baby are to:
- Ask the woman about her health and well-being and that of her baby. This should include asking about her experience of common physical health problems and assessing her psychological state where possible. Any symptoms reported by the woman or identified through clinical observations should be assessed.
- Continue to assess the mother's vital signs, breasts, uterine fundus, lochia, perineum and legs.
- Offer consistent information and clear explanations to empower the woman to take care of her own health and that of her baby, and to recognise symptoms that may require discussion. Encourage the woman and her family to report any concerns in relation to their physical, social, mental or emotional health, discuss issues and ask questions.
- Document in the care plan any specific problems and follow-up. Length of stay in a maternity unit should be discussed between the individual woman

and her midwife, taking into account the health and well-being of the woman and her baby and the level of support available following discharge.
• Administer medications as ordered to relieve discomfort from the episiotomy or from uterine contractions, incisional pain or breast engorgement and assess for therapeutic effectiveness.
• Be sure to document all treatments given, advice given and any medications given in the mother's hospital records.
• Encourage the mother to do her postnatal exercises regularly – the physiotherapist teaches these in hospital but it is vital she carries on with them after discharge. The best time to do them is when she is sitting down, feeding her baby.
• Encourage the mother to rest after delivery and throughout the postnatal period to prevent exhaustion.

A-voiding catheterisation

Assess the woman's urinary elimination – she should void within 6–8 hours after delivery. The postnatal mother has an increased diuresis after delivery and so should pass plenty of urine – failure to do so could indicate:
• bladder trauma – bruising
• lack of return of sensation following epidural or difficult delivery
• a clot at the neck of the bladder following catheterisation trauma
• lack of tone following removal of a urinary catheter

If she doesn't pass urine after 6–8 hours, help her urge to void by administering analgesics as ordered, pouring warm water over the perineum, placing the mother's hands in warm water or running water for her to hear (the sound may encourage the urge to void). She could try a warm bath and be encouraged to void in the water if need be. If all attempts fail, the woman may need to be catheterised.

There is a real danger of urinary retention, other than being very distressing and painful to the woman, causing other complications such as postpartum haemorrhage, infection and renal problems resulting from urinary reflux of urine into the ureters.

Flatus foreshadows function

Finally, assess bowel function. Elimination is typically a good indicator of bowel function. The woman should have a bowel movement 2–3 days after delivery to avoid constipation. However, a woman who has eaten nothing by mouth for 12–24 hours and then has a caesarean birth may not have a bowel movement for several days. In these cases, flatus may be a better indicator of bowel function. Encourage the woman to drink plenty of fluids and eat high-fibre foods to prevent constipation. If necessary, the doctor may order stool softeners or laxatives if the mother has not had a bowel movement by day 4. The woman would be advised to ask her midwife about suppositories or a mini-enema (if constipation persists after taking mild laxatives) and altering her diet and fluid intake. If the woman has haemorrhoids, cool witch hazel compresses may be helpful initially then creams or suppositories. Don't use

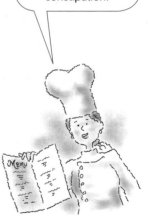

Get a move on! A postnatal mother should drink plenty of fluids and eat high-fibre foods to prevent constipation.

suppositories if the woman has a third or fourth degree tear. The woman may be scared to pass stools and so needs lot of psychological support – particularly if she has a painful perineal area with lots of sutures in place.

Educating the mother in self-care

Because of the short length of stay for most postnatal women, teaching should focus on maternal self-care activities and neonatal care. (See *Postnatal maternal self-care*, page 387.)

Lactation

Lactation refers to the production of breast milk, the preferred source of nutrition for a newborn infant. All mothers experience the physiological changes that occur with lactation and breast milk production regardless of whether they plan to breastfeed.

Physiology of lactation

During pregnancy, a hormone called *prolactin* prepares the woman's breasts to secrete milk. Other hormones (progesterone and oestrogen) interact to suppress milk secretion while developing the breasts for lactation. Oestrogen causes the breasts to grow by increasing their fat content. Progesterone causes lobule growth and develops the alveolar (acinar) cells' secretory capacity.

After birth, the mother's oestrogen and progesterone levels drop abruptly. This drop in hormones triggers the release of prolactin from the anterior pituitary, which starts the cycle of synthesis and secretion of milk. (See *A closer look at lactation*, page 388.)

Breast milk composition

From about the fourth month of pregnancy until the first 3–4 days after delivery, the acinar cells produce and secrete colostrum. Colostrum is a thick, sticky, golden-yellow fluid that contains protein, sugar, fat, water, minerals, vitamins and maternal antibodies. It's easy for the newborn baby to digest because it's high in protein and low in sugar and fat. It also provides completely adequate nutrition for the infant. The high protein level of colostrum aids in the binding of bilirubin and also has a laxative effect, which promotes early passage of the infant's first stool, called *meconium*.

Got milk?

On about the second to fourth postpartum day, colostrum is replaced by mature breast milk. During this time, the woman produces copious amounts of breast milk. The composition of this breast milk changes with each feeding. As the baby breastfeeds, the bluish-white foremilk (containing part skim and part whole milk) primarily provides protein, lactose and

Education edge

Postnatal maternal self-care

When advising the mother about self-care for the postnatal period, be sure to include these topic areas and instructions.

Personal hygiene

- Change perineal pads frequently, removing them from the front to the back and disposing of them in a plastic bag.
- Perform perineal care each time that you urinate or move your bowels.
- Monitor your vaginal discharge; it should change from red to pinkish brown to clear or white before stopping altogether. Notify your midwife or GP if the discharge returns to a previous colour, becomes bright red or yellowish green, suddenly increases in amount or develops an offensive odour.
- Shower daily.

Breasts

- Wear a firm, supportive bra.
- If nipple leakage occurs, use clean gauze pads or nursing pads inside your bra to absorb the moisture.
- Inspect your nipples for cracking, fissures or soreness, and report areas of redness, tenderness or swelling.
- Wash breasts daily with clear water when showering and dry with a soft towel or allow to air dry. Don't use soap on your breasts or nipples because soap is drying.
- If you're breastfeeding and your breasts become engorged, use warm compresses, stand under a warm shower or feed your baby more frequently for relief. If the baby is unable to latch on due to engorgement, using a breast pump should help. If you aren't breastfeeding, apply cool compresses several times per day – cool cabbage leaves work well. Take adequate analgesia.

Activity and exercise

- Balance rest periods with activity, get as much sleep as possible at night and take frequent rest periods or naps during the day.

- Check with your midwife about when to begin exercising.
- Remember to do your postnatal exercises!

Nutrition

- Increase your intake of protein and calories.
- Drink plenty of fluids throughout the day, including before and after breastfeeding.

Elimination

- If you have the urge to urinate or move your bowels, don't delay doing so. Urinate at least every 2–3 hours. This helps keep the uterus contracted and decreases the risk of excessive bleeding.
- Report difficulty urinating, burning or pain to your midwife or GP.
- Drink plenty of liquids and eat high-fibre foods to prevent constipation.
- Follow your midwife's instructions about the use of stool softeners or laxatives.

Sexual activity and contraception

- Remember that breastfeeding isn't a reliable method of contraception. Discuss birth control options with your GP.
- Ask your GP when you can resume sexual activity and contraceptive measures. Most couples can resume having sex within 3–4 weeks after delivery, or possibly as soon as lochia ceases.
- Use a water-based lubricant if necessary.
- Expect a decrease in intensity and rapidity of sexual response for about 3 months after delivery.
- Perform postnatal exercises to help strengthen your pelvic floor muscles. To do this, squeeze your pelvic muscles as if trying to stop urine flow, and then release them.
- Take adequate analgesia to reduce pain and discomfort in the first few weeks after giving birth.

A closer look at lactation

After delivery of the placenta, the drop in progesterone and oestrogen levels stimulates the production of prolactin. This hormone stimulates milk production by the acinar cells in the mammary glands.

Nerve impulses caused by the baby sucking at the breast, travel from the nipple to the hypothalamus, resulting in the production of prolactin-releasing factor. This factor leads to additional production of prolactin and, subsequently, more milk production.

Go with the flow

Milk flows from the acinar cells through small tubules to the lactiferous sinuses (small reservoirs located behind the nipple). This milk, called *foremilk*, is thin, bluish and sugary and is constantly forming. It quenches the baby's thirst but contains little fat and protein.

When the baby sucks at the breast, oxytocin is released, causing the sinuses to contract. Contraction pushes the milk forward through the nipple to the baby. In addition, release of oxytocin causes the smooth muscles of the uterus to contract.

That let-down feeling

Movement of the milk forward through the nipple is termed the *let-down reflex* and may be triggered by things other than the infant sucking at the breast. For example, women have reported that hearing their baby cry or thinking about him causes this reflex.

Once the let-down reflex occurs and the baby has fed for 10–15 minutes, new milk – called *hindmilk* – is formed. This milk is thicker, whiter and contains higher concentrations of fat and protein. Hindmilk contains the calories and fat necessary for the baby to gain weight, build brain tissue and be more content and satisfied between feedings.

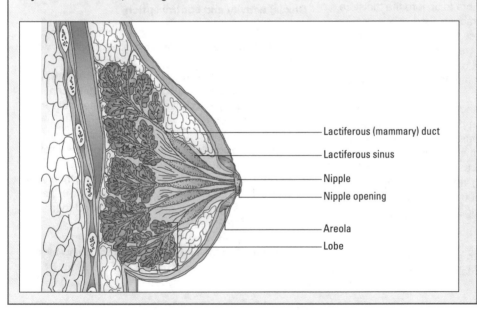

- Lactiferous (mammary) duct
- Lactiferous sinus
- Nipple
- Nipple opening
- Areola
- Lobe

water-soluble vitamins to the baby. Hindmilk, or cream, is produced within the first 10–20 minutes of breastfeeding and contains denser calories from fat. This transitional breast milk is replaced by true or mature breast milk by around day 10 after delivery.

Lactation and the menstrual cycle

After delivery of the placenta, oestrogen and progesterone production ceases. As a result, the pituitary gland increases the production of FSH, which eventually leads to ovulation and resumption of the menstrual cycle.

Here we go again

Lactating women begin menstruating again at various times, anywhere from 2 to 18 months. Ovulation may occur by the end of the first month postpartum, or it may not occur for one or more menstrual cycles. Woman who aren't lactating usually resume menstruating in 6–10 weeks. Approximately half of these women ovulate with the first menstrual cycle.

Neonatal nutrition

Human milk consumed through breastfeeding is considered optimal for babies. Despite this, not all mothers can or choose to breastfeed. Medical conditions, cultural background, anxiety, drug abuse and various other factors can prevent a woman from breastfeeding successfully. Furthermore, some babies can't take in enough breast milk through breastfeeding to meet their nutritional needs. Preterm or high-risk neonates may require additives or fortifiers in their breast milk to meet their unique needs while still receiving all the benefits of regular breast milk.

Breastfeeding

Breastfeeding is considered the safest, simplest and least expensive way to provide complete infant nourishment. The Department of Health recommend breastfeeding exclusively for the first 6 months of the infant's life and then in combination with infant foods until the age of one year.

Contrary to popular belief

Breastfeeding is contraindicated if the mother:
- has herpes lesions on her nipples
- is receiving certain medications, such as sedatives or antidepressants, that pass into the breast milk and may harm the baby
- is on a restricted diet that interferes with adequate nutrient intake and subsequently affects the quality of milk produced
- has breast cancer
- has a severe chronic condition, such as active tuberculosis, human immunodeficiency virus infection or hepatitis.

Here's food for thought. Breastfeeding is the safest, simplest and least expensive way to provide complete infant nourishment.

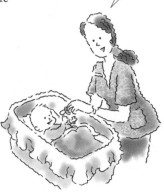

Benefits of breastfeeding

Here are some of the benefits of breastfeeding.

Passive immunity

Human milk provides passive immunity. Colostrum is the first fluid secreted from the breast (occurs within the first few days after delivery) and provides immune factor and protein to the baby. Many components of breast milk protect against infection – it contains antibodies (especially immunoglobulin A) and white blood cells that protect the baby from some forms of infection. Breastfed babies also experience fewer allergies and intolerances.

Easily digestible

Breast milk provides essential nutrients in an easily digestible form. It contains lipase, which breaks down dietary fat, making it easily available to the baby's system.

Brain booster

The lipids in breast milk are high in linoleic acid and cholesterol, which are needed for brain development.

Low protein content

Cow's milk contains proportionally higher concentrations of electrolytes and protein than are needed by human babies. It must be cleared by the immature kidneys and thus isn't recommended until after a baby is at least 12 months old.

Convenient and inexpensive

Breastfeeding saves time and money in buying and preparing formula.

Advantages

Breastfeeding is advantageous for the mother and the baby. (See *Benefits of breastfeeding*.)

Maternal benefits include:
- protection against breast cancer
- assistance in uterine involution due to the release of oxytocin
- empowerment (as the woman learns to master the skill)
- less preparation time and less cost than using infant formula.

More good news about breastfeeding

Breast milk is also highly beneficial for the baby. For example, it reduces the risk of infection because it contains:
- immunoglobulin A – an antibody that prevents foreign proteins from being absorbed by the neonate's GI tract
- lactoferrin – an iron-binding protein that interferes with bacterial growth
- lysozyme – an enzyme that actively destroys bacteria
- leucocytes – WBCs that protect against common respiratory infections
- macrophages – cells that produce interferon, which offers protection from viral invasion.

In addition, breastfeeding is advantageous to the neonate for these reasons:
- Breast milk promotes rapid brain growth because it contains large amounts of lactose, which is easily digested and can be rapidly converted into glucose.
- Breast milk's protein and nitrogen contents provide foundations for neurological cell building.

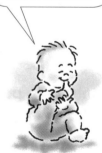

Wow! Breastfeeding is even better than sucking my toes. And it reduces my risk of infection.

- Breast milk contains adequate electrolyte and mineral composition for the baby's needs without overloading his renal system.
- Breastfeeding improves the baby's ability to regulate calcium and phosphorus levels.
- The sucking mechanism associated with breastfeeding reduces dental arch malformations.
- A breastfed baby's GI tract contains large amounts of *Lactobacillus bifidus*, a beneficial bacterium that prevents the growth of harmful organisms.

On the contrary

Breastfeeding may delay ovulation but shouldn't be considered a reliable form of contraception. In addition, evidence doesn't suggest that breastfeeding aids in weight loss after pregnancy.

Maternal nutrition and breastfeeding

Nutritional needs for a woman who's breastfeeding are only slightly different from those during her pregnancy. Folate and iron needs decrease after giving birth, and energy requirements increase.

Fuelling milk production

While breastfeeding, a healthy woman should consume 2,300 to 2,700 calories/day, approximately 500 calories/day more than pre-pregnancy recommendations. If maternal intake is poor, which can occur when a lactating woman is dieting, the nutrient intake in her breast milk may become inadequate.

Water hydrant

Adequate hydration encourages ample milk production, so it's important for new mothers to drink plenty of fluids – 2–3 L/day. The mother should also drink one 150 ml glass of fluid each time she breastfeeds to ensure she stays hydrated. Water and such beverages as fruit juices and milk are good choices to maintain adequate hydration.

Keep contaminants out!

Most substances that the mother ingests are secreted into her milk. Therefore, beverages containing alcohol and caffeine should be limited or avoided because they may be harmful to the neonate. In addition, it's important to check with a paediatrician before taking medication. Some researchers believe that components of the maternal food may contribute to colic or the baby's fussiness.

Breastfeeding assistance

Even women who have previously breastfed can benefit from assistance and instruction. The key is helping the mother to latch the baby on properly. Breastfeeding should occur as soon as possible after birth. However, this may not be possible, especially if the woman is overly fatigued or if a complication has developed.

Sorry, mum, but you're wrong. Breastfeeding will NOT prevent pregnancy!

Eat up! Lactation requires more energy! Now isn't the time for mum to cut calories.

Don't get comfy yet

When assisting with breastfeeding, explain the procedure and provide privacy. Encourage the mother to drink a beverage before and during or after breastfeeding to ensure adequate fluid intake, which maintains milk production. Also encourage her to use the bathroom and change the baby's nappy before breastfeeding begins so that feeding is uninterrupted. Then wash your hands and instruct the mother to do the same.

Now, take a load off

Help the mother find a comfortable position. (See *Breastfeeding positions*.) Then follow these instructions:

• Have the mother expose one breast and rest the nape of the baby's neck in the crook of her arm, supporting his back with her forearm.

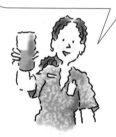

Breastfeeding mums should drink fluids before breastfeeding as well as during or after to ensure adequate intake, which maintains milk production.

Education edge

Breastfeeding positions

The position a mother uses when breastfeeding should be comfortable and efficient. Explain to the mother that changing positions periodically alters the baby's grasp on the nipple and helps to prevent contact friction on the same area. As appropriate, suggest these three popular feeding positions.

Cradle position

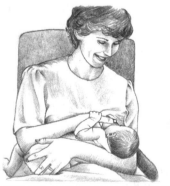

The mother cradles the baby's head in the crook of her arm. Instruct her to place a pillow on her lap for the baby to lie on. Offer to place a pillow behind her back; this provides comfort and may also assist with correct positioning.

Side-lying position

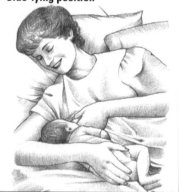

Instruct the mother to lie on her side with her stomach facing the baby's. As the baby's mouth opens, she should pull him toward the nipple. Inform her to place a pillow or rolled blanket behind the baby's back to prevent him from moving or rolling away from the breast.

Football position

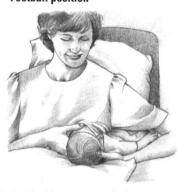

Sitting with a pillow in front of her, the mother places her hand under the baby's head. As the baby's mouth opens, she pulls his head near her breast. This position may be more comfortable for the woman who has had a caesarean birth.

- Inform her that uterine cramping may occur during breastfeeding until her uterus returns to its original size.
- Guiding the mother's free hand, have her place her thumb on top of the exposed breast's areola and her first two fingers beneath it, forming a C. Have her turn the baby so that his entire body faces the breast.
- Tell the mother to stroke her baby's cheek with her finger or the baby's mouth with her nipple. This stimulates the rooting reflex. Emphasise that she should touch the cheek closest to the exposed breast. Touching the other cheek may cause the baby to turn his head towards the touch and away from the breast.
- When the baby opens his mouth and roots for the nipple, instruct the mother to move him onto the breast so that he gets as much of the areola as possible into his mouth. This helps him to exert sufficient pressure with his lips, gums and cheek muscles on the milk sinuses below the areola.
- Show the mother how to check for occlusion of the baby's nostrils by the breast. If this happens, she should reposition the baby to give him room to breathe. The tip of his nose should touch the breast but not be mashed into it. The baby will breathe out of the sides of his nose.
- Suggest that the mother breastfeed for as long as possible each feed and to feed from alternate breasts each time so that one breast always gets completely emptied. Let the baby suck until he comes off himself – the best advice is to never break a good latch. Remember: The baby doesn't start receiving fat-and-protein-rich hind milk until after 15 minutes of feeding.
- If the mother is in pain, it will feel uncomfortable for about 10–15 seconds and it is likely that the baby has not latched on properly or is in a poor position. Take the baby off the breast by instructing the mother to slip a finger into the side of the baby's mouth to break the seal, and then attempt to latch him on again.

The Baby Friendly Initiative (BFI)

The Baby Friendly Initiative (BFI) is a worldwide programme of the World Health Organisation and UNICEF. It was established in 1992 to encourage maternity hospitals to implement the 'Ten Steps to Successful Breastfeeding' and to practise in accordance with the International Code of Marketing of Breastmilk Substitutes. The UNICEF UK Baby Friendly Initiative was launched in the UK in 1994; in 1998 its principles were extended to cover the work of community health care services in the Seven Point Plan for the Promotion, Protection and Support of Breastfeeding in Community Health Care Settings. The BFI works with the health care system to ensure a high standard of care for pregnant women and breastfeeding mothers and babies. They provide support for health care facilities that are seeking to implement best practice, and to offer an assessment and accreditation process that recognises those that have achieved the required standard. More information about the BFI can be accessed from the website: www.babyfriendly.org.uk

Burping basics

Because some babies swallow large amounts of air when feeding, encourage the mother to wind the baby halfway through the breastfeed and again at the end of the feeding. Burping also helps to waken the baby. Before winding the baby, remind the mother to place a protective cover, such as a towel or napkin, under the baby's chin. The most common way to wind a baby is to place him over one shoulder and gently pat or rub his back to help expel ingested air.

A burp is a burp is a burp

Some mothers have trouble supporting the baby's head while patting or rubbing his back. This position may be especially awkward with small babies because they lack the ability to control their heads. In these cases, suggest the sitting position for winding. (See *Sitting up for burping*, page 395.) A third acceptable position is placing the baby prone across the mother's lap.

Taking a breather

When the mother finishes breastfeeding, instruct her to wind the baby, comfort him, then place the baby in the cot, lying on his back. She should let her nipples air dry for about 15 minutes after breastfeeding.

To make sure that both breasts receive equal stimulation, advise the mother to feed the baby on alternate breast each time so that one breast always gets emptied completely. To help her remember, she can put a safety pin on her bra strap on the side last used.

Quelling concerns

Mothers commonly have questions about breastfeeding, including how often the baby should feed, how much the baby is getting and what to do if he is too sleepy to breastfeed. Reassure the mother that breastfeeding schedules aren't carved in stone and that developing a schedule that both she and her baby feel comfortable with takes time.

Feed me, feed me!

During the first few days of life, a baby is usually fed as often as he's hungry, possibly every 2 hours. This helps to ensure that the baby is satisfying his sucking needs and is receiving the necessary fluid and nutrients. Frequent feeding also helps initiate the mother's milk supply because frequent emptying stimulates more milk production.

A baby's behaviour and output helps to determine if he's getting enough breast milk. If he's content between feedings, wets approximately one nappy per day of life and has stool once per day of age, then he's getting enough until the mother's milk comes in. For example, on the first day of life, expect one wet nappy and one stool. On the second day of life, expect two wet nappies and two stools. On the third day of life, expect three wet nappies and

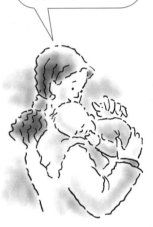

The most common way to burp a baby is to place him over one shoulder and gently pat or rub his back to expel ingested air.

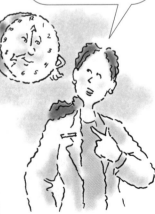

A baby is usually fed every 2 hours, which also helps the mum, because frequent emptying stimulates more milk production.

three stools. More wet nappies or stools than expected is considered good. Once the mother's milk is evident, she can expect to see six to eight wet nappies per day and three to four stools per day. The baby will probably lose up to 1/10th of his birthweight by day 4 but by the time he is 10–14 days old, he will probably have returned to his birthweight and will gain from there on. Breastfed babies can sometimes gain weight at a slower rate, depending on their mother's milk supply and how good they are at feeding!

Whetting his appetite

Sometimes babies seem to be uninterested or fall asleep when breastfeeding. If the baby shows little interest in breastfeeding, assist the mother in keeping him awake. If the baby is sleepy, suggest that the mother try rubbing the baby's feet or unwrapping his blanket. Taking off a layer of clothing, changing the nappy, wetting his face or changing hers or the baby's position may all work. She may also manually express a little milk and allow the baby to taste it. (See *Manual breast milk expression*.) If the baby has little success or interest in breastfeeding for several feedings, refer the mother to a lactation consultant or the breastfeeding coordinator.

Advice from the experts

Sitting up for burping

If the mother indicates that placing the baby over her shoulder for burping is awkward, suggest this alternative:
- Hold the baby in a sitting position on your lap.
- Lean the baby forward against one hand and support his head and neck with the index finger and thumb of that same hand, as shown below.

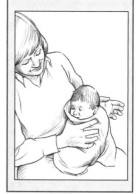

Manual breast milk expression

Manually expressing breast milk can enhance milk production and ensure an adequate supply. It's especially helpful for mothers who have problems with engorgement or those who must be away from their infants for several hours. (A mother who works outside the home or is away on a regular basis may find an electric pump quicker and more efficient.)

Express yourself

To help the mother manually express breast milk, follow these steps:

- Make sure that a clean collection container is available and that you and the mother have washed your hands.
- Explain the procedure to the woman, have her sit in a comfortable position and provide privacy.
- Tell her to place her dominant hand on one breast with the thumb positioned on the top and the fingers below and at the outer limit of the areola.
- Instruct her to press her thumb and fingers inward toward her chest while holding the collection container with her opposite hand directly under the nipple.
- Tell the mother to move her thumb and fingers forward, using gentle pressure in a milking type motion. Caution her not to use too much pressure because this can injure breast tissue. Milk should flow out of the nipple and into the collection container.
- Encourage the mother to move her thumb and fingers around the breast, using the same motion, to ensure complete emptying.
- Advise the mother to cover the container and place the milk in the refrigerator if it will be used within 24 hours; if not, she should freeze it.

Keep up the good work!

Always encourage the mother's breastfeeding efforts. To boost these efforts, urge her to eat balanced meals, to drink at least eight 100 ml glasses of fluid daily and to nap daily for at least the first 2 weeks after giving birth. Answer her questions about breastfeeding and provide instructional materials if available. It can be a good idea to have the new breastfeeding mother placed beside an experienced breastfeeder in the hospital as she can give invaluable support and advice to the novice. Always provide a mother who's breastfeeding with information and instructions related to possible complications. (See Chapter 10, *Complications of the postpartum period*, for more in-depth information on complications.) Contact a lactation consultant as appropriate.

Before discharge, tell the mother about local breastfeeding and parenting support groups – many are available through their own health centre or through the websites of National Childbirth Trust (http://www.nct.org.uk/ info-centre/a-to-z/view/20) and La Leche League International (http://www .laleche.org.uk/).

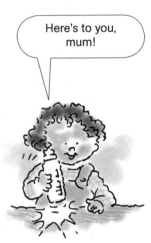

Here's to you, mum!

Daddy dearest

To involve the father, have him change the baby's nappy before feeding or wind the baby afterwards. Even young children can get involved by helping with burping or nappy changes. Dads can feed the baby with expressed breast milk if the opportunity arises.

Bottle-feeding with breast milk

In some cases, a mother may need to be away from her baby but still desires to provide breast milk. The mother may also need to express breast milk when her breasts are engorged. Although breast milk can be expressed by hand, using a breast pump may be the most efficient method.

Expressing milk using a breast pump

Breast pumping involves the use of suction created with a manual pump or a battery-powered or electric pump to stimulate lactation. It's used when the mother and baby are separated or while illness temporarily incapacitates one or the other.

A breast pump can also relieve engorgement, collect milk for a premature baby with a weak sucking reflex, reduce pressure on sore or cracked nipples or reestablish the milk supply. The mother can also use a pump to collect milk when she's unable to manually express it.

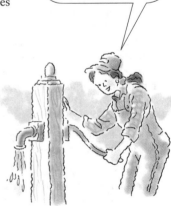

Expression of milk involves the use of suction created with a manual pump or a battery-powered or electric pump to stimulate lactation.

Preparing to pump

Before teaching the mother to use a breast pump:
- Assemble the equipment according to the manufacturer's instructions.
- Explain the procedure to the mother.
- Provide privacy.

- Wash your hands and instruct the mother to wash hers.
- Help the mother into a comfortable position and urge her to relax.

Tell her to drink a beverage before and after expressing. If the mother's breasts are engorged, instruct her to apply warm compresses for 5 minutes or take a warm shower before pumping.

Sometimes, having a picture of her baby or an item of clothing belonging to her baby, can stimulate the flow of breast milk.

Manual pump

To use a manual pump, instruct the mother to place the flange or shield against her breast with the nipple in the centre of the device. Then have her pump each breast by operating the device according to the manufacturer's instructions. She should continue until the breast is empty and then repeat the procedure on the other breast. It's also acceptable to pump for 5 minutes on one side and then switch sides and pump for 5 minutes; then, after 5–10 minutes, she should switch sides again and continue pumping until milk stops flowing from each breast.

Battery-powered or electric pump

To use a battery-powered or electric pump, instruct the mother to set the suction regulator on low. Tell her to hold the collection unit upright to allow milk to flow into it. Have her place the shield against her breast with the nipple in the centre. She should turn on the machine and adjust the suction regulator to a comfortable pressure.

Instruct her to start with the least amount of suction to prevent nipple damage and then gradually increase the suction. Advise her to check the operator's manual to see the pressure setting at which the pump functions most efficiently.

Keep on pumping

Instruct the mother to pump each breast for 15–20 minutes or until the milk stops spraying, which takes longer. She may wish to use a double pump, which allows for pumping both breasts at the same time. Using a double pump is also efficient and will save time if she uses this breastfeeding method.

When she's finished, show the mother how to remove the shield from the breast by inserting a finger between the breast and the shield to break the vacuum seal. Then return the suction regulator to the low setting and turn off the machine.

Freeze, store or enjoy right now?

After using either type of pump, the mother should let her nipples air dry for about 15 minutes. She should also disassemble the removable parts of the pump and clean them according to the manufacturer's directions.

If she plans to store or freeze the milk, have her fill a sterile plastic bottle with milk from the collection unit. Place the milk in the refrigerator or freezer immediately. Always label the collected milk with the date, the time of collection and the amount. Write the baby's name and hospital number on the label, if necessary.

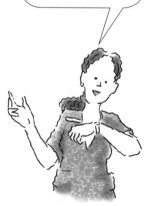

Timing is everything. Store freshly pumped breast milk in the fridge for 3 days or freeze it for up to 6 months. But after it's defrosted (in the fridge, of course), use it within 24 hours.

Bottle-feeding with formula

Formula-feeding is a reliable and nutritionally adequate method of feeding for babies whose mothers are unable to breastfeed or who choose not to. Commercial formulas are designed to mimic human milk but use cows milk as a base; this can cause anxieties for mothers who are concerned about allergies to protein.

Types of formulas

There are two main types of formula:

• Whey-based – Often called 'first' milk. Whey-based milks have nutrients, protein, vitamins and minerals in similar amounts to that found in breast milk. There are slight variations in composition between brands, but there is very little difference between them.

• Casein-based – Often called 'second' milk. The type of protein in casein formula is quite different to that in whey formula. The casein milks are 'older fashioned' types of milks, designed when this was the best the processes could do to modify cow's milk. These casein milks are advertised as being 'more satisfying' or 'for hungrier babies'. There is little evidence to support this and introducing casein milk before 6 weeks can overload the baby's immature kidneys. If a baby seems hungry after feeds, it may be more sensible to offer more frequent feeds with a larger quantity of whey-based milk rather than switching to casein formula. Commercial formulas typically provide 20 calories per ounce when diluted properly and are classified as milk-based, soy-based and elemental. Some of these formulas are lactose-free, so they can be used for babies with galactosaemia or lactose intolerance.

Health food for babies

Soy-based formulas are used for babies who could be allergic to cow's milk protein. Elemental formulas are commonly prescribed for babies who may have protein allergies or fat malnutrition. With these formulas, the amount of fat, protein and carbohydrates is modified. However, all commercial formulas are designed to simulate the nutritional content of human milk.

Commercial formulas may be supplied in one of three forms:

• powdered – to be combined with water
• ready to feed
• disposable, individually prepared bottles.

The powdered form is the least expensive, whereas individually prepared bottles are most expensive but easiest to use. Maternity units tend to use individually prepared bottles. Tell parents about the forms of formula available so they can choose what's most convenient for them.

Formula-feeding assistance

Each day, an infant requires from 60 to 150 ml/kg of milk in 24 hours and 100 to 120 kcal/kg. Because commercial formulas consistently provide 20 calories per 30 ml, only the infant's fluid needs are used to determine the amount of each feeding. Unlike breastfeeding, you can measure the amount of formula

consumed. The amount of milk the baby requires is calculated by multiplying his daily requirements by his birthweight (for the first week), and then dividing by 8 if the baby is feeding 3 hourly and 6 if the baby is feeding 4 hourly. So, for example:
- Day 1 – 60 ml/kg
- Day 2 – 80 ml/kg
- Day 3 – 100 ml/kg
- Day 4 – 120 ml/kg
- Day 5 – 130 ml/kg
- Day 6 – 150 ml/kg
- Day 7 – 180 ml/kg

Until about age 4 months, most infants need 6 feedings per day. After this, the number of feedings drops, but the amount at each feeding increases because the infant starts to eat cereal, fruits and vegetables. Each maternity unit will have a protocol indicating how much fluid babies should receive each day per kilogram.

Pre-feeding prep

When bottle-feeding a baby, or helping the mother with bottle-feeding, know the type of formula that's ordered and how it's supplied. If you're using a commercially prepared formula, check the expiration date, uncap the formula bottle and make sure that the seal isn't broken to ensure sterility and freshness. If the seal is broken, discard the formula. If the seal isn't broken, remove it.

Next, screw on the nipple and cap. Keep the protective sterile cap over the nipple until the baby is ready to feed. If you're preparing formula, follow the manufacturer's directions or the doctor's prescription. Administer the formula at room temperature or slightly warmer. There are many types of teats on the market and each mother will find one that suites her baby – some are orthodontic and mimic the human nipple – some are more suited to smaller babies.

Advice and guidelines are available from the Department of Health on handling, storage and making up of artificial feeds. This information can be accessed from the website: http://www.food.gov.uk/multimedia/pdfs/formulaguidance.pdf

Bottle-feeding blow-by-blow

Teach the mother and other family members to follow these steps when bottle-feeding the baby:
- After washing your hands and preparing the formula, invert the bottle and shake some formula on your wrist to test its temperature and the patency of the teat. The formula should drip freely but not stream out. If the hole is too large, the baby may aspirate formula; if it's too small, the extra sucking effort may tire him before he can empty the bottle.
- Sit comfortably in a semi-reclining position and cradle the baby in one arm to support his head and back. This position allows swallowed air to rise to the top of the stomach where it's more easily expelled.

- Place the teat in the baby's mouth on top of his tongue, but not so far back that it stimulates the gag reflex. He should begin to suck, pulling in as much teat as is comfortable. If he doesn't start to suck, stroke him under the chin or on his cheek, or touch his lips with the teat to stimulate the sucking reflex. Sometimes holding his hand will encourage him to suck.

Tilting does the trick

- As the baby feeds, tilt the bottle upward to keep the teat filled with formula and to prevent him from swallowing air. Watch for a steady stream of bubbles in the bottle. This indicates proper venting and flow of formula.
- If the baby pushes out the teat with his tongue, reinsert the nipple. Expelling the teat is a normal reflex. It doesn't necessarily mean that the baby is full.
- Always hold the bottle for the baby. If left to feed himself, he may aspirate formula or swallow air if the bottle tilts or empties. In older infants, experts also link bottle propping with an increased incidence of otitis media and dental caries.
- Be sure to interact with the baby during feeding, talking and smiling at him. Encourage eye-to-eye contact between mother and baby.
- Burp the baby after each 1 oz of formula because he'll usually swallow some air even when fed correctly. Use the same positions previously described for breastfeeding.
- After feeding and burping the baby, place him on his back as this position reduces the incidence of sudden infant death syndrome. Find out more about how to reduce the risk of sudden infant death syndrome by accessing information from the website: www.fsid.org .uk and also from *Reduce the risk of cot death: An easy guide*. Available from the website: www.dh.gov.uk
- Don't worry if the baby regurgitates some of the feed. Babies are prone to regurgitation because of an immature cardiac sphincter in their stomachs. Regurgitation is merely an overflow and shouldn't be confused with vomiting – a more complete emptying of the stomach accompanied by symptoms not associated with feeding.
- Discard any remaining formula and properly dispose of all equipment.

Too much or not enough

A baby tires if he feeds too long, and his sucking needs aren't met if he doesn't feed long enough. In some cases, you or the mother may need to select a teat of a different size or one with a larger opening to change the duration of the feeding. Additionally, be sure to note how much formula is in the bottle before and after the feeding. Use the calibrations along the side of the container to calculate the amount of formula consumed.

At home, go with the flow

Teach parents and other family members how to prepare and (if required) sterilise bottles, and teats. Advice and guidance on sterilising feeding

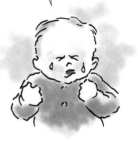

Do I need to say it again? I WANT MILK!

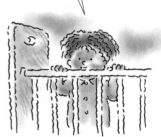

I can't decide. Did I not feed long enough to meet my need to suck, or did I feed too long and now I'm tired?

equipment is available from the website: http://www.babyfriendly.org.uk/page.asp?page=115&category=4

Although most maternity wards have a feeding schedule, advise the mother to switch to a more flexible demand-feeding schedule when at home.

Breast care

A mother who plans to breastfeed after the baby's birth will need to maintain breast tissue integrity. Although postnatal care varies for breastfeeding and nonbreastfeeding women, some guidelines are similar.

For breastfeeding women

Provide these instructions to a woman who's breastfeeding her baby:
- Wash your breasts with water only to avoid washing away the natural oils and keratin.
- If your nipples are sore or irritated, apply cool compresses to them just before breastfeeding. This numbs them, making them less sensitive and easier for the baby to grasp
- To help prevent tenderness, lubricate the nipple with a few drops of expressed breast milk before feeding. Lasinoh cream has been very popular with mothers in recent years.
- Place breast pads over your nipples to collect milk, and replace the pads often to reduce the risk of infection. Breasts often leak during the first few weeks you're breastfeeding.
- Be alert for a slight temperature elevation and an increase in breast size, warmth and firmness 2–5 days after birth. This signals that breast milk is coming in.
- Wear a well-fitting support bra to help control engorgement.
- Apply warm compresses, massage the breasts, take a warm shower or express some milk before feeding if your breasts are engorged and the baby can't latch on to the nipple.

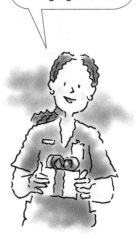

Okay, let's wrap it up. A supportive bra can help minimise engorgement.

For nonbreastfeeding women

Provide these instructions to a woman who isn't breastfeeding her baby:
- Clean your breasts with water only or with soap if necessary.
- Wear a supportive bra to help minimise engorgement and decrease nipple stimulation. Wear the bra at night too.
- To minimise further milk production, avoid stimulating the nipples or manually expressing milk.
- Use analgesics (if ordered).
- Use cool cabbage leaves or a breast binder to minimise engorgement and provide some relief.
- Wear breast pads to collect leakage of milk – change them frequently.

Pain relief

It is vital that the midwife enquires about the mother's state of comfort and ensures that she minimises pain and discomfort in the days following delivery.

Pain will affect how the mother adapts to caring for her new baby, feeding, mobilisation and general psychological state.

If the mother requires analgesia it is important it is given promptly and if necessary, it should be prescribed as a repeat dose at regular intervals. The midwife should always go back and check how effective the analgesia was and take appropriate action if it did not work. It is vital that the mother feels she can ask for, and will receive, adequate pain relief without being judged by professionals in the unit.

Going home?

Mothers are given a lot of information and parentcraft teaching in the short time they are in hospital, so it is important to fragment this by giving a little at a time if possible and adding to it with each session. Teaching the mother about the changes that are taking place in her body are just as important now that she's had her baby, than they were when she was pregnant. She also needs to learn a lot about her new baby, how he feeds, why he is crying, how many wet nappies he should have and many more issues! It is important for the midwife to be sensitive to the mother's learning needs and to take time (if possible!) to make sure the mother understands what she is being told. Leaflets and other information pamphlets will be given to the mother so it is vital that she can read (illiteracy is a growing problem) and that she understands English – if not, an interpreter may be required and if possible, leaflets in that mother's language.

The midwife should enquire about the method of contraception the mother will use when she goes home as some mothers believe that they will not become pregnant until their periods begin again – this is even more true of breastfeeding mothers! The midwife must give the mother advice on the method of contraception that is best suited to her and give her leaflets to take home so that she can discuss this with her partner.

Over to you now!

Once the mother and baby have been examined and are found to be ready for home, all the relevant documentation are completed and they are discharged home to the care of the community midwife in the first instance, and the health visitor in the second instance. The midwife will visit the mother and baby up to 10 days and if the mother needs her to visit for longer due to some problems, e.g. breastfeeding problems, then she will do so.

The health visitor takes over at around 2 weeks when she begins her assessment of the infant into childhood. There should be close liaison between the hospital midwives, community midwives, health visitor and GP to ensure that all necessary care and screening tests are carried out.

Accurate documentation is vital in recording the mother's journey through pregnancy, birth and the postnatal period. Midwives should be concise and adhere to the NMC's guidelines for record-keeping, remembering that they can become legal records and should be treated as such.

The NMC guidelines for record-keeping were updated in 2007, which can be accessed from the website: http://www.nmc-uk.org/aFrameDisplay.aspx?DocumentID=4008

Quick quiz

1. Which option would you identify as a progressive physiological change in the postnatal period?

    A. Lactation
    B. Lochia
    C. Uterine involution
    D. Diuresis

Answer: A. Lactation is an example of a progressive physiological change that occurs during the postnatal period.

2. Where would you expect to assess the uterine fundus in a mother on the second postnatal day?

    A. 2 cm above the level of the umbilicus
    B. At the level of the symphysis pubis
    C. Approximately 2 cm below the umbilicus
    D. 2 cm above the symphysis pubis

Answer: C. The uterus descends at a rate of about 1 cm/day. The fundus of a woman on postnatal day 2 should be 2 cm below the umbilicus.

3. Lactation is stimulated by:

    A. oestrogen.
    B. prolactin.
    C. progesterone.
    D. FSH.

Answer: B. Prolactin is the hormone responsible for stimulating lactation.

4. Which measure would the woman who isn't breastfeeding use to minimise engorgement?

    A. Cool cabbage leaves
    B. Manual expression
    C. Warm showers
    D. Nipple stimulation

Answer: A. For the woman who isn't breastfeeding, cool cabbage leaves help to minimise engorgement.

Scoring

 If you answered all four questions correctly, whoa! You've certainly galloped through this chapter.

If you answered three questions correctly, giddy up! Looks like you've corralled your knowledge of postnatal care.

If you answered fewer than three questions correctly, stay steady. You're sure to be more stable the next time you go over this chapter.

⑩ Complications of the postnatal period

Just the facts

In this chapter, you'll learn:

♦ major complications that can occur during the postnatal period, including risk factors for each

♦ ways to identify complications based on key assessment findings

♦ treatments that are appropriate for each complication

♦ appropriate midwifery interventions for each complication.

A look at postnatal complications

Although the postnatal period is a time of many physiological and psychological changes and stressors, these changes are usually considered good changes – not unhealthy. During this time, the mother, the baby and other family members interact and grow as a family.

A cluster of complications

However, complications can develop due to a wide range of factors, such as blood loss, trauma, infection or fatigue. Some common postnatal complications include postpartum haemorrhage (PPH), postnatal psychiatric disorders, puerperal infection, mastitis and deep vein thrombosis (DVT). Your keen midwifery skills can help to prevent problems or detect them early before they cause more stress or seriously interfere with the parent–infant relationship.

Mastitis

Mastitis is an inflammation of the functional tissue of the breasts that disrupts normal lactation. It occurs postpartum in about 1% of women, mainly in primiparas who are breastfeeding. It occurs only occasionally in nonlactating females. The prognosis for a woman with mastitis is good.

> Postnatal complications can occur for a number of reasons. Some are more complicated than others.

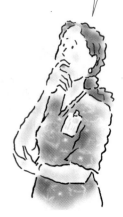

What causes it

Mastitis develops when trauma due to incorrect latching on or removal from the breast allows introduction of organisms from the baby's nose or pharynx into the maternal breast. The pathogen that most commonly causes mastitis is *Staphylococcus aureus*; less frequently, *Staphylococcus epidermidis* and beta-haemolytic streptococci are the culprits. Rarely, mastitis may result from disseminated tuberculosis or the mumps virus.

Predisposing factors include a fissure or abrasion on the nipple, blocked milk ducts and an incomplete let-down reflex, usually due to emotional trauma. Blocked milk ducts can result from wearing a tight-fitting bra or waiting prolonged intervals between breastfeedings.

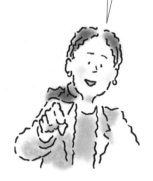

Master the treatment of mastitis adequately and promptly, so it can't progress to breast abscess.

What to look for

Mastitis may develop anytime during lactation, but it usually begins 1–4 weeks postpartum with fever (38.3°C, or higher in acute mastitis), chills, malaise and flu-like symptoms. Mastitis is generally unilateral and localised, but, in some cases, both breasts or the entire breast is affected.

Inspection and palpation may uncover redness, swelling, warmth, hardness, tenderness, nipple cracks or fissures and enlarged axillary lymph nodes. Unless mastitis is treated adequately, it may progress to breast abscess.

Which kind is it?

Mastitis must be differentiated from normal breast engorgement, which generally starts with the onset of lactation (days 2–5 postpartum). During this time, the breasts undergo changes similar to those in mastitis and body temperature may also be elevated.

Engorgement may be mild, causing only slight discomfort, or severe, causing considerable pain. A severely engorged breast can prevent a baby from feeding properly because he can't latch on to the nipple of the swollen, rigid breast.

What tests tell you

Cultures of expressed breast milk are used to confirm generalised mastitis; cultures of breast skin can be used to confirm localised mastitis. These cultures are also used to determine antibiotic therapy. Differential diagnosis should exclude breast engorgement, breast abscess, viral syndrome and a clogged duct.

How it's treated

The first thing you must be sure of is that the baby is latching on and feeding well for the breast – and most importantly, that the breast is being emptied.

Antibiotic therapy, the primary treatment for mastitis, usually consists of either amoxacillen 250 mg TID, cefalexin 250 mg or erythromycin 250 mg TID. For women who are allergic to penicillin azithromycin (Zithromax) or vancomycin (Vancocin) may be used. Although symptoms usually subside after 24–48 hours of antibiotic therapy, antibiotic therapy should continue for 10 days.

Other appropriate measures include analgesics for pain and, on the rare occasions when antibiotics fail to control the infection and mastitis progresses to breast abscess, incision and drainage of the abscess.

What to do

Here's what you should do to treat a mother with mastitis:
- Explain mastitis to the mother and why infection control measures are necessary.
- Establish infection control measures for the mother and baby to prevent the spread of infection to other nursing mothers.
- Obtain a complete client history, including a drug history, especially allergy to penicillin.
- Administer antibiotic therapy, as ordered.
- Assess and record the cause and amount of discomfort. Give analgesics, as needed.
- Reassure the mother that breastfeeding during mastitis won't harm her baby because often he's the source of the infection.
- Tell the mother to offer the baby the affected breast first to promote complete emptying and prevent clogged ducts. However, if an open abscess develops, she must stop breastfeeding with this breast and use a breast pump until the abscess heals. She should continue to breastfeed on the unaffected side.
- Suggest applying a warm, wet towel to the affected breast or taking a warm shower to relax and improve her ability to breastfeed. Cold compresses may also be used to relieve discomfort.
- Advise the mother to wear a supportive bra.
- Provide good skin care.
- Show the mother how to position the baby properly to prevent cracked or sore nipples.
- Tell the mother to empty her breast as completely as possible with each feed.
- Tell the mother to get plenty of rest and drink sufficient fluids to help combat fever.

Before your breastfeeding mother leaves the hospital, teach her about breast care and how to prevent mastitis. (See *Preventing mastitis*, page 407.)

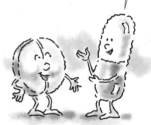

Whadda ya say we treat our friend mastitis here to our own kind of therapy, eh?

Postpartum haemorrhage (PPH)

The WHO defines PPH as:
- Primary PPH is defined as the loss of blood estimated to be >500 ml, from the genital tract, within 24 hours of delivery (commonest obstetric haemorrhage).
- Secondary PPH is defined as abnormal bleeding from the genital tract, from 24 hours after delivery until 6 weeks postpartum.

Education edge

Preventing mastitis

With today's shortened hospital stays for childbirth, postnatal teaching is more important than ever. If the mother is breastfeeding, be sure to include these instructions about breast care and preventing mastitis when giving information to the mother:

- Wash your hands after using the bathroom, before touching your breasts and before and after every breastfeeding.
- If necessary, apply a warm compress or take a warm shower to help facilitate milk flow.
- Position the baby properly at the breast, and make sure that he grasps the nipple and entire areola area when feeding.

- Empty the breast as completely as possible at each feeding.
- Alternate feeding positions and rotate pressure areas.
- Release the baby's grasp on the nipple before removing him from the breast.
- Expose your nipples to the air for part of each day.
- Drink plenty of fluids, eat a balanced diet and get sufficient rest to enhance the breastfeeding experience.
- Don't wait too long between feedings or wean the infant abruptly.

The danger of PPH due to uterine atony (lax uterus) is greatest during the first hour after birth. During this time, the placenta has detached, leaving the highly vascular yet denuded uterus widely exposed. The risk continues to be high for 24 hours after birth.

After vaginal birth, blood loss of up to 500 ml is considered acceptable, although this amount may vary among health care facilities. The acceptable range for blood loss after caesarean birth is usually between 1,000 and 1,200 ml. The Confidential Enquiry into Maternal and Child Health (CEMACH) report reported 14 women in the period 2003–2005 dying from haemorrhage following childbirth.

Complicating the matter

A woman who has a birth complicated by any of these factors should be observed for the possibility of developing a PPH:
- placental abruption
- missed abortion
- placenta praevia
- uterine infection
- placenta accreta
- uterine inversion
- severe pre-eclampsia
- amniotic fluid embolism
- intrauterine fetal death
- precipitous labour
- macrosomia

Relaxation is risky

Risk factors for uterine atony include:

- polyhydramnios
- delivery of a macrosomic baby, usually more than 4.1 kg (9 lb)
- use of magnesium sulphate during labour
- multiple gestation
- delivery that was rapid or required operative techniques, such as forceps or vacuum suction

- injury to the cervix or birth canal, such as from trauma, lacerations or haematoma development
- use of oxytocin to initiate or augment labour or prolonged use of tocolytic agents
- dystocia (dysfunctional labour)
- previous history of postpartum haemorrhage
- use of deep analgesia or anaesthesia
- infection, such as chorioamnionitis or endometritis.

- multiple gestation
- prolonged labour
- multiparity.

What causes it

Uterine atony, lacerations, retained placenta or placental fragments and disseminated intravascular coagulation (DIC) are the leading causes of PPH.

Relax – don't do it!

The primary cause of PPH, especially early PPH, is uterine atony (uterine relaxation). When the uterus doesn't contract properly, vessels at the placental site remain open, allowing blood loss. Any condition that interferes with the ability of the uterus to contract can lead to uterine atony and, subsequently, PPH. (See *Relaxation is risky.*)

Blame it on lacerations

Lacerations of the cervix, birth canal or perineum can also lead to PPH. Cervical lacerations may result in profuse bleeding if the uterine artery is torn. This type of haemorrhage usually occurs immediately after delivery of the placenta, while the mother is still in the delivery area. Suspect lacerations when bleeding persists but the uterus is firm.

Stuck on you

Entrapment of a partially or completely separated placenta by an hourglass-shaped uterine constriction ring (a condition that prevents the entire placenta from expelling) can cause placental fragments to be retained in the uterus (retained products). Poor separation of the placenta is common in preterm births of 20–24 weeks' gestation.

You're kidding. Relaxation is bad? When the uterus relaxes, blood loss can occur, causing postpartum haemorrhage.

The reason for abnormal adherence is unknown but it may result from the implantation of the zygote in an area of defective endometrium. This abnormal implantation leaves a zone of separation between the placenta and the decidua. If the fragment is large, bleeding may be apparent in the early postnatal period. If the fragment is small, however, bleeding may go unnoticed for several days, after which time the woman suddenly has a large amount of bloody vaginal discharge.

To clot or not to clot

DIC is a fourth cause of PPH. Any woman is at risk for DIC after childbirth. However, it's more common in women with placental abruption, missed abortion, placenta praevia, uterine infection, placenta accreta, uterine inversion, severe pre-eclampsia, amniotic fluid embolism or intrauterine fetal death.

What to look for

Bleeding is the key assessment finding for PPH. It can occur suddenly in large amounts or over time, as seeping or oozing of blood. Expect a woman with PPH to saturate perineal pads more quickly than usual.

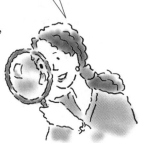

Uh oh. Is that blood I see? Bleeding is the key assessment finding for postpartum haemorrhage.

Soft and boggy

When uterine atony is the cause, the uterus feels soft and relaxed. The bladder may be distended, displacing the uterus to the right or left side of midline and preventing it from contracting properly. The fundus may also be pushed upward.

A cut above

When a laceration is the cause of PPH, you may notice bright-red blood with clots oozing continuously from the site and a uterus that remains firm.

Left behind

Bleeding caused by a retained placenta or placental fragments usually starts as a slow trickle, oozing or frank haemorrhage. In the case of retained placental fragments, also expect to find the uterus soft and noncontracting.

The fourth culprit: DIC

When the woman's bleeding is continuous and uterine atony, lacerations and retained placenta or fragments have been ruled out, coagulation problems may be the cause of the bleeding.

The shocking truth

If blood loss is sufficient, the woman exhibits signs and symptoms of hypovolaemic shock, such as increasing restlessness, light-headedness and dizziness as cerebral tissue perfusion decreases. Inspection may also reveal pale skin, decreased sensorium, increased pulse rate and rapid, shallow respirations. Urine output usually falls below 25 ml/hour. Palpation may disclose rapid, thready peripheral pulses and cool skin that becomes cold and clammy.

Auscultation of blood pressure usually detects a mean arterial pressure below 60 mmHg and a narrowing pulse pressure. Capillary refill at the nail beds is delayed 3–5 seconds.

What tests tell you

Diagnostic testing reveals a decrease in haemoglobin level and haematocrit. The woman's haemoglobin level typically decreases 1–1.5 g/dl and haematocrit drops 2–4% from baseline. If the woman has retained placental fragments, you may also find that serum human chorionic gonadotropin levels are elevated.

Coagulating the matter

When DIC is the cause of PPH, platelet and fibrinogen levels are decreased and clotting times (prothrombin time [PT] and partial thromboplastin time [PTT]) are prolonged. Blood tests also reveal decreased fibrinogen levels and fragmented red blood cells (RBCs). Fibrinolysis increases and then decreases. Coagulation factors are decreased, with decreased antithrombin III, an increased d-dimer test and a normal or prolonged euglobulin lysis time.

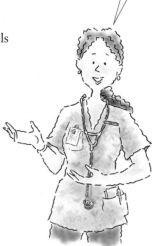

Treating postpartum haemorrhage involves correcting the underlying cause, controlling blood loss and minimising hypovolaemic shock.

How it's treated

Treatment of PPH focuses on:
- correcting the underlying cause
- instituting measures to control blood loss
- minimising the extent of hypovolaemic shock.
   It is vital to alert the whole obstetric emergency team and involve the laboratories and the blood transfusion service.

Pump up the tone

For the woman with uterine atony, rub up a contraction by massaging the fundus of the uterus. The goal is to increase uterine tone and contractility to minimise blood loss. If clots are present, they should be expressed. If the woman's bladder is distended, this will prevent uterine contraction so she should be catheterised if she cannot pass urine. If these efforts are ineffective or fail to maintain the uterus in a contracted state, ergometrine 0.5 mg may be given I.M. or I.V. (slowly), to produce sustained uterine contractions. Syntocinon 5–10 IU may be given I.M. or 10–20 IU in an infusion, misoprostil or carboprost 0.25 mg can also be given I.M. to promote strong, sustained uterine contractions. At this point, it is advisable to gain I.V. access with a wide-bore cannula so that blood samples can be taken and blood products can be transfused if necessary.

Source search

If the uterus is firm and contracted and the bladder isn't distended, the source of the bleeding must still be identified. Perform visual or manual inspection of the perineum, vagina, uterus, cervix and rectum. A laceration requires sutures. If a haematoma is found, treatment may involve observation, cold therapy, ligation of the bleeding vessel or evacuation of the haematoma. Depending on the extent of fluid loss, replacement therapy may be indicated.

Remove the stragglers

Retained placental fragments typically are removed manually or, if manual extraction is unsuccessful, via dilatation and curettage (D&C). If the placenta is adhered to the uterine wall or has implanted into the myometrium, a hysterectomy may need to be performed to stop uterine bleeding.

Supportive to specific

Successful management of DIC requires prompt recognition and adequate treatment of the underlying disorder. Treatment may be supportive (for example, when the underlying disorder is self-limiting) or highly specific. If the woman isn't actively bleeding, supportive care alone may reverse DIC. Active bleeding may require administration of blood, fresh-frozen plasma, platelets or packed RBCs to support haemostasis.

Heparin therapy for DIC is controversial. It may be used early in the disease to prevent microclotting but may be considered a last resort in the woman who's actively bleeding. If thrombosis occurs, heparin therapy is usually mandatory. In most cases, it's administered in combination with transfusion therapy.

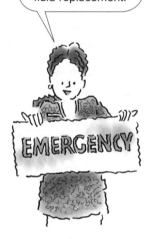

Emergency treatment of DIC relies on prompt and adequate blood and fluid replacement.

Making up for lost fluids

Emergency treatment relies on prompt and adequate blood and fluid replacement to restore intravascular volume and to raise blood pressure and maintain it above 60 mmHg. Rapid infusion of lactated Ringer's solution and, possibly, albumin or other plasma expanders may be needed to expand volume adequately until whole blood can be matched.

What to do

Close, frequent assessment in the hour following delivery is crucial to prevent complications or allow early identification and prompt intervention should haemorrhage occur.

Here are other steps you should take in case of PPH:

• Assess the woman's fundus and lochia every 15 minutes for 1 hour after birth to detect changes. Notify the senior doctor if the fundus doesn't remain contracted or if lochia increases.

• Rub up a contraction, as indicated, to assist with uterine involution. Stay with the woman, frequently reassessing the fundus to ensure that it remains firm and contracted. Keep in mind that the uterus may relax quickly when massage is completed, placing the woman at risk for continued haemorrhage.

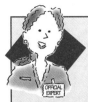

Advice from the experts

Managing low blood pressure

If the mother's systolic blood pressure drops below 80 mmHg, increase the oxygen flow rate and notify the doctor immediately. Systolic blood pressure below 80 mmHg usually results in inadequate coronary artery blood flow, cardiac ischaemia, arrhythmias and further complications of low cardiac output.

Another ominous sign

Notify the doctor and increase the infusion rate if the mother has a progressive drop in blood pressure (30 mmHg or less from baseline) accompanied by a thready pulse. This usually signals inadequate cardiac output from reduced intravascular volume. Assess the mother's level of consciousness. As cerebral hypoxia increases, the mother becomes more restless and confused.

- If you suspect PPH, keep perineal pads to estimate blood loss.
- Turn the woman onto her side and inspect under the buttocks for pooling of blood.
- Inspect the perineal area closely for oozing from possible lacerations.
- Monitor vital signs frequently for changes, noting trends such as a continuously rising pulse rate and a drop in blood pressure. Report changes immediately. (See *Managing low blood pressure.*)
- Assess intake and output, and report urine output less than 30 ml/hour. Encourage the woman to void frequently to prevent bladder distention from interfering with uterine involution. If she can't void, you may need to insert an indwelling urinary catheter.

A shocking development

Here are the steps you should take if the woman develops signs and symptoms of hypovolaemic shock:
- Begin an I.V. infusion, delivered through a large-bore (14G–18G) catheter.
- Administer colloids (albumin) and blood products as ordered.
- Monitor the woman for fluid overload.
- Monitor for signs and symptoms of infection, such as increased temperature, foul-smelling lochia or redness and swelling of the incision.
- Record blood pressure, pulse and respiratory rates and peripheral pulse rates every 15 minutes until stable.
- Monitor cardiac rhythm continuously.
- During therapy, assess skin colour and temperature and note changes. Cold, clammy skin may signal continuing peripheral vascular constriction and progressive shock.
- Monitor capillary refill and skin turgor.
- Watch for signs of impending coagulopathy, such as petechiae, bruising and bleeding or oozing from gums or venipuncture sites.

- Anticipate the need for fluid replacement and blood component therapy, as ordered.
- Obtain arterial blood samples to measure arterial blood gas (ABG) levels. Administer oxygen by nasal cannula, face mask or airway to ensure adequate tissue oxygenation. Adjust the oxygen flow rate as ABG measurements indicate.
- Obtain venous blood specimens as ordered for a complete blood count, electrolyte measurements, typing and crossmatching and coagulation studies.
- If the woman has received I.V. Syntocinon for treatment of uterine atony, continue to assess the fundus closely. The action of Syntocinon, although speedy, is short in duration, so atony may recur. Monitor for nausea and vomiting.
- Provide emotional support to the woman, and explain all procedures to help alleviate fear and anxiety.
- Monitor the woman's level of consciousness (LOC) for signs of hypoxia (decreased LOC).
- Prepare the woman for possible treatments, such as bimanual massage, surgical repair of lacerations or D&C.

Puerperal infection

Infection during the puerperal period is a common cause of childbirth-related death. In the UK, 18 women died from genital tract infections in the period 2003–2005. Statistics on causes of maternal deaths are available from the CEMACH website. http://www.cemach.org.uk/

Puerperal infection affects the uterus and structures above it with a characteristic fever pattern. It can result in endometritis, parametritis, pelvic and femoral thrombophlebitis and peritonitis.

The prognosis is good in most cases with early diagnosis and treatment. There are also certain precautions you can take up to prevent puerperal infection. (See *Preventing puerperal infection*.)

Preventing puerperal infection

Here are some steps that you can take up to help prevent puerperal infection in the postpartum woman:

- Adhere to standard precautions at all times.
- Maintain aseptic technique when assisting with or performing a vaginal examination. Limit the number of vaginal examinations performed during labour. Wash your hands thoroughly after each client contact.

- Instruct all pregnant women to contact their midwife or maternity unit immediately when their membranes rupture. Warn them to avoid intercourse after rupture of or leakage from the amniotic sac.
- Keep the episiotomy site clean, and teach the woman how to maintain good perineal hygiene.
- Screen personnel and visitors to keep people with active infections away from mothers in maternity units.

What causes it

Microorganisms that commonly cause puerperal infection include group A, B or G haemolytic streptococcus; *Gardnerella vaginalis*; *Chlamydia trachomatis* and coagulase-negative staphylococci. Less common causative agents are *Clostridium perfringens, Bacteroides fragilis, Klebsiella, Proteus mirabilis, Pseudomonas, S. aureus* and *Escherichia coli*.

Normal unless predisposed

Most of these organisms are considered normal vaginal flora. However, they can cause puerperal infection in the presence of the following predisposing factors:
- prolonged (more than 24 hours) or premature rupture of the membranes
- prolonged (more than 24 hours) or difficult labour, allowing bacteria to enter while the fetus is still in utero
- frequent or unsterile vaginal examinations or unsterile delivery conditions
- delivery requiring the use of instruments, which may traumatise the tissue, providing an entry portal for microorganisms
- internal fetal monitoring, which may introduce organisms when electrodes are placed
- retained products of conception (such as placental fragments), which cause tissue necrosis and provide an excellent medium for bacterial growth
- haemorrhage, which weakens the woman's overall defences
- maternal conditions, such as anaemia, diabetes mellitus, immunosuppression or debilitation from malnutrition, that lower the woman's ability to defend against microorganism invasion
- caesarean birth (places woman at a 30–50% increased risk for puerperal infection)
- existence of localised vaginal infection or other type of infection at delivery, which allows direct transmission of infection
- bladder catheterisation
- episiotomy or lacerations
- history of urinary tract infection
- pneumonia
- venous thrombosis.

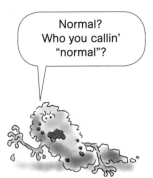

Normal?
Who you callin'
"normal"?

What to look for

A characteristic sign of puerperal infection is fever (a temperature of at least 38°C) that occurs during the first 10 days postpartum (except during the first 24 hours) and lasts for 2 consecutive days. The fever can spike as high as 40.6°C and is commonly accompanied by chills, headache, malaise, restlessness, loss of appetite and anxiety.

Care to accompany me?

Accompanying signs and symptoms depend on the extent and site of infection and may include:
• localised perineal infection – pain, elevated temperature, oedema, redness, firmness and tenderness at the wound site; sensation of heat; burning on urination; discharge from the wound or separation of the wound
• endometritis – heavy, sometimes foul-smelling lochia; tender, enlarged uterus; backache; severe uterine contractions persisting after childbirth; temperature greater than 38°C, chills and increased pulse rate
• parametritis (pelvic cellulitis) – vaginal tenderness and abdominal pain and tenderness (pain may become more intense as infection spreads).

Spreading far and wide

The inflammation may remain localised, may lead to abscess formation or may spread through the blood or lymphatic system. Widespread inflammation may cause these conditions, signs and symptoms:
• septic pelvic thrombophlebitis – severe, repeated chills and dramatic swings in body temperature; lower abdominal or flank pain and, possibly, a palpable tender mass over the affected area, which usually develops near the second postpartum week
• peritonitis – rigid, boardlike abdomen with guarding (usually the first sign); elevated body temperature; tachycardia (greater than 140 beats/minute); weak pulse; hiccups; nausea; vomiting; diarrhoea and constant, possibly excruciating, abdominal pain.

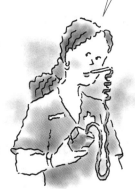

A characteristic sign of puerperal infection is a temperature of at least 38°C that lasts for 48 hours.

What tests tell you

Development of the typical clinical features – especially fever for 48 hours or more after the first postpartum day – suggests a diagnosis of puerperal infection. Uterine tenderness is also highly suggestive. Typical clinical features usually suffice for a diagnosis of endometritis and peritonitis. In parametritis, vaginal examination shows induration without purulent discharge.

You're so cultured

A culture of lochia, incisional exudate (from caesarean incision or episiotomy), uterine tissue or high vaginal swab that reveals the causative organism may help confirm the diagnosis. However, such cultures are generally contaminated with vaginal flora and aren't considered helpful. A sensitivity test is also done to determine if the proper antibiotic has been administered. Blood cultures are performed for a temperature above 38.3°C.

White cell uprising

Normal white blood cell (WBC) count during pregnancy is 5,000–15,000 µl. WBCs can increase to 30,000 µl during labour due to the stress response and decreases after recovery. A sudden increase of 30% above the baseline WBC count over a 6-hour period or the presence of bands in the differential WBC count is a sign of infection after birth. Erythrocyte sedimentation rate may also be elevated.

How it's treated

Treatment of puerperal infection usually begins with I.V. infusion of a broad-spectrum antibiotic. This controls the infection and prevents its spread while you await culture results. After identifying the infecting organism, the doctor may prescribe a more specific antibiotic. (An oral antibiotic may be prescribed after discharge.)

Ancillary measures include analgesics for pain, antiseptics for local lesions and antiemetics for nausea and vomiting from peritonitis.

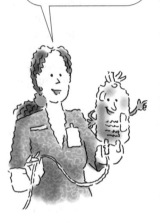

Treatment of puerperal infection usually begins with I.V. infusion of a broad-spectrum antibiotic.

Stick to the standards

A mother with a contagious disease is usually placed in a private room and should be isolated, but not from her baby. The baby should be isolated from other babies and should remain in the room with his mother. If the mother isn't contagious, she doesn't need to be isolated but you should follow standard precautions. Follow the guidelines from your cross infection advisor to determine whether isolation precautions are necessary.

A break from breastfeeding?

Whether the mother can continue breastfeeding, if applicable, depends on the type of antibiotic she's receiving and her physical ability to breastfeed. A mother can't breastfeed if she's receiving metronidazole (Flagyl) or acyclovir (Zovirax). If she plans to breastfeed after her course of antibiotics, help her to express breast milk, but discard the milk produced while she's on the medication. The mother will need lots of encouragement and support at this time as this can be devastating for her.

Standard precautions are a must, even if the mother isn't contagious.

Support, surgery and drugs

Supportive care includes bed rest, adequate fluid intake, I.V. fluids when necessary and measures to reduce fever. Surgery may also be necessary to remove remaining products of conception or retained placental fragments or to drain local lesions such as an abscess in parametritis.

If the mother develops septic pelvic thrombophlebitis, treatment consists of heparin anticoagulation for about 10 days in conjunction with broad-spectrum antibiotic therapy.

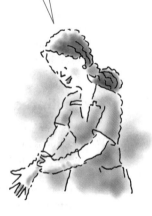

What to do

If your postnatal mother develops an infection, perform these interventions:
• Monitor vital signs every 4 hours (or more frequently depending on her condition).
• Assess capillary refill and skin turgor as well as mucous membranes.

- Assess intake and output closely.
- Enforce strict bed rest.
- Provide a high-calorie, high-protein diet to promote wound healing.
- Provide extra fluids, unless otherwise contraindicated.
- Encourage the woman to void frequently, which empties the bladder and helps to prevent infection.
- Inspect the perineum often. Assess the fundus and palpate for tenderness (subinvolution may indicate endometritis). Note the amount, colour and odour of vaginal drainage and document your observations.
- Encourage the woman to change perineal pads frequently, removing them from front to back. Help her change pads, if necessary. Be sure to wear gloves when helping the woman change a perineal pad.
- Administer antibiotics and analgesics, as ordered. Assess and document the type, degree and location of pain as well as the woman's response to analgesics. Give her an antiemetic to relieve nausea and vomiting, as needed.
- Provide bidet and warm or cool compresses for local lesions.
- Change bedlinens, perineal pads and underpads frequently.
- Provide warm blankets and keep the mother warm.
- Thoroughly explain all procedures to the woman and her family. Offer reassurance and emotional support.
- If the mother is separated from her baby, reassure her often about his progress. Encourage the father to talk with the mother about the baby's condition. Having a midwife/nurse from the neonatal unit to speak to the mother can be comforting.

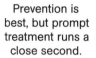

Prevention is best, but prompt treatment runs a close second.

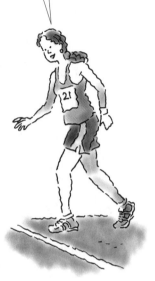

Deep vein thrombosis

DVT, also called *deep vein thrombophlebitis* which can develop into a deep vein thrombosis, is an inflammation of the lining of a blood vessel that occurs in conjunction with clot formation. It typically occurs at the valve cusps because venous stasis encourages the accumulation and adherence of platelets and fibrin.

Thrombophlebitis usually begins with localised inflammation (phlebitis), but this rapidly provokes thrombus formation. Rarely, venous thrombosis develops without associated inflammation of the vein.

Any vein will do

DVT can affect small veins, such as the lesser saphenous vein, or large veins, such as the iliac, femoral, pelvic and popliteal veins and the vena cava. It's more serious than superficial vein thrombophlebitis because it affects the veins deep in the leg musculature that carry 90% of the venous outflow from the leg.

What causes it

DVT may be idiopathic, but it's more likely to occur along with certain diseases, treatments, injuries or other factors.

Risky business

Risk factors for developing DVT in the postnatal period include:
- history of varicose veins
- obesity
- previous DVT
- multiple gestations
- increased age (older than age 30)
- family history of DVT
- smoking
- caesarean birth
- multiparity.
- These risk factors are compounded by specific occurrences during labour and delivery. For example, blood clotting increases postnatally as a result of elevated fibrinogen levels. Also, pressure from the fetal head during pregnancy and delivery causes veins in the lower extremities to dilate, leading to venous stasis. Finally, lying in the lithotomy position for a long time with the lower extremities in stirrups promotes venous pooling and stasis.

Bad news × 2

During the postnatal period, two major types of DVT may occur: femoral or pelvic. Pelvic DVT runs a long course, usually 6–8 weeks. (See *Comparing femoral and pelvic DVT*, page 419.)

What to look for

The signs and symptoms for femoral and pelvic DVT differ, but both types require careful assessment.

Femoral DVT

With femoral thrombophlebitis, the woman's temperature increases around the 10th day postnatally. Other signs and symptoms include malaise, chills, pain, stiffness or swelling in the leg or in the groin.

With leg swelling, the affected extremity appears reddened or inflamed, oedematous below the level of the obstruction and possibly shiny and white. This white appearance may be related to an accompanying arterial spasm, which results in a decrease in arterial circulation to the area. When measured, the thigh and calf of the affected leg are typically larger than the unaffected extremity.

Man, Homan oh man!

Pain may occur in the calf of the affected leg when the foot is dorsiflexed. This finding – a positive Homans' sign – suggests DVT, but isn't a reliable indicator. Even if the woman is negative for Homans' sign, the possibility of an obstruction can't be ruled out. NICE guidelines discourage active use of the Homan's signs in testing for DVT – active dorsiflexion could lead to embolisation of a clot.

Comparing femoral and pelvic DVT

This table outlines the major differences between femoral and pelvic deep vein thrombosis (DVT), including the vessels affected, time of onset, assessment findings and treatment.

Characteristic	Femoral DVT	Pelvic DVT
Vessels affected	• Femoral • Saphenous • Popliteal	• Ovarian • Uterine • Hypogastric
Onset	Approximately postpartum day 10	Approximately postpartum day 14–15
Assessment findings	• Associated arterial spasm, making leg appear milky-white or drained • Oedema • Fever • Malaise • Diminished peripheral pulses • Positive Homans' sign • Chills • Pain • Redness and stiffness of affected leg • Shiny white skin on extremity	• Extremely high fever • Tachycardia • Chills • General malaise • Possible pelvic abscess • Abdominal and flank pain
Treatment	• Bed rest • Elevation of affected extremity • Never massaging affected area • Anticoagulants • Moist heat applications • Analgesics	• Complete bed rest • Anticoagulants • Antibiotics • Incision and drainage if abscess develops

What's your sign?

A positive Rielander's sign (palpable veins inside the thigh and calf) or Payr's sign (calf pain when pressure is applied on the inside of the foot) also suggests femoral DVT.

Pelvic DVT

The woman with pelvic DVT appears acutely ill with a sudden onset of a high fever, severe repeated chills and general malaise. In most cases, body temperature fluctuates widely. The woman may complain of lower abdominal or flank pain, and you may be able to palpate a tender mass over the affected area.

What tests tell you

Diagnosis of DVT is based on these characteristic test findings:
• Doppler ultrasonography identifies reduced blood flow to a specific area and obstruction to venous flow, particularly in iliofemoral DVT.
• More sensitive than ultrasonography in detecting DVT, plethysmography shows decreased circulation distal to the affected area. This apparatus measures blood flow and circulation to specific parts/organs of the body.
• Venography usually confirms the diagnosis and shows filling defects and diverted blood flow.
• If pulmonary thromboembolism is suspected, a chest x-ray should be taken.

How it's treated

Treatment for DVT includes bed rest, with elevation of the affected arm or leg; application of warm, moist compresses and administration of analgesics, antibiotics and anticoagulants. After the acute episode subsides, the woman may begin to ambulate while wearing antiembolism stockings TED stockings (applied before she gets out of bed). It is vital that she is measured for the right size of stockings and is taught how to put them on properly.

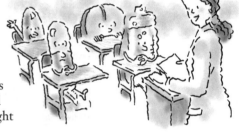

Drug therapy for DVT typically includes anticoagulants, starting with heparin and then changing to another anticoagulant such as warfarin.

Bring on the meds

Common practice in the United Kingdom is to use low molecular weight heparin during pregnancy, with either low molecular weight heparin or warfarin for 6–12 weeks after the birth. Practice, however, still varies widely, with some centres using unfractionated heparin. Guidelines prepared by the haemostasis and thrombosis task force recommend that women receive heparin for at least 4 days and treatment should not be discontinued until the international normalised ratio (INR) has been in the therapeutic range for 2 consecutive days. According to these guidelines, a woman with a first episode of a proximal vein thrombosis should receive anticoagulants for 6 months, with a target INR of 2.5. The issue of length of anticoagulation is still under debate.

Heparin is given subcutaneously in two divided doses and should be titrated against the woman's booking or most recent weight. There should be clear local guidelines for dosages and monitoring.

Kicking the treatment up a notch

Rarely, DVT may cause complete venous occlusion, which requires venous interruption through simple ligation, vein plication or clipping. Embolectomy may be done if clots are being shed to the pulmonary and systemic vasculature and other treatments are unsuccessful.

Caval interruption with transvenous placement of an umbrella filter can trap emboli, preventing them from travelling to the pulmonary vasculature. If the woman develops a pulmonary embolism, heparin may be initiated until the embolism resolves, then subcutaneous heparin or an oral anticoagulant may be continued for 3–6 months.

Pelvic DVT in particular

In addition, treatment for pelvic DVT focuses on complete bed rest and administration of antibiotics along with anticoagulants. If the woman develops a pelvic abscess, a laparotomy for incision and drainage may be done. Because this procedure may cause tubal scarring and may interfere with fertility, the woman may need additional surgery later to remove the vessel before becoming pregnant again.

Hidden enemy

Thromboembolic disorders are now the main cause of maternal death in the UK. CEMACH have highlighted the failures in diagnosing and treating women effectively who have DVTs and other thromboembolic conditions. Access the most recent statistics on the CEMACH website: http://www. cemach.org.uk/

Diagnosis of DVT and pulmonary embolism is particularly unreliable in pregnancy due to the normal physiological changes that occur in pregnancy and in the puerperium.

Venous thrombolic embolism is 10 times more common in pregnant women than nonpregnant women and although it can occur at any stage during pregnancy, the puerperium is the time of highest risk. Guidelines on diagnosis and management of thromboembolic disorders in pregnancy are available on the RCOG website: www.rcog.org.uk/

What to do

Prevention of DVT is key. Assess the woman for risk factors, and teach her ways to reduce her risk. (See *Preventing DVT*, page 422.)

In addition, because postpartum DVT commonly results from an endometrial infection:

- be alert to signs and symptoms of endometritis
- notify the doctor if signs and symptoms of endometritis occur
- institute treatment promptly, as ordered.

Fighting back

To combat DVT, take the following measures:

- Enforce bed rest as ordered, and elevate the woman's affected arm or leg. If you use pillows for elevation of a leg, place the pillows so that they support its entire length to avoid compressing the popliteal space.
- Apply warm compresses to increase circulation to the affected area and to relieve pain and inflammation.
- Give analgesics to relieve pain as ordered.
- Assess uterine involution and note changes in fundal consistency such as the inability to remain firm or contracted.

Education edge

Preventing DVT

Incorporate these instructions in your information-giving to reduce a woman's risk of developing deep vein thrombosis (DVT):

- Check with your midwife about using the 'all fours' position, squatting, side lying or back lying (supine recumbent) positions for birth. These alternative positions reduce the risk of blood pooling in the lower extremities.
- If you must use the lithotomy position for birth, ask the midwife to pad the stirrups well so that you put less pressure on your calves.
- Change positions frequently if on bed rest.
- Avoid deeply flexing your legs at the groin or sharply flexing your knees.

- Don't stand in one place for too long or sit with your knees bent or legs crossed. Elevate your legs slightly to improve venous return.
- Don't wear garters or constrictive clothing.
- Wiggle your toes and perform leg lifts while in bed to minimise venous pooling and help increase venous return.
- Use a sequential compression device or wear TED stockings during and after caesarean birth until you're ambulating. Make sure your leg is measured to ensure you get the right size of stockings.
- Walk as soon as possible after birth.
- Wear antiembolism (TED stockings) or support stockings as ordered. Put them on before getting out of bed in the morning.

- Monitor vital signs closely, at least every 4 hours or more frequently if indicated. Report changes in pulse rate or blood pressure as well as temperature elevations.
- Administer I.V. anticoagulants as ordered, using an infusion monitor or pump to control the flow rate, if necessary. Have an anticoagulant antidote, such as protamine sulphate (for heparin therapy), readily available.
- Because neither heparin nor warfarin is excreted in significant amounts in breast milk, breastfeeding is allowed.
- If the mother is hospitalised, have her express breast milk for her baby.
- Administer antibiotic and antipyretic therapy for the woman with pelvic DVT.
- Mark, measure and record the circumference of the affected extremity at least once daily, and compare it to the other extremity. To ensure accuracy and consistency of serial measurements, mark the skin over the area and measure at the same spot daily.
- Obtain coagulation studies, such as INR, PTT and PT, as ordered.

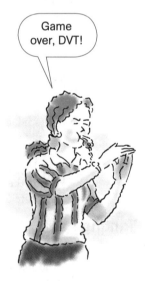

Game over, DVT!

On the lookout for lochia

- Monitor the mother for increased amounts of lochia. Encourage her to change perineal pads frequently, and estimate the amount of blood loss.
- Watch for signs and symptoms of bleeding, such as tarry stools, coffee-ground vomitus and ecchymoses. Note oozing of blood at I.V. sites, and assess gums for excessive bleeding. Report positive findings to the doctor immediately.

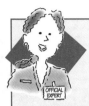

Advice from the experts

Dealing with pulmonary embolism

A woman with deep vein thrombosis is at high risk for developing a pulmonary embolism. Be alert for the classic signs and symptoms of pulmonary embolism, such as:

- chest pain
- dyspnoea
- tachypnoea
- tachycardia
- haemoptysis
- sudden changes in mental status
- hypotension.

   Also, be vigilant in monitoring for these problems, which may occur along with the classic signs and symptoms:

- chills
- fever
- abdominal pain
- signs and symptoms of respiratory distress, including tachypnoea, tachycardia, restlessness, cold and clammy skin, cyanosis and retractions.

Nip it in the bud

A pulmonary embolism is a life-threatening event that can lead to cardiovascular collapse and death. You should intervene at once if pulmonary embolism is suspected. Follow these steps:

- Elevate the head of the bed to improve the work of breathing.
- Administer oxygen via face mask at 8–10 L/minute, as ordered.
- Begin I.V. fluid administration, as ordered.
- Monitor oxygen saturation rates continuously via pulse oximetry.
- Obtain arterial blood gas samples for analysis as ordered to evaluate gas exchange.

- Assess vital signs frequently, as often as every 15 minutes.
- Anticipate the need for continuous cardiac monitoring to evaluate for arrhythmias secondary to hypoxaemia and for insertion of a pulmonary artery catheter to evaluate haemodynamic status and gas exchange.
- Administer emergency drugs, such as dopamine (Intropin) for pressure support and morphine for analgesia, as ordered.
- Expect the woman to be transferred to the intensive care unit.
- Administer analgesics without aspirin for pain relief.
- Administer anticoagulants or thrombolytics, as ordered.

- Assess the mother for signs and symptoms of pulmonary emboli, such as crackles, dyspnoea, haemoptysis, sudden changes in mental status, restlessness and hypotension. (See *Dealing with pulmonary embolism*.)
- Provide emotional support to the woman and her family, and explain all procedures and treatments.
- Prepare the woman for surgery, if indicated.
- Emphasise the importance of follow-up blood studies to monitor anticoagulant therapy.
- If the woman is discharged on heparin therapy, teach her or a family member how to give subcutaneous injections. If additional assistance is required, arrange for a home health care referral and follow-up.
- Teach the woman how to properly apply and use antiembolism stockings. Tell her to report complications, such as toes that are cold or blue.
- To prevent bleeding, encourage the woman to avoid medications that contain aspirin and to check with the doctor before using over-the-counter

medications. Teach her the signs and symptoms of bleeding, such as easy bruising or blood in the urine or stool.

• Tell her to use a soft toothbrush and an electric razor to prevent tissue damage and bleeding.

• Advise her to use contraception because oral anticoagulants are teratogenic.

• Tell the woman not to increase her vitamin K intake while taking oral anticoagulants because vitamin K counteracts the anticoagulant effects.

• Stress that the woman should report her history of DVT to the doctor if she becomes pregnant again so that preventative measures can be started early.

Postnatal psychiatric disorders

Three distinct psychiatric disorders have been recognised during the postnatal period: postnatal blues (or baby blues), postnatal depression and postnatal psychosis.

'Baby blues' are the most common of the postnatal psychiatric disorders and the least severe. Approximately 50% of all postpartum women experience some form of baby blues – these usually occur within 3–5 days after birth. They are a normal, hormonally generated postnatal occurrence that is thought to foster maternal–neonatal attachment. Mothers who have delivered prematurely, and those who have an infant in the newborn intensive care unit, are at particularly high risk.

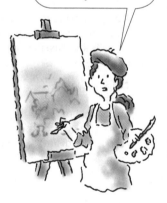

I think I'm definitely in my blue period. About 50% of all postnatal women experience some form of baby blues.

From blue to black

Postnatal depression and postnatal psychosis are mood disorders widely recognised by obstetricians, psychologists and psychiatrists. Approximately 1:10 women develop postnatal depression and 1:1,000 women develop postnatal psychosis in the UK annually; these are only the reported cases – many women may slip through the net if they are not diagnosed or do not seek help. http://www.mind.org.uk/

Postnatal depression

Postnatal depression affects as many as 15% of new mothers. This number may be higher because many cases probably aren't reported due to the stigma of a psychiatric illness. Not only does postnatal depression interfere with the mother–infant relationship, it is also thought to interfere with child development and the relationship the child has with other children, family and friends.

What causes it

The exact cause is unknown, but some antenatal risk factors may contribute to the development of postnatal depression.

A major key

A major risk factor for developing postnatal depression is a previous history of depression or a psychiatric illness before or during the pregnancy. Anxiety during the pregnancy, a teenage pregnancy, multiple births, lack of social support, stressful life situations other than the pregnancy and conflict with a spouse or significant other during the pregnancy can also be major risk factors.

A minor key

Some minor risk factors include the socioeconomic status of the mother and obstetric complications.

The result

Untreated depression during pregnancy can lead to poor self-care; noncompliance with antenatal care; a negative effect on maternal–infant bonding; a higher risk of obstetric complications; drug, tobacco or alcohol abuse; termination of the pregnancy and suicide.

What to look for

Some distinct signs and symptoms help distinguish postnatal depression from postnatal 'baby blues', including:
- feeling sad or down for prolonged periods
- decreased interest in normal activities
- appetite problems and weight changes
- anxiety and agitation
- difficulty sleeping
- fatigue and reduced energy
- feeling guilty or worthless
- feelings of suicide or thoughts of harming the infant.

What tests tell you

There are no specific diagnostic tests for postnatal depression, but women can be screened during the antenatal period. Many health visitors use the Edinburgh Postnatal Depression Scale (EPDS) as a screening method. This is a self-report questionnaire which is both easy to complete and acceptable to the mother. Evidence from a number of research studies has confirmed the tool to be both reliable and sensitive in detecting depression, and it has been validated for use in the community.
- New mothers usually complete it 6–8 weeks postpartum.
- A score of 11-12/30 has a sensitivity of 76.7% and specificity of 92.5%.
- It should be confirmed by interview and mental state examination.

The EPDS can be accessed in full from the website: http://www.patient.co.uk/showdoc/40002172/

The NICE guidelines for antenatal and postnatal mental health were published in 2007 and are available on their website. They recommend that at the initial booking visit and postnatally, health care professionals should ask two questions:

1. During the past month, have you often been bothered by feeling down, depressed or hopeless?
2. During the past month, have you often been bothered by having little interest or pleasure in doing things?

A third question should be considered if the woman answers 'yes' to either of the initial questions. – Is this something you feel you need or want help with?

By asking these two questions, it is hoped that at-risk women may be identified and given the right support and treatment.

You can view the NICE guidelines on the website: http://www.nice.org.uk/Guidance/CG45

How it's treated

Treatment can usually be accomplished on an outpatient basis. Selective serotonin reuptake inhibitors are prescribed as these agents are thought to be safe for breastfeeding women.

Cognitive behavioural therapy and counselling may also prove beneficial.

What to do

* Advise the postnatal mother about the warning signs of postnatal depression and provide resource material.
* Include information about postnatal depression as part of the mother's discharge plan.
* Encourage the woman to verbalise her feelings about the pregnancy.
* Help the woman understand that it's normal to feel sadness or a lack of enthusiasm about motherhood.
* Instruct the woman and her family that postnatal depression can occur at any time after delivery.
* Advise the family of the warning signs of postnatal depression. Inform them that it's important not to ignore even the subtlest of signs. Urge them to immediately report these signs to the midwife, health visitor or general practitioner.
* Assist the woman in contacting a support group that can help to alleviate her feelings of isolation.

Postnatal psychosis is a medical emergency and requires immediate hospitalisation.

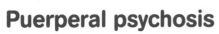

Puerperal psychosis

Puerperal psychosis usually appears within the first 2–3 weeks after birth but can occur as early as the first or second day. This condition affects about 1–2 women in every 1,000 births and is an emergency situation that requires immediate intervention.

What causes it

The exact cause is unknown but some predisposing factors may contribute to the development of postnatal psychosis. These include changing hormone levels, lack of support systems, low sense of self-esteem, financial difficulties and major life changes.

What to look for

Signs and symptoms of puerperal psychosis may be similar to those of any psychosis. For example, the woman may experience symptoms associated with schizophrenia, bipolar disorder or major depression. She may also experience:
- feelings that her baby is dead or defective
- hallucinations that may include voices telling her to harm the baby or herself
- severe agitation, irritability or restlessness
- poor judgment and confusion
- feelings of worthlessness, guilt, isolation or over concern with the baby's health
- sleep disturbances
- euphoria, hyperactivity or little concern for self or infant.

What tests tell you

There are no specific diagnostic tests for puerperal psychosis, but women can be screened during the antenatal period. Some studies have shown that women who were depressed antenatally were more likely to develop postnatal depression. http://www.nhs.uk/news/2008/06June/Pages/Depressionduringpregnancy.aspx

How it's treated

Puerperal psychosis is a medical emergency and requires immediate hospitalisation. Medications such as antipsychotics and antidepressants are used. It may also be necessary to institute suicide precautions. The family should also be involved in the woman's treatment plan.

What to do

- Advise the mother about the warning signs of postnatal depression and psychosis. Provide resource material.
- Include information about postnatal depression and psychosis as part of the woman's discharge plan.
- Advise the woman and her family that postnatal depression and psychosis can occur at any time after delivery.
- Advise the family of the warning signs of postnatal depression and psychosis. Inform them that it's important not to ignore even the subtlest of signs. Urge them to immediately report these signs to the midwife, health visitor or general practitioner.

More information on postnatal depression can be accessed from the following websites:

http://www.mind.org.uk/
http://www.depression-in-pregnancy.org.uk/
http://www.psychotherapy.org.uk/

Quick quiz

1. What's considered the major cause of early (primary) postpartum haemorrhage?

    A. Uterine atony
    B. Perineal laceration
    C. Retained placental fragments
    D. DIC.

Answer: A. Although all of the above complications are possible causes of postpartum haemorrhage, uterine atony (relaxation of the uterus) is considered the primary and most common cause of early postpartum haemorrhage.

2. Which finding would lead you to suspect that a woman has developed hypovolaemic shock secondary to postpartum haemorrhage?

    A. Respiratory rate of 22 breaths/minute
    B. Pale-pink, moist skin
    C. Urine output below 25 ml/hour
    D. Bounding peripheral pulses

Answer: C. A urine output below 25 ml/hour suggests hypovolaemic shock secondary to decreased renal perfusion. Other findings include rapid and shallow respirations; pale, cold, clammy skin; rapid, thready peripheral pulses; mean arterial pressure below 60 mmHg and narrowed pulse pressure.

3. Which factor predisposes a mother to a puerperal infection?

    A. External fetal monitoring during labour
    B. Rupture of membranes 15 hours ago
    C. Labour lasting 20 hours
    D. Caesarean birth

Answer: D. A caesarean birth increases a woman's risk for puerperal infection by as much as 20 times. The use of internal fetal monitoring, prolonged (more than 24 hours) or premature rupture of membranes and prolonged (more than 24 hours) or difficult labour also increase the risk for puerperal infection.

4. A woman reports foul-smelling lochia with strong uterine contractions persisting after birth. Her temperature has been elevated, ranging from 39 to 40°C, for the past 2 days. Her uterus is firm but tender and her abdomen is soft with no guarding noted. You would suspect:

    A. localised perineal infection.
    B. peritonitis.
    C. endometritis.
    D. parametritis.

Answer: C. Endometritis may cause heavy, foul-smelling lochia; a tender, enlarged uterus; backache; severe uterine contractions that persist after childbirth and elevated temperature for 2 or more days after the first 24 hours.

5. Which microorganism most commonly causes mastitis?
   A. *Staphylococcus aureus*
   B. *Staphylococcus epidermis*
   C. Beta-haemolytic streptococcus
   D. Mumps virus

Answer: A. Although all are possible causative organisms, *Staphylococcus aureus* is the most common. Mastitis caused by the mumps virus is rare.

6. If the mother has DVT, for which complication should you watch?
   A. Endometritis
   B. Pulmonary embolism
   C. Haematoma
   D. Mastitis

Answer: B. A possible life-threatening complication of DVT, pulmonary embolism occurs when the clot breaks off and travels to the pulmonary vascular bed, interfering with gas exchange.

Scoring

☆☆☆ If you answered all seven questions correctly, great going! You've summed it up totally.

☆☆ If you answered five or six questions correctly, fantastic! You've added immeasurably to your knowledge of the subject.

☆ If you answered fewer than five questions correctly, no problem. Count on doing better when you read through the chapter once more.

11 Neonatal assessment and care

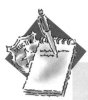

Just the facts

In this chapter, you'll learn:

♦ changes that occur in the newborn infant after birth

♦ the proper way to perform newborn assessment

♦ nursing interventions critical to neonatal care.

Adapting to extrauterine life

After birth, a baby must quickly adapt to extrauterine life, even though many of his body systems are still developing. During this time of adaptation, the midwife must be aware of normal neonatal physiological characteristics and assessment findings in order to detect possible problems and initiate appropriate interventions. (See *Physiology of the neonate*, page 431.)

Respiratory system

The major adaptation for the newborn infant is that he must breathe on his own rather than depend on fetal circulation. At birth, air is substituted for the fluid that filled the baby's respiratory tract in the alveoli during gestation. In a normal vaginal delivery, some of this fluid is squeezed out during birth. After delivery, the fluid is absorbed across the alveolar membrane into the capillaries.

At first breath

The onset of the baby's breathing is stimulated by several factors:
- low blood oxygen levels
- increased blood carbon dioxide (CO_2) levels
- low blood pH
- temperature change from the warm uterine environment to the cooler extrauterine environment.

Physiology of the neonate

This chart provides a summary of the physiological characteristics of a neonate after birth, including adaptations the baby must make to cope with extrauterine life.

Body system	Physiology after birth
Respiratory	• Onset of breathing occurs as air replaces the fluid that filled the lungs before birth.
Cardiovascular	• Functional closure of fetal shunts occurs. • Transition from fetal to postnatal circulation occurs.
Renal	• System doesn't mature fully until after the first year of life; fluid imbalances may occur.
Gastrointestinal	• System continues to develop. • Uncoordinated peristalsis of the oesophagus occurs. • The neonate has a limited ability to digest fats.
Thermogenic	• The neonate is susceptible to rapid heat loss due to acute change in environment and thin layer of subcutaneous fat. • Nonshivering thermogenesis occurs. • The presence of brown fat (more in mature babies; less in preterm babies) warms the neonate by increasing heat production.
Immune	• The inflammatory response of the tissues to localised infection is immature.
Haematopoietic	• Coagulation time is prolonged.
Neurological	• Presence of primitive reflexes and time in which they appear and disappear indicate the maturity of the developing nervous system.
Hepatic	• The neonate may demonstrate jaundice.
Integumentary	• The epidermis and dermis are thin and bound loosely to each other. • Sebaceous glands are active.
Musculoskeletal	• More cartilage is present than ossified bone.
Reproductive	• Females may have a mucoid vaginal discharge and pseudomenstruation due to maternal oestrogen levels. • In males, testes descend into the scrotum. • Small, white, firm cysts called epithelial pearls may be visible at the tip of the prepuce. • Scrotum may be oedematous if the neonate presented in breech position.

Noise, light, touch, smell and other sensations related to the birth process may also influence the baby's initial breathing.

Delicate and developing

Although the newborn infant can breathe on his own, his respiratory system isn't as developed as an adult's. Babies are obligatory nose breathers. In addition, babies have a relatively large tongue whereas the trachea and glottis are small.

Other significant differences between a neonate's respiratory system and an adult's system include:

- airway lumens that are narrower and collapse more easily
- respiratory tract secretions that are more abundant
- mucous membranes that are more delicate and susceptible to trauma
- alveoli that are more sensitive to pressure changes
- a capillary network that's less developed
- rib cage and respiratory musculature that are less developed.

Cardiovascular system

The baby's first breath triggers several cardiopulmonary changes that help transition from fetal circulation to postnatal circulation. During this transition, the foramen ovale, ductus arteriosus and ductus venosus close. These closures allow blood to start flowing to the lungs.

Ovale to no avail

When the newborn baby takes his first breath, the lungs inflate. When the lungs are inflated, pulmonary vascular resistance to blood flow is reduced and pulmonary artery pressure drops. Pressure in the right atrium decreases, and the increased blood flow to the left side of the heart increases the pressure in the left atrium. This change in pressure causes the foramen ovale (the fetal shunt between the left and right atria) to close. Increased blood oxygen levels then influence other fetal shunts to close.

From ducts to ligaments

The ductus arteriosus, located between the aorta and pulmonary artery, eventually closes and becomes a ligament. The ductus venosus, between the left umbilical vein and the inferior vena cava, closes because of vasoconstriction and lack of blood flow, then it also becomes a ligament. The umbilical arteries and vein and the hepatic arteries also constrict and become ligaments.

Renal system

After birth, the renal system is called into action because the baby can no longer depend on the placenta to excrete waste products. However, renal system function doesn't fully mature until after the first year, which means that the baby is at risk for chemical imbalances. The baby's limited ability to excrete drugs because of renal immaturity, coupled with excessive fluid loss, can rapidly lead to acidosis and fluid imbalances.

Gastrointestinal system

At birth, the baby's gastrointestinal (GI) system isn't fully developed because normal bacteria aren't present in the digestive tract. The lower intestine contains meconium, which usually starts to pass within 24 hours. It appears greenish black and viscous.

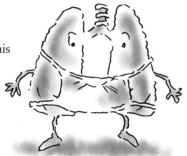

Careful! A neonate's mucous membranes are more susceptible to trauma than an adult's.

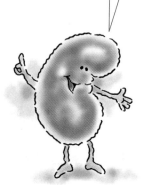

Hey, I'm new to the job. Give me a chance to mature or I might easily develop acidosis and fluid imbalances.

Ongoing developments

As the GI system starts to develop, these characteristics appear:
• audible bowel sounds 1 hour after birth
• uncoordinated peristaltic activity in the oesophagus for the first few days of life
• limited ability to digest fats because amylase and lipase are absent at birth
• frequent regurgitation because of an immature cardiac sphincter.

Thermogenic system

Among the many adaptations that occur after birth, the baby must regulate his body temperature by producing and conserving heat. This can be difficult for the baby because he has a thin layer of subcutaneous fat and his blood vessels are closer to the surface of the skin. In addition, the baby's vasomotor control is less developed, his body surface area-to-weight ratio is high and his sweat glands have minimal thermogenic function until he's 4 weeks or older.

Where's the heat?

The baby's body also has to work against four routes of heat loss:

convection – the flow of heat from the body to cooler air

radiation – the loss of body heat to cooler, solid surfaces near (but not in direct contact with) the neonate, for example – incubator walls

evaporation – heat loss that occurs when liquid is converted into vapour – if the baby's skin was wet he could lose heat when currents of air move past him

conduction – the loss of body heat to cooler substances in direct contact with the baby, for example, cold hands, weigh scales and stethoscopes.

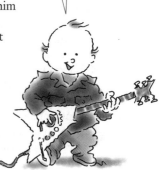

I'd like to heat things up a little. This next number is something I like to call thermogenesis.

Warming things up

To maintain body temperature, the baby must produce heat through a process called *nonshivering thermogenesis*. This involves an increase in his metabolism and oxygen consumption. Thermogenesis mainly occurs in the heart, liver and brain. Brown fat (brown adipose tissue) is another source of thermogenesis that's unique to the neonate.

Immune system

The neonatal immune system depends largely on three immunoglobulins: IgG, IgA and IgM.

Fighting infection with shear numbers

IgG (which can be detected in the fetus at 18 weeks' gestation) consists of bacterial and viral antibodies. It's the most abundant immunoglobulin and is found in all body fluids. In utero, IgG crosses from the placenta to the fetus, so he is receiving immunity from his mum. After birth, the baby produces his own IgG during the first 3 months while the leftover maternal antibodies in his body break down.

The enforcer of bacterial growth

IgA, an immunoglobulin that limits bacterial growth in the GI tract, is produced gradually. Maximum levels of IgA are reached during childhood. The baby obtains IgA from maternal colostrum and breast milk. It is also found in the baby's tears after 2 weeks of age.

First responder

IgM, found in blood and lymph fluid, is the first immunoglobulin to respond to infection. It's produced at birth, and by the age of 9 months the IgM level in the neonate reaches the level found in adults.

Still in training

Even though these immunoglobulins are present in the newborn infant, the inflammatory response of the tissues to localised infection is still immature. All neonates, especially preterm neonates, are at high risk for infection during the first several months of life.

Other means of protection for the baby come in the following forms:
• White blood cells – phagocytes, neutrophils, basophils, eusonophils, macrophages and lymphocytes. The lymphocytes are divided into two groups – B lymphocytes and T lymphocytes. Both of these not only fight infection but also create memory cells and antibodies so that if the same pathogen enters the baby's body second time, it will be recognised and an immediate immune response will ensue.
• Skin and hair – These protect the sensitive areas of the body.
• Mucous membranes – These secrete mucus which bathes the respiratory, GI tract and urinary tract. This mucus also protects and fights against infection.
• High pH level of the gastric secretions and urine protects the GI tract and bladder by killing bacteria.
• Inflammatory response – Once pathogens enter the body, an inflammatory response is initiated which releases white blood cells and chemicals that kill bacteria. It also causes a rise in temperature, redness, swelling and pain in the localised area which assist in dealing with the infection.

Haematopoietic system

In the neonatal haematopoietic system, blood volume accounts for 80–85 ml/kg of body weight. Immediately after the birth, the baby's blood volume averages 300 ml; however, it can drop to as low as 100 ml depending on how long the baby remains attached to the placenta via the umbilical cord. In addition, neonatal blood has a prolonged coagulation time because of decreased levels of vitamin K.

Vitamin K deficiency and HDN

Vitamin K helps blood to clot and is essential to prevent serious bleeding. Babies do not get enough vitamin K from their mothers during pregnancy, or when they are breastfeeding. Without vitamin K, they are at risk of getting a rare disorder called haemorrhagic disease of the newborn (HDN), which can cause bleeding into the brain and may result in brain damage or even death. This can be prevented by giving new babies extra vitamin K. By the age of about 6 months, they have built up their own supply.

How is vitamin K given?

The easiest and most reliable way, as highlighted by current research, is to give babies vitamin K by injection – a single injection just after birth will protect a baby for many months. Vitamin K can also be given by mouth, but this is a less effective route because vitamin K is not absorbed well when given by mouth and the effect does not last long. Also, three doses are usually needed to give enough protection – particularly if the baby is breastfed. The first dose is given at birth, the second between 4 and 7 days and the third when the baby is 4 weeks old. Babies fed mainly on formula products do not usually need the third dose. If the baby vomits within 1 hour of swallowing vitamin K, he will need to have another dose. Most hospitals advise I.M. vitamin K now.

Can all babies have vitamin K?

All babies need to have vitamin K. Very small or premature babies may need smaller doses – but the neonatologist can advise about this. Vitamin K by mouth is not suitable for some babies:

• Babies who are premature or sick should be given the vitamin by injection as they have lower levels of vitamin K and are at higher risk of haemorrhagic disease of the newborn.

• If the mother chooses vitamin K by mouth but her baby is unwell when a dose is due, the baby may need to have the injection instead.

• If, while pregnant, the mother took medication for epilepsy, blood clots or tuberculosis, she should tell her doctor or midwife. Her baby may not be able to absorb vitamin K by mouth and may need the injection instead.

It is vital that every mother is given all the information available about vitamin K so that she can make an informed decision about whether she wants her baby to have it. Mothers should be given information verbally or given literature to read as consent should be sought before vitamin K is given to the baby.

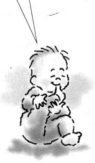

My reflexes are primitive – neurologically speaking, that is.

Neurological system

The neurological system at birth isn't completely integrated, but it's developed enough to sustain extrauterine life. Most functions of this system are primitive reflexes. The full-term baby's neurological system should produce equal strength and symmetry in responses and reflexes. Diminished or absent reflexes may indicate a serious neurological problem, and asymmetrical responses may indicate that trauma, such as nerve damage, paralysis or fracture, occurred during birth.

Hepatic system

Jaundice (yellowing of the skin) is a major concern in the neonatal hepatic system. It's caused by hyperbilirubinaemia, a condition that occurs when serum levels of unconjugated bilirubin increase because of increased red blood cell lysis, altered bilirubin conjugation or increased bilirubin reabsorption from the GI tract.

A mellow yellow

Jaundice resulting from physiological hyperbilirubinaemia is a mild form of jaundice that appears after the first 24 hours of extrauterine life and usually disappears in 7 days (9 or 10 days in preterm babies). However, if bilirubin levels rise, pathological conditions such as bilirubin encephalopathy may develop.

Shades of an underlying condition

Jaundice resulting from pathological hyperbilirubinaemia is evident at birth or within the first 24 hours of extrauterine life. It may be caused by haemolytic disease, liver disease or severe infection. Prognosis varies depending on the cause.

Integumentary system

At birth, all of the structures of the integumentary system are present, but many of their functions are immature. The epidermis and dermis are bound loosely to each other and are very thin. In addition, the sebaceous glands are very active in early infancy because of maternal hormones. (See *Protecting babies from the sun.*) Premature babies are particularly at risk of skin damage due to the very thin layer of immature epidermis and the nature of the environment in which they are nursed.

Education edge

Protecting babies from the sun

Babies are more susceptible to the harmful effects of the sun because the amount of melanin (pigment) in the skin is low at birth. Teach parents the importance of avoiding sun exposure by giving them these tips:

- Keep a hat with a visor on the baby when outside.
- Make sure that the hood of the pram covers the baby.
- Be especially careful in the car. Sun roofs and windows may expose the baby to too much sun. Use commercially available window shades and visors.

Musculoskeletal system

At birth, the skeletal system contains more cartilage than ossified bone. The process of ossification occurs very rapidly during the first year of life. The muscular system is almost completely formed at birth.

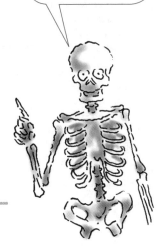

Here's an interesting fact: At birth, the skeletal system contains more cartilage than ossified bone.

Reproductive system

The ovaries of the female infant contain thousands of primitive germ cells. These germ cells represent the full potential for ova. The number of ova decreases from birth to maturity by about 90%. After birth, the uterus undergoes involution and decreases in size and weight because, in utero, the fetal uterus enlarges from the effects of maternal hormones.

For 97% of male infants at term, the testes descend into the scrotum before birth. Babies who are less than 36 weeks' gestation may well have undescended testes. Spermatogenesis does not occur until puberty.

Neonatal assessment

Neonatal assessment includes initial and ongoing assessments, a head-to-toe physical examination and neurological and behavioural assessments.

Initial assessment

The initial newborn examination involves assessment of the baby's ability to adapt from fetal to neonatal state, examining the baby for abnormalities and keeping accurate records. To complete an initial assessment, follow these steps:
- For infection control purposes, all caregivers should wash their hands and wear gloves when assessing or caring for the newborn infant.
- Carry out a quick initial assessment by using the Apgar scoring system.
- Ensure a proper airway and administer oxygen as needed.
- Dry the baby on his mother's abdomen and make sure he has a warm, dry towel over him. If he appears well – initiate skin-to-skin (STS) care on his mother's chest.
- Apply a cord clamp and monitor for abnormal bleeding from the cord; check the number of cord vessels.
- Examine the baby for gross abnormalities and clinical manifestations of suspected abnormalities.
- Continue to assess the baby by using the Apgar score criteria even after the 5-minute score is received.
- Observe the baby passing urine and meconium and document.
- Apply identification bands to the mother and the baby, with the baby's hospital number and birth details, (two bands) before they leave the delivery room. A cot card should also be completed and it should stay with the baby.
- Promote bonding between mother and baby by putting the baby to his mother's breast or continuing STS contact.

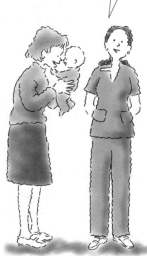

Mother and infant bonding can be helped by skin-to-skin contact.

Recording the Apgar score

Use this chart to determine the neonatal Apgar score at 1 minute and 5 minute intervals after birth. For each category listed, assign a score of 0–2, as shown. A total score of 7–10 indicates that the baby is in good condition; 4–6, fair condition (the baby may have moderate central nervous system depression, muscle flaccidity, cyanosis and poor respirations); 0–3, danger (the baby needs immediate resuscitation, as ordered). Each component should be assessed at 1, 5, 10, 15 and 20 minutes after delivery, as necessary. Resuscitation efforts such as oxygen, endotracheal intubation, chest compressions, positive pressure ventilation or nasal continuous positive airway pressure and epinephrine administration should also be documented.

Sign	Apgar score		
	0	1	2
Heart rate	Absent	Less than 100 beats/minute	More than 100 beats/minute
Respiration	Absent	Weak cry, hypoventilation	Good crying
Muscle tone	Flaccid	Some flexion	Active motion
Reflex irritability	No response	Grimace or weak cry	Cry or active withdrawal
Colour	Pallor, cyanosis	Pink body, blue extremities	Completely pink

Apgar scoring

During the initial examination of a baby, expect to calculate an Apgar score and make general observations about his appearance and behaviour. Developed by anaesthetist Dr Virginia Apgar in 1952, Apgar scoring evaluates the newborn's heart rate, respiratory effort, muscle tone, reflex irritability and colour. Evaluation of each category is performed 1 minute after birth and again at 5 minutes after birth. Each item has a maximum score of 2 and a minimum score of 0. The final Apgar score is the sum total of the five items; a maximum score is 10.

Evaluation at 1 minute quickly indicates the baby's initial adaptation to extrauterine life and whether resuscitation is necessary. The 5-minute score gives a more accurate picture of his overall status. (See *Recording the Apgar score*.) If the baby requires active resuscitation and is not adapting normally to extrauterine life, continue to make Apgar scores every 5 minutes until such times as the baby is transferred to the neonatal unit.

First and foremost

Assess heart rate first. If the umbilical cord still pulsates, you can palpate the baby's heart rate by placing your fingertips at the junction of the umbilical cord and the skin. The baby's cord stump continues to pulsate for several hours and is an easy place (next to the abdomen) to check heart rate. You

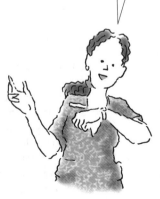

Got a minute? An easy place to check heart rate is the baby's cord stump. Be sure to count for a full minute.

can also place two fingers or a stethoscope over the baby's chest at the fifth intercostal space to obtain an apical pulse. For accuracy, the heart rate should be counted for 1 full minute or more.

Second to one

Next, check the baby's respiratory effort, the second most important Apgar sign. Assess his cry, noting its volume and vigour. Then auscultate his lungs using a stethoscope. Assess his respirations for depth and regularity. If the baby exhibits abnormal respiratory responses, begin neonatal resuscitation according to the guidelines of the UK Resuscitation Council who provide the Neonatal Life Support courses. Then use the Apgar score to judge the progress and success of resuscitation efforts. Further information on neonatal resuscitation is available from the NLS website: http://www.resus.org.uk/pages/nls.pdf

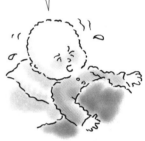

Stop trying to straighten my arms and legs or I'll tell my mummy!

Move along to the muscles

Determine muscle tone by evaluating the degree of flexion in the baby's arms and legs and their resistance to straightening. This can be done by extending the limbs and observing their rapid return to flexion – the baby's normal state.

Assess reflex irritability by evaluating the baby's cry for presence, vigour and pitch. Initially, he may not cry, but you should be able to elicit a cry when you administer his vitamin K injection. The usual response is a loud, angry cry. A high-pitched or shrill cry is abnormal.

Now add a little colour

Finally, observe skin colour for cyanosis. A newborn baby usually has a pink body with blue extremities. This condition, called acrocyanosis, appears in about 85% of normal neonates 1 minute after birth. Acrocyanosis results from decreased peripheral oxygenation caused by the transition from fetal to independent circulation. When assessing a nonwhite infant, observe for colour changes in the mucous membranes of the mouth, conjunctivae, lips, palms and soles.

Gestational age and birthweight

Perinatal mortality and morbidity are related to gestational age and birthweight. Classifying an infant by both weight and gestational age provides a more accurate method for assessing mortality risk and offers guidelines for treatment. The infant's age and weight classifications should also be considered during future assessments.

How old are you now?

The clinical assessment of gestational age classifies a baby as *preterm* (37 completed weeks gestation), *term* (37–42 weeks' gestation) or *post-term* (42 weeks' gestation or longer). The Ballard scoring system uses physical and neurological findings to estimate a baby's gestational age within 1 week, even in extremely preterm babies. This evaluation can be done at any time between birth and 42 hours after birth, but the greatest reliability is between 30 and 42 hours after birth. (See *Ballard gestational-age assessment tool*.)

Too small, too big, just right

Normal birthweight is 2,500 g (5 lb, 8 oz) or greater. A baby is considered to have a low birthweight if he weighs between 1,500 g (3 lb, 5 oz) and 2,499 g.

Ballard gestational-age assessment tool

To use this tool, evaluate and score the neuromuscular and physical maturity criteria, total the score and then plot the sum in the maturity rating box to determine the neonate's corresponding gestational age.

Posture

With the baby supine and quiet, score as follows:

- Arms and legs extended = 0
- Slight or moderate flexion of hips and knees = 1
- Moderate to strong flexion of hips and knees = 2
- Legs flexed and abducted, arms slightly flexed = 3
- Full flexion of arms and legs = 4

Square window

Flex the hand at the wrist. Measure the angle between the base of the thumb and the forearm. Score as follows:

- >90° = −1
- 90° = 0
- 60° = 1
- 45° = 2
- 30° = 3
- 0° = 4

Arm recoil

With the baby supine, fully flex the forearm for 5 seconds, then fully extend by pulling the hands and releasing. Observe and score the reaction according to the following criteria:

- Remains extended 180° or displays random movements = 0
- Minimal flexion (140–180°) = 1
- Small amount of flexion (110–140°) = 2
- Moderate flexion (90–110°) = 3
- Brisk return to full flexion <90°) = 4

Popliteal angle

With the baby supine and the pelvis flat on the examining surface, use one hand to flex the leg and then the thigh. Then use the other hand to extend the leg. Score the angle attained:

- 180° = −1
- 160° = 0
- 140° = 1
- 120° = 2
- 100° = 3
- 90° = 4
- <90° = 5

Scarf sign

With the baby supine, take his hand and draw it across the neck and as far across the opposite shoulder as possible. You may assist the elbow by lifting it across the body. Score according to the location of the elbow:

- Elbow reaches or nears level of opposite shoulder = −1
- Elbow crosses opposite anterior axillary line = 0
- Elbow reaches opposite anterior axillary line = 1
- Elbow at midline = 2
- Elbow doesn't reach midline = 3
- Elbow doesn't cross proximate axillary line = 4

Heel to ear

With the baby supine, hold his foot with one hand and move it as near to the head as possible without forcing it. Keep the pelvis flat on the examining surface. Score as shown in the chart.

Ballard gestational-age assessment tool *(continued)*

Neuromuscular maturity

Neuromuscular maturity sign	Score							Record score here
	−1	0	1	2	3	4	5	
Posture 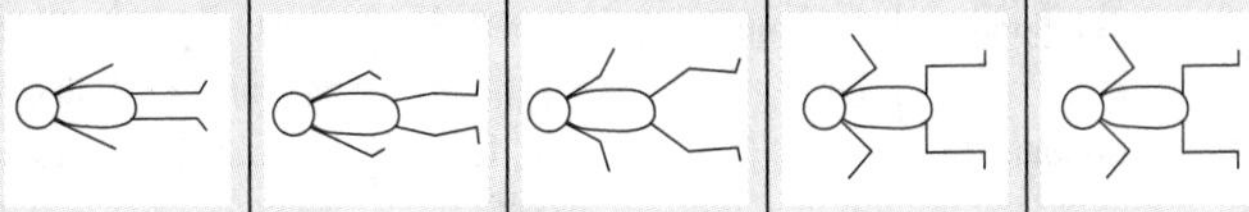	—						—	
Square window (wrist) 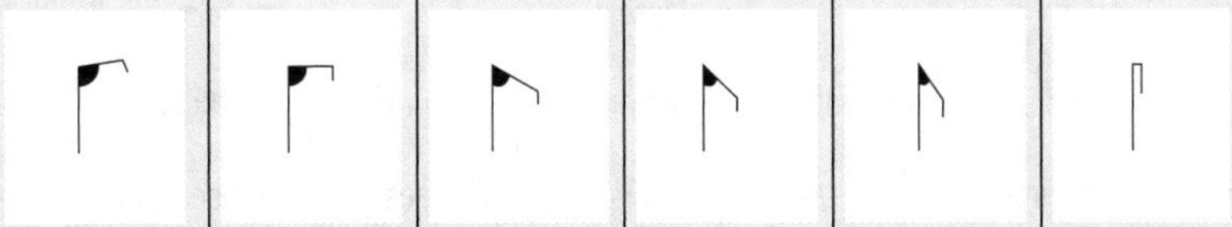	>90°	90°	60°	45°	30°	0°	—	
Arm recoil 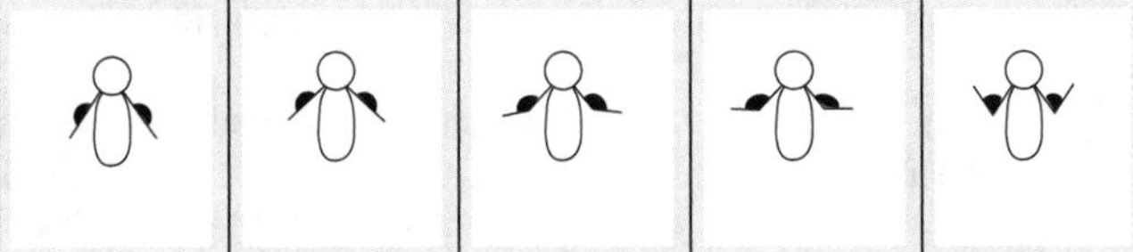	—	180°	140°–180°	110°–140°	90°–110°	<90°	—	
Popliteal angle 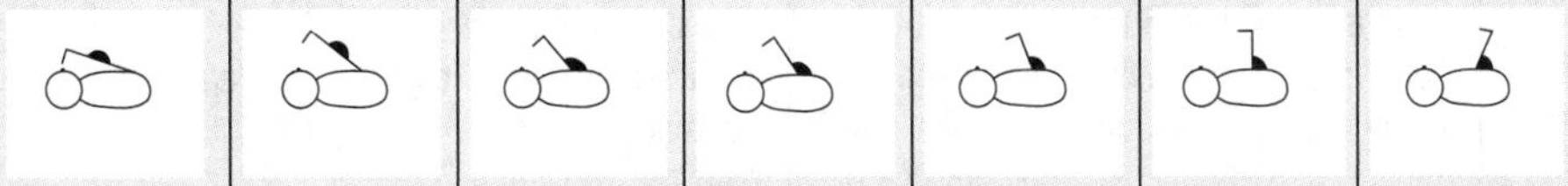	180°	160°	140°	120°	100°	90°	<90°	
Scarf sign 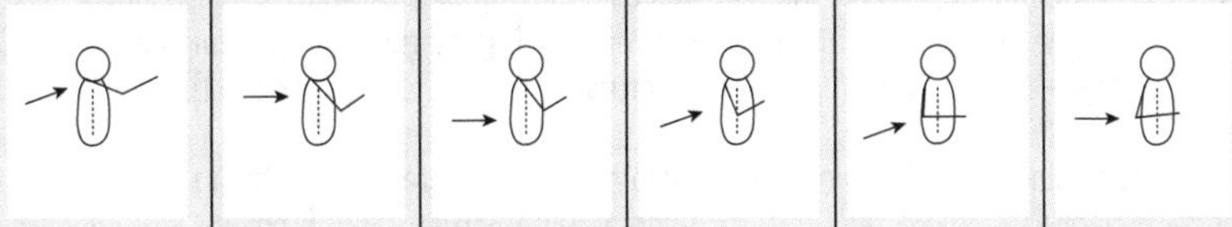							—	
Heel to ear 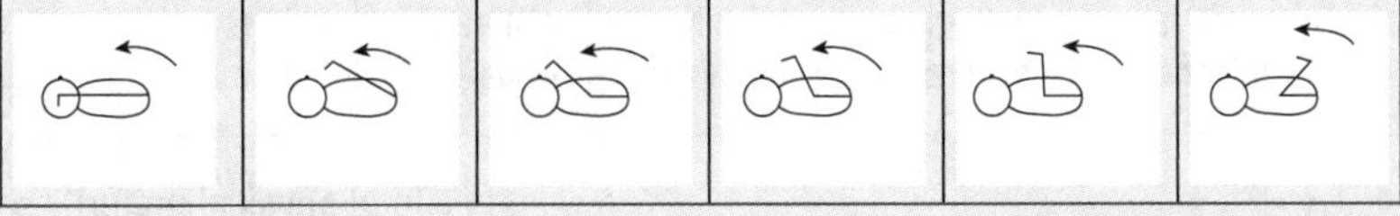							—	
						Total neuromuscular maturity score		

(continued)

Ballard gestational-age assessment tool (continued)

Physical maturity

Physical maturity sign	Score							Record score here
	−1	0	1	2	3	4	5	
Skin	Sticky, friable, transparent	Gelatinous, red, translucent	Smooth, pink; visible vessels	Superficial peeling or rash; few visible vessels	Cracking; pale areas; rare visible vessels	Parchment-like; deep cracking; no visible vessels	Leathery, cracked, wrinkled	
Lanugo	None	Sparse	Abundant	Thinning	Bald areas	Mostly bald	—	
Plantar surface	Heel-toe 40–50 mm: −1; <40 mm:−2	>50 mm; no crease	Faint red marks	Anterior transverse crease only	Creases over anterior two-thirds	Creases over entire sole	—	
Breast	Imperceptible	Barely perceptible	Flat areola; no bud	Stippled areola; 1–2-mm bud	Raised areola; 3–4-mm bud	Full areola; 5–10-mm bud	—	
Eye and ear	Lids fused, loosely: −1; tightly: −2	Lids open; pinna flat, stays folded	Slightly curved pinna; soft, slow, recoil	Well-curved pinna; soft but ready recoil	Formed and firm; instant recoil	Thick cartilage; ear stif	—	
Genitalia (male)	Scrotum flat, smooth	Scrotum empty; faint rugae	Testes in upper canal; rare rugae	Testes descending; few rugae	Testes down; good rugae	Testes pendulous; deep rugae	—	
Genitalia (female)	Clitoris prominent; labia flat	Prominent clitoris; small labia minora	Prominent clitoris; enlarging minora	Majora and minora equally prominent	Majora large; minora small	Majora cover clitoris and minora	—	

Total physical maturity score

Ballard gestational-age assessment tool *(continued)*

Maturity rating

Score		Total maturity score	−10	−5	0	5	10	15	20	25	30	35	40	45	50

Total maturity score	−10	−5	0	5	10	15	20	25	30	35	40	45	50
Gestational age (weeks)	20	22	24	26	28	30	32	34	36	38	40	42	44

Score

Neuromuscular _____

Physical _____

Total _____

Gestational age (weeks)

By dates _____

By ultrasound _____

By score _____

Adapted with permission from Ballard, J.L., *et al.* 'New Ballad Score, expanded to include extremely premature infants', *Journal of Pediatrics* 119(3):417–423, 1991. Used with permission from Mosby-Year Book, Inc.

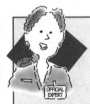

Advice from the experts

Caring for a preterm baby

When caring for a preterm baby, be alert for problems – even if the baby is of average size. A preterm baby who's an appropriate weight for his gestational age is more prone to respiratory distress syndrome, apnoea, patent ductus arteriosus (PDA) with left-to-right shunt and infection. A preterm baby who's small for his gestational age is more likely to experience asphyxia, hypoglycaemia and hypocalcaemia.

A baby of very low birthweight ranges between 1,000 g (2 lb, 3 oz) and 1,499 g. A baby weighing less than 1,000 g has an extremely low birthweight.

Postnatal growth charts are used to assess the baby based on head circumference, weight, length and gestational age. Babies who are small for gestational age (SGA) have a birthweight less than the 10th percentile for that gestational age, on postnatal growth charts; weight appropriate for gestational age signifies a birthweight within the 10th and 90th percentiles and weight large for gestational age means a birthweight greater than the 90th percentile. (See *Caring for a preterm baby*.)

Reviewing normal neonatal vital signs

This list includes the normal ranges for neonatal vital signs.

Respiration

- 40–60 breaths/minute

Heart rate (apical)

- 110–160 beats/minute

Temperature

- Rectal: 35.6–37.5°C
- Axillary: 36.4–37.2°C

Blood pressure

- Systolic: 60–80 mmHg
- Diastolic: 40–50 mmHg

Ongoing assessment

Ongoing newborn physical assessment includes observing and recording vital signs and administering prescribed medications. To perform ongoing assessment, follow these steps:

- Assess the baby's vital signs.
- Measure and record the baby's vital statistics.
- Monitor the baby's intake and output – he should pass urine and meconium within 24–48 hours.
- Administer prescribed medications such as vitamin K.

Vital signs

Measuring vital signs establishes the baseline of any neonatal assessment. Vital signs include the respiratory rate, heart rate (taken apically) and the first temperature. Temperature readings are axillary to avoid injuring the rectal mucosa. Blood pressure readings are usually assessed by an electronic vital signs monitor. (See *Reviewing normal neonatal vital signs*.)

Determining respiratory rate

Observe respirations first, before the baby becomes active or agitated. Watch and count respiratory movements for 1 minute and record the result – it is easier to watch the baby's abdominal movements when counting. A normal respiratory rate is usually between 40 and 60 breaths/minute. Also, note any signs of respiratory distress, such as cyanosis, tachypnoea, sternal retractions, grunting, nasal flaring or periods of apnoea. Short periods of apnoea (less than 15 seconds) are characteristic of the neonate in the first 24 hours when he is still trying to adapt and open up his lungs fully. (See *Counting neonatal respirations*.)

Assessing heart rate

Use a paediatric stethoscope to determine the baby's apical heart rate. Place the stethoscope over the apical impulse on the fourth or fifth intercostal space at the left midclavicular line over the cardiac apex. To ensure an accurate measurement, count the beats for at least 1 minute. A normal heart rate ranges from 110 to 160 beats/minute. Variations during sleeping and waking states are normal.

Advice from the experts

Counting neonatal respirations

When counting a baby's respiratory rate, observe abdominal excursions rather than chest excursions. Auscultation of the chest or placing the stethoscope in front of the mouth and nares are other ways to count respirations.

Taking an axillary temperature

To take an axillary temperature, make sure that the axillary skin is dry. Place the thermometer in the axilla and hold it along the lateral aspect of the baby's chest between the axillary line and the arm. Hold the thermometer in place until the temperature registers. Normal axillary temperature is 36.4–37.2°C. If a temperature probe is being used from an electronic monitor, it will record within a few seconds, if a TempaDOT is being used (a paper strip with coded dots on it), it needs to be kept in place for at least 3 minutes before it will register an accurate reading.

Reassess axillary temperature in 15–30 minutes if the first measurement registers outside the normal range. If the temperature remains abnormal, notify the doctor.

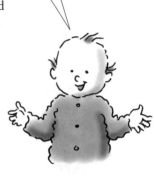

You're not really going to put the thermometer there, are you?

The low-down on low temperatures

Decreased temperatures by the axillary route could suggest:
- prematurity
- infection
- low environmental temperature
- inadequate clothing
- dehydration.

Why it may be high

Possible reasons for increased temperatures include:
- infection
- high environmental temperature
- excessive clothing
- proximity to heating unit or direct sunlight
- drug addiction
- dehydration.

Rectal temperatures are not considered safe due to the risk of perforation or rectal damage. There are additional risks associated with the use of glass mercury thermometers.

Determining blood pressure

If possible, measure a baby's blood pressure when he's in a quiet or relaxed state. Make sure that the blood pressure cuff is small enough for the baby (cuff width should be about one-third of the baby's arm – if the cuff is too small the reading will be high and if too big the reading may be lower), then wrap the cuff one or two fingerbreadths above the antecubital or popliteal area. With the stethoscope held directly over the chosen artery, hold the cuffed extremity firmly to keep it extended and inflate the cuff no faster than 5 mmHg/second.

Normal systolic readings are 60–80 mmHg and normal diastolic readings are 40–50 mmHg. A drop in systolic blood pressure (about 15 mmHg) during the first hour after birth is common. A good 'rule of thumb' is that the baby's mean arterial pressure (MAP) is roughly the same as their gestational age ±5. Crying and movement result in blood pressure changes. If you are using electronic apparatus such as a Dinamap, you may need to take a second reading to allow the machine to calibrate itself to the baby – this is only necessary if you are using the same machine for every baby in the Neonatal Unit (NNU). If the machine is linked to the baby all the time, then the first reading is adequate.

From top to bottom

Compare blood pressures in the upper and lower extremities at least once to detect cardiac problems if this is suspected. Remember that blood pressure readings from the thigh will be approx. 10 mmHg higher than the arm. If the blood pressure reading in the thigh is the same or lower than the arm, notify the practitioner. This could indicate coarctation of the aorta, a congenital heart defect, and should be investigated further.

Size and weight

Size and weight measurements establish the baseline for monitoring growth. Size and weight measurements can also be used to detect such disorders as failure to thrive and hydrocephalus. (See *Average neonatal size and weight*.) It is vital that all measurements are plotted on the baby's centile chart.

Average neonatal size and weight

In addition to weight, anthropometric measurements include head and chest circumferences and head-to-heel length. Together, these measurements serve as a baseline and show whether neonatal size is within normal ranges or whether there may be a significant problem or anomaly – especially if values stray far from the mean.
   Average initial anthropometric ranges are:

- head circumference – 33–35.5 cm
- chest circumference – 30.5–33 cm
- head to heel – 46–53 cm
- weight – 2,500–4,000 g (5 lb, 8 oz to 8 lb, 13 oz).

Head circumference

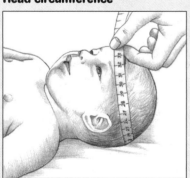

Chest circumference

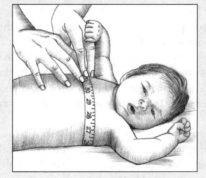

Head-to-heel length

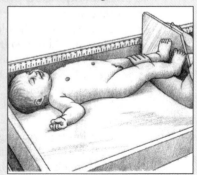

It's personal!

All measurements are recorded in the baby's personal child health record (PCHR) book – otherwise known as the 'Red Book'. This book is filled in by the midwife in delivery suite and on discharge from hospital the midwife who checks the baby will fill her findings also. Every entry from then on is made in the appropriate pages – this book is the child's health record and is completed by the community midwife and the health visitor until the child is at school. All immunisations, hospital treatments, growth record and developmental information are stored in this book.

Measuring head circumference

Head circumference reflects the rate of growth of the head and its contents. To measure head circumference, slide the tape measure under the baby's head at the occiput and draw the tape around snugly, just above the eyebrows. Normal neonatal head circumference is 33–36 cm. Cranial moulding or caput succedaneum from a vaginal delivery may affect this measurement.

Measuring head-to-heel length

Fully extend the baby's legs with the toes pointing up. Measure the distance from the heel to the top of the head. A length board may be used if available. Normal length is 46–53 cm.

Weighing the newborn baby

A baby should be weighed at birth and then in the postnatal ward after the scale has been calibrated. Remove the nappy and place the baby in the middle of the scale tray. Keep one hand poised over the baby at all times; never leave him unattended on the scale. Be careful to prevent heat loss during the procedure.

Average weight is 2,500–4,000 g (5 lb, 8 oz to 8 lb, 13 oz).

Return the baby to the cot or examination table. Be sure to document if the baby had any clothing or equipment on him (such as an I.V.). Take the baby's weight on the same scale, if possible and always before a feed. Most babies in the postnatal ward are only weighed on admission and on the third or fourth postnatal day – it is important to ascertain that the baby is thriving, but not weighed so frequently as to make the mother overanxious. The baby will be weighed by the community midwife when she visits him at home.

Head-to-toe assessment

The baby should receive a thorough physical examination of each body part. However, before each body part is examined, assess the general appearance and posture of the baby. Neonates usually lie in a symmetrical, flexed position – the characteristic 'fetal position' – as a result of their position while in utero.

Skin

The term baby has beefy red skin for a few hours after birth. Then the skin turns to its normal colour. It commonly appears mottled or blotchy, especially on the extremities.

Findings can be skin deep

Common findings in a neonatal assessment may include:
• acrocyanosis (caused by vasomotor instability, capillary stasis and high haemoglobin level) for the first 24 hours after birth
• milia (clogged sebaceous glands) on the nose or chin
• lanugo (fine, downy hair) appearing after 20 weeks of gestation on the entire body, except the palms and soles
• vernix caseosa (a white, cheesy protective coating composed of desquamated epithelial cells and sebum)
• erythema toxicum neonatorum (a transient, maculopapular rash)
• telangiectasia (flat, reddened vascular areas) appearing on the neck, upper eyelid or upper lip
• sudamina or miliaria (distended sweat glands), which cause minute vesicles on the skin surface, especially on the face
• Mongolian spots (bluish black areas of pigmentation more commonly noted on the back and buttocks of dark-skinned babies [regardless of race]).

Make general observations about the appearance of the baby's skin in relationship to his activity, position and temperature. Usually, the baby is redder when crying or hot. He may also have transient episodes of cyanosis with crying. Cutis marmorata is transient mottling when the baby is exposed to cooler temperatures.

Ready? Set? Waaah!

Roll with it, baby

Palpate the skin to assess skin turgor. To do this, roll a fold of skin on the baby's abdomen between your thumb and forefinger. Assess consistency, amount of subcutaneous tissue and degree of hydration. A well-hydrated infant's skin returns to normal immediately upon release.

Head

The newborn baby's head is about a quarter of his body size. Six bones make up the cranium:
• the frontal bone
• the occipital bone
• two parietal bones
• two temporal bones.

Bands of connective tissue, called sutures, lie between the junctures of these bones. At the junction of the sutures are wider spaces of membranous tissues, called fontanelles.

Fontanelle facts

The neonatal skull has two fontanelles. The anterior fontanelle is diamond shaped and located at the juncture of the frontal and parietal bones. It measures approx. 3 cm long and 2 cm wide. The anterior fontanelle closes in about 12–18 months. The posterior fontanelle is triangle shaped. It's located at the juncture of the occipital and parietal bones and measures about 2 cm across. The posterior fontanelle closes in approx. 8 weeks.

The fontanelles should feel soft to touch but shouldn't be depressed. A depressed fontanelle indicates dehydration. In addition, fontanelles shouldn't bulge. Bulging fontanelles require immediate attention because they may indicate increased intracranial pressure (ICP). Pulsations in the fontanelles reflect the peripheral pulse. The anterior fontanelle may bulge a little when the baby is crying.

Moulding under the pressure

Moulding refers to asymmetry of the cranial sutures due to difficulties during vaginal delivery; it isn't normally seen in babies born by caesarean delivery. There are two types of cranial abnormalities:

Cephalhaematoma occurs when blood collects between a skull bone and the periosteum. It's caused by pressure during delivery or trauma resulting from an instrumental delivery and tends to spontaneously resolve in 3–6 weeks. A cephalhaematoma doesn't cross cranial suture lines. This condition can cause great discomfort to the baby and he may need analgesia. The midwife also needs to watch out for signs of mild cerebral irritation in the baby. In severe cases of cephalhaematoma, the baby may develop jaundice from the excessive bruising caused by breakdown of damaged red blood cells.

Caput succedaneum is a localised oedematous area due to the presenting part of the skull being pushed through a partially dilated cervix during labour. It can also cause mild discomfort to the baby, but disappears spontaneously in 4–7 days and can cross cranial suture lines.

Heads up!

The degree of head control the infant has should also be evaluated during this part of the examination. If babies are placed down on a firm surface, they'll turn their heads to the side to maintain an open airway. They also attempt to keep their heads in line with their body when raised by their arms. Although head lag is normal in the neonate, marked head lag is seen in neonates with Down syndrome or brain damage and in hypoxic infants.

Eyes

Babies tend to keep their eyes tightly shut – especially when nursed in a brightly lit room. Observe the lids for oedema, which is normally present for the first few days of life. The eyes should also be assessed for symmetry in size and shape. Here are some common findings of neonatal eye examination:
• The neonate's eyes are usually blue or grey because of scleral thinness. Permanent eye colour is established within 3–12 months.
• Lacrimal glands are immature at birth, resulting in tearless crying for up to 2 months.
• The neonate may demonstrate transient strabismus (crossed eyes).

- The doll's eye reflex (when the head is rotated laterally, the eyes deviate in the opposite direction) may persist for up to 10 days.
- Subconjunctival haemorrhages may appear from vascular tension changes during birth.
- The corneal reflex is present but generally isn't elicited unless a problem is suspected.
- The pupillary reflex and the red reflex are present.

Nose

Observe the baby's nose for:
- shape
- symmetry
- placement
- patency
- bridge configuration.

Because babies are obligatory nose breathers for the first few months of life, nasal passages must be kept clear to ensure adequate respiration – they instinctively sneeze to remove obstruction. (See *Monitoring for respiratory distress*.)

Mouth and pharynx

The newborn's mouth usually has scant saliva and pink lips. Inspect the mouth for its existing structures. The palate is usually narrow and highly arched. Inspect the hard and soft palates for clefts – this means looking into the mouth with a torch and also feeling the soft and hard palate with your finger.

Pearls of wisdom on pearls

Epstein's pearls (pinhead-size, white or yellow, rounded elevations) may be found on the gums or hard palate. These are caused by retained secretions and disappear within a few weeks or months. The frenulum of the upper lip may be quite thick. Precocious teeth may also be apparent. The pharynx can be best assessed when the baby is crying. Tonsillar tissue generally isn't visible.

Ears

Assess the baby's ears for:
- symmetry
- placement on head
- amount of cartilage
- open auditory canal
- hearing.

The neonate's ears are characterised by incurving of the pinna and cartilage deposition. The pinna is usually flattened against the side of the head from pressure in utero. The top of the ear should be above or parallel to an imaginary line from the inner to the outer canthus of the eye. Low-set ears are associated with several syndromes, including chromosomal abnormalities.

Advice from the experts

Monitoring for respiratory distress

Nasal flaring is a serious sign of air hunger from respiratory distress. If you assess nasal flaring or seesaw respirations; pale, grey skin; periods of apnoea or bradycardia, alert the doctor. These may be signs of respiratory distress syndrome.

Weighing the evidence

Universal neonatal hearing screening

Considerable data have been collected to support the early screening of neonates for detecting hearing loss and providing early intervention in those infants determined to have hearing loss.

All babies have their hearing tested in the postnatal ward as part of the NHS Infant Screening programme.

- All infants should have hearing screening using a physiological measure.
- Babies who receive routine care should have access to hearing screening during their hospital birth admission.

- Babies born at home should have access to hearing screening before 1 month of age.
- All neonates who require neonatal intensive care should receive hearing screening before discharge.
- All infants who don't pass the initial screen and any subsequent re-screening will begin appropriate audiological and medical evaluations to confirm the presence of hearing loss before 3 months of age.

Before you go

Procedures to screen for hearing in neonates have become common practice before a neonate leaves the hospital. Testing can detect permanent bilateral or unilateral sensory or conductive hearing loss.

Now hear this!

Auditory assessment is performed by noninvasive, objective, physiological measures that include otoacoustic emissions or auditory brainstem response. Both testing methods are painless and can be performed while the baby rests. Newborn babies quite often don't pass the test due to the amount of vernix and fluid in the inner ear – this should clear within a few days when the test can be repeated, or alternatively, at 3 months of age.

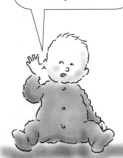

Say what? Auditory assessment can include otoacoustic emissions or auditory brainstem response.

Neck

The newborn's neck is typically short and weak with deep folds of skin. Observe for:
- range of motion
- shape
- abnormal masses.

Also, palpate each clavicle and sternocleidomastoid muscle. Note the position of the trachea. The thyroid gland generally isn't palpable.

Chest

Inspect and palpate the chest, noting:
- shape
- clavicles

- ribs
- nipples
- breast tissue
- respiratory movements
- amount of cartilage in rib cage.

The neonatal chest is characterised by a cylindrical thorax (because the anteroposterior and lateral diameters are equal) and flexible ribs. Slight intercostal retractions are usually seen on inspiration. The sternum is raised and slightly rounded, and the xiphoid process is usually visible as a small protrusion at the end of the sternum.

It is important to check the clavicles for fractures – they are the most commonly fractured bones in newborn babies. Often this is spontaneous, or due to excessive traction at delivery – particularly in the macrosomic infant. The infant may be unable to move his arm on the affected side, or may cry if it is moved. When a Moro reflex is performed, he will be unable to extend and flex his arm on the affected side.

Breast engorgement from maternal hormones may be apparent, and the secretion of 'witch's milk' may occur. Supernumerary nipples may be located below and medial to the true nipples.

Lungs

Normal respirations of the neonate are abdominal with a rate between 30 and 50 breaths/minute. After the first breaths to initiate respiration, subsequent breaths should be easy and fairly regular. Occasional irregularities may occur with crying, sleeping and feeding.

Hush little baby, don't say a word

It's easiest to auscultate the lung fields when the baby is quiet. Bilateral bronchial breath sounds should be heard. Crackles soon after birth represent the transition of the lungs to extrauterine life.

Heart

The newborn's heart rate is normally between 110 and 160 beats/minute. Because babies have a fast heart rate, it's difficult to auscultate the specific components of the cardiac cycle. Heart sounds during the neonatal period are generally of higher pitch, shorter duration and greater intensity than in later life. The first sound is usually louder and duller than the second, which is sharp in quality. Murmurs are commonly heard, especially over the base of the heart or at the third or fourth intercostal space at the left sternal border, due to incomplete functional closure of the fetal shunts.

The apical impulse (point of maximal impulse) is at the fourth intercostal space and to the left of the midclavicular line.

Abdomen

Neonatal abdominal assessment should include:
- inspection and palpation of the umbilical cord – look for umbilical hernias
- evaluation of the size and contour of the abdomen

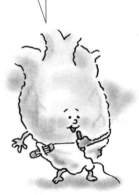

I'm so excited to be here, my heart's beating fast – between 110 and 160 beats/minute.

- auscultation of bowel sounds
- assessment of skin colour
- observation of movement with respirations
- palpation of internal organs
- checking of the groin area for inguinal hernias.

Stop, look, listen . . .

The neonatal abdomen is usually cylindrical with some protrusion. Bowel sounds are heard a few hours after birth. A scaphoid appearance indicates a diaphragmatic hernia. The umbilical cord is white and gelatinous with two arteries and one vein and begins to dry within 1–2 hours after delivery.

. . . and feel

The liver is normally palpable 2.5 cm below the right costal margin. Sometimes the tip of the spleen can be felt, but a spleen that's palpable more than 1 cm below the left costal margin warrants further investigation. Both kidneys should be palpable; this is easiest done soon after delivery, when muscle tone is lowest. The suprapubic area should be palpated for a distended bladder. The baby should void within the first 24 hours of birth.

Femoral pulses should also be palpated at this point in the examination. Inability to palpate femoral pulses could signify coarctation of the aorta or any cardiac condition which has a reduced left ventricular outflow. A bounding femoral pulse may indicate a PDA.

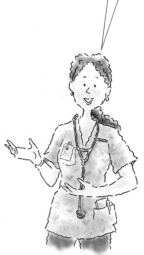

Palpate femoral pulses while examining the neonate. If they're weak or absent this could indicate coarctation of the aorta, a congenital heart defect.

Genitalia

Characteristics of a male infant's genitalia include rugae on the scrotum and testes descended into the scrotum. Scrotal oedema may be present for several days after birth due to the effects of maternal hormones or it could be a hydrocele. The midwife should check the term baby to make sure the testes have descended – if they have not, the baby should be reviewed within a month.

The urinary meatus should be checked for location – it is located in one of three places:

 at the penile tip (normal)

 on the dorsal surface (epispadias)

 on the ventral surface (hypospadias).

In the female neonate, the labia majora cover the labia minora and clitoris. These structures may be prominent due to maternal hormones or prematurity. Vaginal discharge may also occur and the hymenal tag is present.

Extremities

The extremities should be assessed for range of motion, symmetry and signs of trauma. All newborn infants are bow-legged and have flat feet. The hips should be assessed for dislocation, suggestive of developmental dysplasia of the hip. Hyperflexibility of joints is characteristic of Down syndrome. Some babies may have abnormal extremities. They may be polydactyl (more than five digits on an extremity) or syndactyl (two or more digits fused together). Also look for fingers or toes that overlap as this can be suggestive of certain genetic syndromes.

Note the nails

The nail beds should be pink, although they may appear slightly blue due to acrocyanosis. Persistent cyanosis indicates hypoxia or vasoconstriction.

Reading palms

The palms should have the usual creases. A bilateral transverse palmar crease, called a *Simian crease*, suggests a possibility of Down syndrome.

Expect resistance

Assess muscle tone. Extension of any extremity is usually met with resistance and, upon release, returns to its previously flexed position.

Spine

The neonatal spine should be straight and flat. It is important to look and feel carefully along the spine – from the occiput to the coccyx, checking that there are no breaks in the continuity. Look for tufts of hair, cysts or any unusual skin lesions. The anus should be patent without any fissure, you may be lucky enough to see the baby actually pass meconium – this enables you to check that it is actually coming from his anal sphincter. Dimpling at the base of the spine is commonly associated with spina bifida – if there is a sinus or dimple, and you cannot see where it ends – or it appears to track deeper into the baby's back, it is wise to have this x-rayed or an ultrasonic scan done to rule out spinal defects. The shoulders, scapulae and iliac crests should line up in the same plane.

Neurological assessment

An examination of the reflexes provides useful information about the neonate's nervous system and his state of neurological maturation. Some reflexive behaviours in the newborn are necessary for survival whereas other reflexive behaviours act as safety mechanisms.

Reflex revelations

Normal infants display several types of reflexes. Abnormalities are indicated by absence, asymmetry, persistence or weakness in these reflexes:
* rooting – when the infant's cheek is stroked, he turns his head in the direction of the stroke
* sucking – this begins when a nipple or finger is placed in the infant's mouth

- Moro reflex – when the infant's head is lifted in one hand and lowered into the other; the arms and legs symmetrically extend and then abduct while the thumb and forefinger spread to form a 'C' – the infants arms come back towards his centre and he closes his fingers as he does so
- atonic neck reflex (ATNR, fencing position) – when the infant's head is turned while he's lying in a supine position, the extremities on the same side straighten and those on the opposite side flex
- Babinski's reflex – when the sole on the side of the infant's small toe is stroked, the toes fan upward
- grasping – when a finger is placed in the outer aspect of the infant's hand, his fingers grasp tightly enough to be pulled to a sitting position
- pacing – when the infant is held up against the edge of a table and his shins touch the edge, he automatically lifts his legs up to 'step' unto the surface
- stepping – when the infant is held upright with the feet touching a flat surface, he responds with stepping movements
- startle – a loud noise such as a hand clap elicits neonatal arm abduction and elbow flexion and the baby's hands stay clenched
- trunk incurvature (Galant reflex) – when a finger is run laterally down the baby's spine, the trunk flexes and the pelvis swings towards the stimulated side
- blinking – the baby's eyelids close in response to bright light
- acoustic blinking – both eyes of the baby blink in response to a loud noise
- Perez reflex – when the baby is suspended prone in one of the practitioner's hands and the thumb of the other hand is moved firmly up the baby's spine from the sacrum, the baby's head and spine extend, the knees flex, the neonate cries and he may empty his bladder.

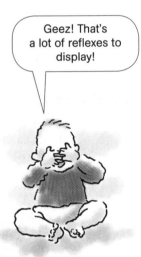

Geez! That's a lot of reflexes to display!

Behavioural assessment

Behavioural characteristics are an important part of neonatal development. To assess whether a baby is exhibiting normal behaviour, be aware of the newborn baby's principal behaviours of sleep, wakefulness and activity (such as crying) as well as his social capabilities and ability to adapt to certain stimuli.

Factors that affect behavioural responses include:
- gestational age
- time of day
- stimuli
- medication.

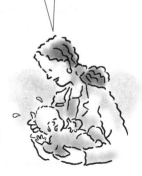

Absent, weak or constant crying indicates neonatal brain damage

Why cry?

The baby should begin life with a strong cry. Variations in this initial cry can indicate abnormalities. For example, a weak, groaning cry or grunt during expiration usually signifies respiratory disturbances. Absent, weak or constant crying suggests brain damage. A high-pitched shrill cry may be a sign of increased ICP. A hoarse cry may be suggestive of hypothyroidism.

Are you sleeping, are you sleeping?

Another aspect of behavioural assessment is observing the baby's sleep–wake cycles (the variations in his consciousness). The midwife should assess how the baby handles transitions from one state in the cycle to the next. Six specific sleep-activity states have been defined:

1. deep sleep – regular breathing, eyes closed, no spontaneous activity
2. light sleep – eyes closed, rapid eye movements (REMs), random movements and startles, irregular breathing, sucking movements
3. drowsy – eyes open, dull, heavy eyelids, variable activity, delayed response to stimuli
4. alert – bright, seems focused, minimal motor activity
5. active – eyes open, considerable motor activity, thrusting movements, briefly fussy
6. crying – high motor activity.
   Sleep–wake cycles are highly influenced by the environment.

Social senses

Neonates possess sensory capabilities that indicate their readiness for social interaction. An absence of these behavioural responses is cause for concern:

- sensitivity to light – a baby opens his eyes when the lights are dim and his responses to movement are noticeable
- selective listening – a baby tends to exhibit selective listening to his mother's voice
- response to touch – a baby responds to touch, such as calming when touched softly, suggesting that he's ready to receive tactile messages
- taste preferences – a series of studies have demonstrated that babies prefer sweet fluids to those that are sour or bitter – colostrum and breast milk are sweet!
- sense of smell – studies have shown that babies prefer pleasant smells and that they have the ability to learn and remember odours. Every baby will recognise the scent of his mother's breast milk.

Filtering stimuli

Each infant has a unique temperament and varies in his ability to handle stimuli from the external world. Through habituation, the infant can control the type and amount of stimuli processed, which decreases his response to constant or repeated stimuli. An infant presented with new stimuli becomes wide-eyed and alert but eventually shows decreased interest. Habituation enables him to respond to select stimuli, such as human voices, that encourage continued learning about the social world.

The ability to habituate depends on the babies:

- state of consciousness
- hunger
- fatigue
- temperament.

Factor this in

These factors also affect behaviours:
- consolability – the ability of the infant to console himself or be consoled
- cuddliness – the infant's response to being held
- irritability – how easily an infant is upset
- crying – the ability of the infant to communicate different needs with his cry.

Neonatal care

Physical care for the neonate includes:
- skin care/nappy area
- eye care
- umbilical cord care
- maintaining a stable body temperature
- protecting from infection and injury
- maintaining a patent airway
- maintaining normal blood glucose (BG) levels
- encouraging mother–infant attachment.

Skin care

Skin care is an important aspect of neonatal care. The first bath should not be performed for at least 12 hours – this gives the baby time to regulate his body temperature. It is important not to wash the newborn baby's skin too soon as vernix is a rich source of vitamin K and has antibacterial properties, both of which provide the baby with protection against haemorrhagic disease and infection. It is important to explain this to mothers so they do not complain about it being left in the skin creases.

Glove up

Wear gloves when touching the baby before the first bath and for all subsequent nappy changes. Don't use bath products on the eyes but these may be used on the baby's body, especially on the hair to remove blood. Be careful to remove all of the blood to minimise transmission of blood-borne pathogens to the baby or health care providers. Running a fine comb gently through the hair will help remove blood.

Hot or cold?

The temperature of the bath water should be 38°C when run. Check the baby's temperature before bathing to make sure he is not hypothermic – if his temperature is less than 36.4°C then postpone the bath till later.

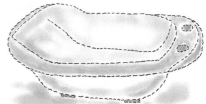

Bundle up

When the baby's temperature is within normal limits, dress him in a vest, babygro and nappy. If the baby is low birthweight, he should have a hat as well. When the baby is in his cot, make sure he is lying on his back with his feet at the foot of the cot. Place any blankets over him loosely so they do not constrict his movement.

The nappy area should be well cleaned at every nappy change and inspected regularly to prevent breakdown of the skin. Baby girls should always be cleaned from front to back to prevent urinary tract infections. Baby wipes should be avoided in the early days as they contain chemicals which might be abrasive on the newborn's skin.

Creams can be used to act as a barrier or to treat damaged skin, but only use these sparingly – applied too thick, they can cause more problems by preventing the skin from breathing.

Thermoregulation

Because the neonate has a relatively large surface-to-weight ratio, reduced metabolism per unit area and small amounts of insulating fat, he's susceptible to hypothermia. Babies keep warm by metabolising brown fat, which has a greater concentration of energy-producing mitochondria in its cells, enhancing its capacity for heat production. This kind of fat is unique to babies. Brown fat metabolism is effective, but only within a very narrow temperature range.

Without careful external thermoregulation, babies may become chilled, which can result in:

- hypoxia
- acidosis
- hypoglycaemia
- pulmonary vasoconstriction
- reduced surfactant production
- poor weight gain
- death.

Keep it neutral

The object of thermoregulation is to provide a neutral thermal environment that helps the neonate maintain a normal core temperature with minimal oxygen consumption and caloric expenditure. The core temperature varies with the neonate but is about 36.6°C. Cold stress and its complications can be prevented with proper interventions. (See *Understanding thermoregulators*, page 459.)

To maintain thermoregulation, you may need:

- radiant warmer or incubator (if necessary)
- blankets
- skin probe
- thermometer

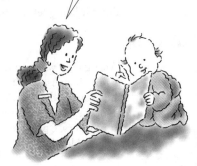

See? It says right there: Core temperature for neonates is about 36.6°C

Understanding thermoregulators

Thermoregulators preserve neonatal body warmth in various ways. A radiant warmer maintains the baby's temperature by radiation. An incubator maintains the baby's temperature by conduction and convection.

Temperature settings

Radiant warmers and incubators have two operating modes: nonservo and servo. The midwife manually sets temperature on nonservo equipment; a probe on the baby's skin controls temperature settings on servo models.

Other features

Most thermoregulators come with alarms. Incubators have the added advantage of providing a stable, enclosed environment, which protects the baby from evaporative heat loss.

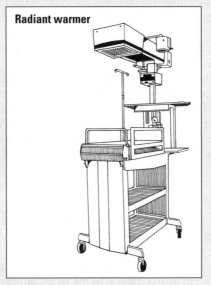
Radiant warmer

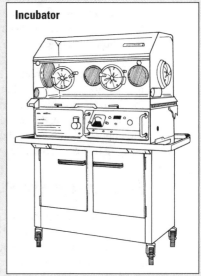
Incubator

- clothing, including a cap
- heated mattress
- STS availability.

While you wait

While preparing for the infant's birth, turn on the radiant warmer in the delivery room and set it to the desired temperature. Warm the blankets or towels under a heat source.

After the arrival

In the birthing room:
- If the baby is well – dry him, then place him STS with his mother for as long as possible – cover them both with a blanket to keep them warm; this is also called 'Kangaroo care'.
- If his temperature is low, place him under the radiant warmer, wrap him in warm towels, then cover his head with a cap to prevent heat loss.
- Perform required procedures quickly and wrap him in the warmed blankets. If his condition permits, give him to his parents to promote bonding and initiate breastfeeding if possible.

If the baby is warm, keep him with his mother (STS) and transport both to the postnatal ward onto the mother's bed.

If the baby's temperature is unstable – particularly if he is low birthweight – he may have to be placed in an incubator.

In the postnatal ward:
• Continue to nurse the baby in his cot, beside his mother. Avoid nursing interventions which mean exposing the baby or allowing him to cool.
• Some maternity units check the newborn baby's temperature for 8–12 hours after delivery to make sure the baby is maintaining his core temperature.
• If the baby is premature, or is unable to maintain a normal temperature, he may need to be nursed in an open cot with a heated mattress or an incubator beside his mother. He will need his temperature monitored closely. Use an adhesive pad to attach the temperature control probe to his skin in the upper-right abdominal quadrant. Don't cover the device with anything because this could interfere with the servo-control.

Servo-control

This mode of temperature control means that after applying the skin probe, you select the skin temperature and the probe reflects what the actual skin temperature of the baby is. If the baby's temperature falls below the set temperature, the incubator generates and circulates more heat – this continues until the baby's temperature comes up to the temperature you have preset.
• Check the baby's temperature on admission and record. If the baby is low birthweight, premature or SGA, check axillary temperatures on a regular basis until the temperature stabilises, then every 4–8 hours to ensure stability. (See *Preventing heat loss*, page 461.) Sometimes taking a temperature too often actually defeats the object as it means disturbing and exposing the baby for short periods. If a baby has an unstable temperature or a persistently high or low temperature – check for signs of infection, which can cause hyperthermia or hypothermia.

Incubator involvement

Apply a skin probe to a baby in an incubator as you would for a baby in a radiant warmer. Move the incubator away from cold walls or objects. Perform all required procedures quickly and do not have the portholes open longer than you need to.

When moving the baby from an incubator to an open cot, the baby must be weaned from the incubator by slowly reducing the temperature to that of the nursery. Check periodically for hypothermia. When the baby's temperature stabilises, dress him, put him in a cot and cover him with a blanket. Also, be sure to instruct the parents on the importance of maintaining body temperature (see *Maintaining the neonate's body temperature*, page 461) and keeping their nursery at home within the normal temperature range.

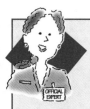

Advice from the experts

Preventing heat loss

Follow these steps to prevent heat loss in the newborn infant.

Conduction

- Preheat the radiant warmer bed and linen.
- Warm hands, stethoscopes and other instruments before use.
- Before weighing the baby, pad the scale with a paper towel or a preweighed, warmed sheet.

Convection

- Place the baby's cot out of a direct line with an open window, fan or air-conditioning vent.

Evaporation

- Dry the baby immediately after delivery.
- When bathing the baby, expose only one body part at a time, wash each part thoroughly and then dry him immediately.

Radiation

- Keep the baby and examination tables away from outside windows and air conditioners.

Education edge

Maintaining the neonate's body temperature

To help parents understand the importance of maintaining the neonate's temperature, instruct them to:

- keep the baby wrapped in a blanket and out of drafts when he isn't in the cot
- avoid placing the cot next to a window, a fan, an air conditioner or an air-conditioning vent

- keep the stockinette cap/hat on his head because a baby loses considerable heat through his head – do not keep the hat during STS care
- remove any wet linens from on or around the baby as soon as possible
- avoid placing the baby on a cold surface such as a change mat without placing a towel or blanket down first.

Noteworthy items

In your baby's notes, be sure to document:
- the name and temperature of the heat source used
- the baby's temperature and the method used to record the temperature
- complications resulting from use of thermoregulatory equipment.

Eye care

Babies' eyes are checked daily to look for early signs of infection. Often babies can have sticky eyes which will clear up when cleaned with cool, boiled water. If the discharge is persistent or purulent, a swab should be taken, cleaning should continue and antibiotic cream or drops should be applied if prescribed. All babies have their Red Reflex checked prior to leaving hospital but the midwife still needs to look for any unusual features in the baby's eyes – particularly their colour – jaundice can be very evident by looking at the sclera.

The babies should have their eyes cleaned daily with cotton wool and clean water. The mother should be taught to wipe from the inside of the eye to the outside so as to avoid sweeping dirt into the tear duct. It is vital that the mother is taught the importance of washing her hands well before touching the baby's eyes.

Cord care

The baby's cord is inspected daily and the findings recorded in the baby's notes. The cord should not be handled if possible – usually the baby will have a bath which is sufficient for cleaning. The cord is inspected for:

- signs of separation (when there is still an umbilical stump)
- any bleeding
- discharge
- odour
- redness where the cord joins the skin.

If the skin around the cord looks red or there is cellulitis, the cord should be swabbed and the baby started on antibiotics right away – a cord infection can lead to septicaemia in a short space of time.

The umbilical cord may have a clamp on it – some midwives remove this on Day 3 – some will leave it to fall off with the cord stump. Community midwives usually continue to visit the baby until the cord is separated and looks clean and healed.

Protecting the newborn from infection

The newborn has a very immature immune system and so needs to be protected till such times as his body affords him some immunity. The midwife should check the baby daily for at least 10 days, and record her findings in the baby's hospital and community notes.

Daily examination of the following should be conducted:
- skin – for spots, rashes, abrasions or dry area which could crack and become infected
- skin folds – red areas, abrasions
- eyes – for discharge
- fingers and toes – ragnails or nailbed infections (paronychia)
- cord – for bleeding, discharge, odour or redness of adjoining skin
- breasts – for engorgement or inflammation (hormonal effects)
- nappy area – for redness or breaking of skin.

Catch it early!

Daily examination will hopefully alert the midwife to early signs of infection; the appropriate investigations should therefore be carried out and treatment commenced. But prevention is better than cure and all babies should be nursed in an environment that is clean and safe. To prevent infection in the neonates, the precautions that need to be taken are:

- place each baby in his individual cot
- do not place the baby on his mother's bed
- sterilise all feeding utensils
- use clean sheets and clothing
- do not share equipment between babies
- strict handwash before handling the baby
- discourage the practice of visitors lifting the baby.

Monitoring feeding

The baby's feeding method, amount taken and tolerance of feeds should all be recorded on the feeding chart so that both the mother and the midwife can review the previous 24 hours fluid intake. If a baby is breastfeeding, the frequency of feeds, the duration and tolerance should all be recorded. If the baby is being fed artificially, the amount should be calculated, intake and tolerance recorded. Any vomiting or possetting should be marked clearly on the chart so the midwife can ascertain how well the baby is coping with the fluid given and investigate possible reflux problems if the baby is vomiting large amounts back – this presents a danger of aspiration of the feed into the lungs.

As well as recording the fluid intake, the midwife needs to assess how well the baby actually feeds. Is the suck reflex present? Does he have a strong suck or does he tire easily without finishing his feed? Is his suck/swallow coordination present or does he choke on any regurgitated milk?

Look at the big picture!

When checking the feeding chart, the midwife should not take each feed as a separate entity but look at the 24 hour picture. The baby may take a few of his feeds quite close together but then have a long period when he doesn't feed at all. It can be difficult to ascertain whether the breastfed baby has had his quota of milk for the 24 hours and so the midwife must use other factors to reassure the mother that her baby is getting enough – these factors will apply to the bottle-fed baby as well:

- does the baby suck well during the feed?
- does he settle for at least 2 hours after his feed?
- does he wake for feeds or does he need to be awakened?
- when he is awake – is he alert?
- are his lips and tongue moist?
- is there turgor of his skin – sign of dehydration?
- is his anterior fontanelle sunken/depressed – sign of dehydration?
- is he having wet and dirty nappies? Urine dilute?

Hazards of oxygen therapy

No matter which system delivers the oxygen, oxygen therapy is potentially hazardous to a baby. The gas must be warmed and humidified to prevent hypothermia and dehydration. Given in high concentrations over prolonged periods, oxygen can cause retinopathy of prematurity, leading to blindness. With low oxygen concentration, hypoxia and central nervous system damage may occur. Also, depending on how it's delivered, oxygen can contribute to bronchopulmonary dysplasia.

Other worries

Here are some other possible complications of oxygen therapy in neonates:

- Infection or 'drowning' can result from overhumidification. Overhumidification, in turn, allows water to collect in tubing, providing a growth medium for bacteria or suffocating the baby.
- Hypothermia can increase oxygen consumption and can result from administering cool oxygen.
- Metabolic and respiratory acidosis may follow inadequate ventilation.
- Pressure ulcers may develop on the neonate's head, face and around the nose during prolonged oxygen therapy.
- A pulmonary air leak (pneumothorax, pneumomediastinum, pneumopericardium, interstitial emphysema) may arise spontaneously with respiratory distress or result from forced ventilation.
- Decreased cardiac output may result from excessive continuous positive airway pressure.

Monitoring output

Usually on the baby's feeding chart, the midwife will teach the mother to record the contents of her baby's nappy – the urine and stools. Initially, the first stools are recorded – known as meconium. Over the next few days the stools will change colour and consistency, turning to a yellowish/brown colour and becoming more formed. Breastfed babies may have softer stools that resemble mustard grains.

The baby's urinary output should also be monitored – particularly the first sample – just to make sure he has actually passed urine! His urine should be dilute – pale in colour and odour free. Assessing output can be difficult as the gel contained in disposable nappies, absorb the urine making it 'disappear'. Nappies may have to be weighed in an effort to estimate the urine content.

If babies vomit – all vomitus should be recorded so that if it becomes problematic, the midwife can estimate how much fluid the baby is losing at each feed.

Monitoring blood glucose levels

The midwife must monitor closely the baby's ability to take milk and metabolise it in order to maintain his normal BG levels. She must bear in mind that some babies are more at risk of developing hypoglycaemia than others – premature and SGA babies, babies of diabetic mothers, babies who cannot regulate their body temperature and babies with metabolic disorders.

Diagnosing hypoglycaemia by BG levels is controversial – many neonatologists debate what the normal range of BG levels should be.

Definitive values range from <1 to <4 mmol/L.

Currently, data would show that BG level less than 2.4 mmol/L should be avoided (especially for at-risk infants). When BG levels fall to low-enough levels to produce symptoms, it indicates true cellular glucose deficiency.

Hypoglycaemia

Clinical features of hypoglycaemia are the following:
- Onset is usually in the first 6 hours of life.
- Many neonates can be asymptomatic – especially preterm babies.
- Pallor.
- Lethargy – apathy – refusal to feed.
- Abnormal, high-pitched cry.
- Apnoeas, irregular respirations.
- Hypotonia.
- Tremors, jitteriness.
- Eye rolling; seizures.

Testing for hypoglycaemia

It is normally done by a midwife using a 'glucometer'. A capillary sample is taken usually from the heel and the result is instantaneous – this should always be recorded.

The limitations of this technique are that when whole blood is used, glucose levels in red blood cell is 10–15% lower than in plasma so it is better to take a venous sample rather than a capillary sample.

The actual procedure of taking and measuring the sample may vary so the best method is sending a sample of blood to lab for analysis of plasma glucose levels. If the midwife is concerned about the baby's condition or the BG result, she should notify the neonatologist at once as well as keep the mother informed of the results.

Prevention is better than cure!

- Early identification prevents major problems.
- Feeding should be commenced early.
- Frequent feeds should be given.
- Neutral thermal environment should be maintained at all times.
- Bolus of IV Dextrose 10% (3–5 ml/kg) should be given slowly if BG is low.
- BG should be checked in 15 minutes and followed up with IV infusion if normal levels are not sustained.

Monitoring weight gain

The baby should be weighed on admission to the postnatal ward and again on the third postnatal day – depending on what unit policy is. The mother will need reassurance about weight loss as most babies will lose about a tenth of their birthweight in the first few days and will take up to 10–14 days to return to their birthweight before they start to gain. Some midwives believe it is better not to weigh the baby till later on in the week – particularly if the mother is breastfeeding and is anxious. This is a clinical judgement the midwife makes when she knows the mother and the baby.

Midwifery examination of the newborn (prior to discharge)

All babies have a final examination carried out to ensure that he/she is in good health and ready for home. However, even after being examined by a midwife, doctor or advanced neonatal nurse practitioner, problems can develop after discharge from hospital. It is vital that the parents understand that while the practitioner has not detected any major defects, the baby's overall condition has the potential to alter dramatically – particularly in relation to his heart. In some instances, the baby's PDA can close later than normal, highlighting a more serious cardiac disorder like coarctation, and the baby's condition may deteriorate. This could occur anytime from 5 days to 3 months of age.

Newborn screening involves a detailed head-to-toe examination, neurological assessment, eye examination, hip screening, hearing test and cardiovascular assessment. The head-to-toe examination has already been described so let's look at the other aspects:

Neurological assessment

The baby's colour, muscle tone and behaviour are assessed – much of this can be done as you are undressing the baby or handling him. The baby undergoes a range of exercises which assess his reflexes – in other words – how his neurological system reacts to various stimuli. These reflexes have already been described, but it is important to understand the relevance of these to the overall examination of the baby. If he doesn't respond to the stimuli in the normal way, it could mean that he has either a neurological problem or perhaps a muscular one. Some forms of paralysis or reduced movement are as a result of musculoskeletal problems such as myotonia dystrophia, birth traumas like fractured clavicle or abnormal muscular development.

When the reflexes and neurological testing has been done, the methods and tests used should all be recorded in the notes and the responses elicited.

Eye examination

The eye examination is also a part of the neurological tests. The baby's eyes should be checked for:

- any obvious defects in size, shape or position
- trauma, swelling, subconjunctival haemorrhages
- colour of the sclera – yellow can mean jaundice, blue could be indicative of osteogenesis imperfecta
- the canthus (inner fold of skin where the tear duct is) – if it slants downwards and the outside canthus slants upwards, this could mean the baby has Down syndrome. Be sure to consider the baby's ethnic origin before making assumptions!

Eye-to-eye

The baby's eyes should be examined using an ophthalmoscope in a darkened room. Never force the eyes open – changing the baby's position can help – or get mum to hold the baby over her shoulder and look into his eyes. Hold the ophthalmoscope about 10–15 cm away from his eyes and adjust it so you're getting a round-shaped light shining onto your hand.

'PEARL'

Check for pupillary reflex – do the pupils constrict when you shine the light into the eye and dilate when you move it away? Are they both equal and reactive to light? (PEARL)

Next, you check for the Red Reflex. As you shine the light into the baby's eye, you should see a reddish disc image reflecting back (a bit like the photos you see of people with 'red-eye' present).

In some babies, this may look slightly paler, for example, Black babies or Asian babies. You should always check that the optic disc looks complete and round. Any deviation from normal should be reported to a paediatrician and the eyes should be checked again.

Eye problems such as retinoblastoma and cataracts (white discolouration of the eye) can be detected by carrying out this eye examination.

Hip screening

Developmental dysplasia of the hips is a term used to explain hip instability in an infant. The femur (long bone of the thigh) and acetabulum (part of the hip where the femur attaches) can become unstable, leading to long-term problems of the hip.

Is that a 'clunk'?

At first, the symptom is only an abnormal 'clunk' sound heard during a manoeuvre the midwife performs at a newborn examination. Within a few weeks, symptoms can include different leg lengths, inability to fully move the hip and asymmetrical skin folds of the thighs. Multiple factors include breech delivery, abnormal position in the uterus and response to hormonal factors influencing the laxity of the ligaments surrounding the hips.

The diagnosis is made by performing a physical examination followed by an x-ray or ultrasound of the hips in suspicious cases. The midwife checks for developmental dysplasia of the hip by carrying out two manoeuvres, Barlow's and Ortolani's manoeuvres; looking for discrepancies in leg length; checking for limited motion of the hip joint and observing for asymmetrical skin folds in the thighs.

- Barlow manoeuvre checks to see if the hip can be dislocated.
- Ortolani manoeuvre checks to see if a dislocated hip can be relocated.

A 'clunk' sound during either of these manoeuvres is suspicious and an x-ray or ultrasound of the hip should be carried out to confirm the diagnosis. Ultrasound is becoming more popular and is now the study of choice.

Cardiovascular assessment

The baby's colour is checked for cyanosis – if he goes blue when he feeds or cries, then it can be a warning sign of cardiac problems. Assessment is carried out by:

- Observing the precordium for any signs of palpitations or visible pulses.
- Localising the heart sounds – are they where they should be? What is the heart rate? (110–160 beats/minute is normal).
- Focusing on one element at a time: first heart sound, second heart sound, systolic interval and diastolic intervals.
- Listening for murmurs – these can sound like extra heart sounds. The commonest cause of a murmur in a term baby is a PDA which hasn't closed yet.
- Checking the pulses – you can check both brachial and femoral – the femoral are the most important. If a baby has reduced or absent femoral pulses this could mean he has a cardiac anomaly such as coarctation of the aorta; bounding femoral pulses could indicate PDA.
- Checking the baby's oxygen saturation levels and blood pressure – in some maternity units, these are checked before discharge.

Hearing test

All newborn babies have their hearing checked before leaving the hospittal – if it is not normal, they come back within a week to have it rechecked; any problems are referred to an audiology clinic.

Testes

Early diagnosis and management of the undescended testicle are needed to preserve fertility and improve early detection of testicular malignancy. Physical examination of the testicles can be difficult; if one or both testicles are undescended the baby should be rechecked within 1 month. Observation is not recommended beyond 1 year of age because it delays treatment, lowers the rate of surgical success and probably impairs spermatogenesis. Therapy for an undescended testicle should begin between 6 months and 2 years of age and may consist of hormone or surgical treatment.

Newborn screening

In the UK, midwives, doctors and advanced neonatal nurse practitioners carry out newborn examinations routinely. Regular updates and continued education is needed to enable them to maintain their knowledge and skills. The *Newborn and 6–8 week Infant Physical Examination Digital Toolbox* has been prepared for the UK National Screening Committee by the Cambridgeshire-based partnership of HSHS (formerly known as Homerton School of Health Studies) and Jill Rogers Associates (JRA). The toolbox contains listings of journal articles, books and reports, CD-ROMS/videos, websites and simulators relevant to the physical examination of the newborn and 6–8 week infant. The website address is http://www.nipetoolbox.screening.nhs.uk/toolbox/

Metabolic screening

Bloodspot screening delivers screening to newborn babies, enabling the prevention of severe disability associated with phenylketonuria (PKU), homocystinuria and congenital hypothyroidism (CHT). The programme has been expanded to screen for additional conditions including sickle cell disorders (SCD) and cystic fibrosis (CF) and national programmes are currently being introduced led by the UK Newborn Screening Programme Centre. In February 2007, the NSC also recommended that all newborn babies in England should be offered screening for medium chain acyl CoA dehydrogenase deficiency (MCADD) by March 2009. For more information on bloodspot screening, access the website at http://www.screening.nhs.uk/bloodspot/index.htm

Immunisation

Most immunisations (also known as vaccinations) are given during childhood and are usually given by injection. The immunisation programme for children mainly takes place over the course of 5 years; the first injection is given at 2 months of age. Immunisations are used to protect children from diseases such as tetanus, polio, pneumococcal infections, diphtheria, meningitis C, measles, mumps and rubella (MMR) – they are often given more than once to make sure the protection continues. The general practitioner usually carries out the injections and these are always recorded in the baby's PCHR book.

Quick quiz

1. Which factor doesn't stimulate the onset of breathing?
  A. Decreased CO_2 levels
  B. Increased CO_2 levels
  C. Decreased blood pH
  D. Decreased blood oxygen levels

Answer: A. Decreased CO_2 levels don't stimulate breathing.

2. Which option correctly describes the normal anatomy of the umbilical cord?
  A. One artery and one vein
  B. One artery and one ligament
  C. Two arteries and one vein
  D. One artery and two veins

Answer: C. The umbilical cord should consist of two arteries and one vein.

3. Apgar scoring evaluates:
  A. heart rate, respiratory rate, colour, blood pressure and temperature.
  B. heart rate, respiratory effort, muscle tone, reflex irritability and colour.
  C. respiratory rate, blood pressure, reflex irritability, muscle tone and temperature.
  D. temperature, heart rate, colour, muscle tone and blood pressure.

Answer: B. Apgar scoring involves evaluating the baby's heart rate, respiratory effort, muscle tone, reflex irritability and colour.

4. A sign of respiratory distress in a neonate is:
  A. acrocyanosis.
  B. nasal flaring.
  C. abdominal movements.
  D. short periods of apnoea (less than 15 seconds).

Answer: B. Nasal flaring is a sign of respiratory distress in the neonate. Acrocyanosis, abdominal movements and short periods of apnoea are all normal findings.

5. Which finding is normal for a neonate's fontanelles?
  A. They're soft to touch.
  B. They're depressed.
  C. They're bulging.
  D. They're closed.

Answer: A. The fontanelles should feel soft to the touch.

6. During which sleep–wake cycle does the neonate experience REM?
   A. Deep sleep
   B. Light sleep
   C. Drowsy
   D. Crying

Answer: B. During light sleep the eyes are closed and the neonate experiences REM, random movements and startles, irregular breathing and sucking movements.

7. Poor thermoregulation can result in:
   A. hypoxia.
   B. acidosis.
   C. hyperglycaemia.
   D. increased surfactant production.

Answer: A and B. Babies consume more oxygen when cold and this can result in hypoxia, leading to acidosis.

8. Which screening tests are done for babies in the UK?
   A. Congenital hypothyroidism
   B. Phenylketonuria
   C. Rubella antibody
   D. Cystic fibrosis
   E. Sickle cell disorders

Answer: A, B, D and E. All are carried out in the UK.

Scoring

☆☆☆ If you answered all eight questions correctly, give yourself a high five! Then toddle on over to the next chapter!

☆☆ If you answered six or seven questions correctly, stand tall! There's no holding you back!

☆ If you answered fewer than five questions correctly, roll with the punches! Get a leg up by revisiting this chapter!

12 High-risk neonatal conditions

Just the facts

In this chapter, you'll learn:

♦ characteristics of selected neonatal disorders

♦ tests used to diagnose certain high-risk neonatal conditions

♦ medical treatments and therapies for high-risk neonatal conditions

♦ nursing interventions for high-risk neonatal conditions.

A look at the high-risk neonate

A neonate is considered to be high risk if he has an increased chance of dying during or shortly after birth or has a congenital or perinatal problem that requires prompt intervention. As medicine continues to develop more treatments for perinatal problems, high-risk neonates are more likely to survive. Many of these babies have few or no residual effects from the crisis that marked their first hours after birth.

High-risk neonates may be nursed in various settings:
- Neonatal Intensive care units
- Special care baby units
- Transitional care units within the maternity unit
- Paediatric intensive care units
- Infant surgical units
- Palliative care units

The staffs who care for babies in these units are often made up from a variation of skilled professionals such as midwives, nurses, sick children's nurses, nursery nurses and auxiliary nurses. Doctors, radiographers, physiotherapists and clinical pharmacologists are also involved in the day-to-day management of many conditions.

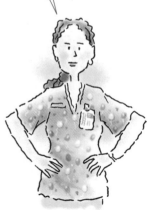

Because they feel a sense of loss, parents may have difficulty bonding with a high-risk neonate.

Of all these people, the most important are the parents – they may feel their role is a small one, but it is they who will form a lasting attachment to their infant and will be encouraged to provide love, support, stimulation and of course mum can provide breast milk!

A shaky start

Parents of high-risk neonates may experience grief and difficulty coping as they adjust to their baby's condition. They may also feel a sense of loss and have difficulty bonding because their baby isn't the perfect, healthy baby they anticipated. The family of a baby with a chronic illness or congenital anomaly must find ways to cope with long-term grief and develop strategies to provide the special care the condition will require (and perhaps to balance these care needs with those of other children). If the infant is stillborn or dies within a few hours or days after birth, family members must complete their bonding with the infant, then detach themselves gradually so they can focus again on the family's life and needs.

A big part of the midwife/nurse's role in the neonatal unit is supporting the parents and the family in what is very difficult time. Some units will have a designated professional to counsel and advise the parents, some may require psychological counselling to assist them through the initial grieving period and then the readjustment and acceptance of their baby's ongoing condition. It is helpful if one or two staff are the main carers so that parents have the opportunity to build relationships and trust in those midwives/nurses.

Some parent support groups are excellent at providing information and support to parents of sick or premature babies, such as:
- BLISS – http://www.bliss.org.uk/
- Tinylife – http://www.tinylife.org.uk/help.html
- Born Too Soon – http://www.borntoosoon.org.uk/
- For parents by parents – http://www.forparentsbyparents.com/

Many organisations are formed locally to give assistance to parents in their own area but some are national, such as BLISS. They are particularly helpful in assisting parents in practical ways, such as financial help with travelling expenses, accommodation, loaning out breast pumps and just forming friendships with other parents.

Nursing goals

Although the baby's condition dictates the specifics of nursing care, the main nursing goals for all high-risk neonates are to:
- ensure oxygenation, ventilation, thermoregulation, nutrition and fluid and electrolyte balance
- prevent and control infection
- encourage parent–infant bonding
- provide developmental care.

Drug addiction

Neonatal drug addiction and its associated signs and symptoms of withdrawal result from addictive drug use by the infant's mother during pregnancy. As in all aspects of health care, care for the drug-addicted infant should be provided in a nonjudgmental manner, especially because the neonate is an innocent victim of substance abuse by another person.

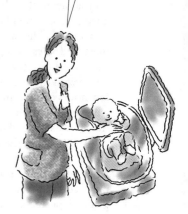

Low birthweight and respiratory problems are some of the complications seen in drug-addicted babies.

Low-down on drug effects

Pregnant women who use addictive drugs are at higher risk for:
- placental abruption
- spontaneous abortion
- preterm labour
- precipitous labour
- psychotic responses.
  Complications seen in the neonate may include:
- urogenital malformations
- cerebrovascular complications
- low birthweight
- decreased head circumference
- respiratory problems
- death.

What causes it

Neonatal drug addiction can occur if the mother uses addictive drugs while pregnant. These drugs have teratogenic effects, causing abnormalities in embryonic or fetal development.

What to look for

Intrauterine drug exposure may cause obvious physical anomalies, neurobehavioural changes or withdrawal. Signs and symptoms of a baby's drug dependence vary and may include physical and behavioural changes. These changes depend on:
- specific drug or combination of drugs used
- dosage
- route of administration
- metabolism and excretion by the mother and fetus
- timing of drug exposure
- length of drug exposure.

Benzodiazepines

Diazepam, a benzodiazepine, is one of the most commonly prescribed drugs in the world. It easily crosses the placental barrier to the fetus and is eliminated slowly by the fetus. Withdrawal signs and symptoms may appear hours to

Opiate withdrawal syndrome

Be alert for these signs and symptoms of opiate withdrawal in the neonate.

Central nervous system

- Seizures
- Tremors
- Irritability
- Increased wakefulness
- High-pitched cry
- Increased muscle tone
- Increased deep tendon reflexes
- Increased Moro reflex
- Increased yawning
- Increased sneezing
- Rapid changes in mood
- Hypersensitivity to noise and external stimuli
- Sleep disturbances
- Sweating

GI system

- Poor feeding
- Uncoordinated and constant sucking
- Vomiting
- Diarrhoea
- Dehydration
- Poor weight gain

Autonomic nervous system

- Increased sweating
- Nasal stuffiness
- Fever
- Mottling
- Temperature instability
- Increased respiratory rate
- Increased heart rate

weeks after birth and may persist for months. Common signs and symptoms of withdrawal include:
- hypothermia
- hyperbilirubinaemia
- central nervous system (CNS) depression.

Opiates

Clinical presentation of opiate withdrawal in the neonate can last 2–3 weeks. Withdrawal signs and symptoms generally include dysfunction of the CNS and GI system. (See *Opiate withdrawal syndrome*.)

Heroin

Neonates who have been exposed to heroin generally have low birthweights and are small for gestational age. They may also exhibit these signs and symptoms:
- jitters and hyperactivity
- shrill and persistent cry
- frequent yawning or sneezing
- increased deep tendon reflexes
- decreased Moro reflex
- poor feeding and sucking
- increased respiratory rate
- vomiting
- diarrhoea

- hypothermia or hyperthermia
- increased sweating
- abnormal sleep cycle.

Methadone

Withdrawal from methadone resembles that from heroin but tends to be more severe and prolonged. It includes:

- increased incidence of seizures
- disturbed sleep patterns
- higher birthweight in babies who are appropriate size for gestational age
- higher risk of sudden infant death syndrome.

Marijuana

Neonates born to mothers who used marijuana while pregnant tend to be born at earlier gestations. An increased incidence of precipitous labour and meconium staining also occurs in this population of neonates. These babies may exhibit tremors, jitteriness and impaired sleep. When the mother abuses marijuana and alcohol during pregnancy, there's a fivefold increase in the risk of fetal alcohol syndrome (FAS).

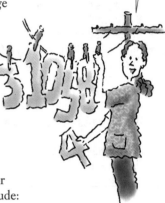

The risk of FAS increases fivefold if a mother abuses marijuana and alcohol during pregnancy.

Amphetamines

Women who use amphetamines while pregnant may have preterm babies or babies of low birthweight. Other characteristics these babies may have include:

- drowsiness
- jitters
- respiratory distress soon after birth
- frequent infections
- poor weight gain
- emotional disturbances
- delays in gross motor and fine motor development in early childhood
- heart murmurs
- transient bradycardia and tachycardia.

What tests tell you

The signs and symptoms of addiction and withdrawal may be mistaken for other common neonatal problems, especially if the mother's drug use is unknown. You'll need to differentiate between neonatal drug withdrawal and CNS irritability caused by infectious or metabolic disorders, such as hypoglycaemia, hypomagnesaemia or hypocalcaemia. You'll also need to rule out hyperthyroidism, CNS haemorrhage and anoxia.

Assessing the systems

The neonatal abstinence scoring system is a scoring tool that can be used for term babies. It assesses and scores areas of response in babies with CNS, metabolic, vasomotor, respiratory and GI disturbances. The higher the overall score, the more likely the need for medication administration for withdrawal. The test is repeated at specific intervals based on previous scores.

When it's withdrawal

If the clinical signs and symptoms are consistent with drug withdrawal, obtain specimens of urine and meconium for drug testing. Meconium testing can detect drug use over a 20-week period. Be aware that urine screening may have a high false-negative rate because only babies with recent exposure test positive. Also keep in mind that although meconium drug testing isn't conclusive if results are negative, this method is more reliable than urine testing.

How it's treated

Initial treatment of the baby who's experiencing withdrawal should be supportive. This includes:
* swaddling
* holding the baby
* pacifiers
* reducing environmental stimuli (lights, noise)
* frequent, small feedings of hypercaloric (24 calories/ounce) formula
* observing sleep habits
* observing for temperature instability, weight gain or loss or changes in clinical status that might suggest another disease process
* fluid and electrolyte replacement
* infection control
* respiratory care.

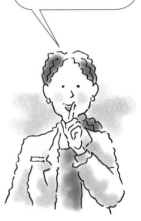

> Reducing environmental stimuli and swaddling are some of the initial treatments for supporting babies experiencing withdrawal.

Treating drugs with drugs

Indications for pharmacological therapy include:
* seizures
* poor feeding
* diarrhoea
* vomiting leading to weight loss and dehydration
* inability to sleep
* fever unrelated to infection.
    If pharmacological therapy is needed, specific therapy from the same drug class is preferred. (See *Drugs for withdrawal*; *Narcan and drug withdrawal*.)

Weighing the evidence

Narcan and drug withdrawal

Over the years, it has become common practice to administer naloxone (Narcan) in the birthing room to a baby who's exhibiting central nervous system depression and whose mother recently received an opioid.

Naloxone is contraindicated in a neonate whose mother is a known or suspected opioid abuser because of the potential for neonatal seizures, which can develop as a result of the abrupt withdrawal of the drug.

Drugs for withdrawal

Drugs used to treat withdrawal include:

* chlorpromazine
* clonidine
* diazepam
* methadone
* morphine
* paregoric
* phenobarbital
* tincture of opium.

What to do

Nursing interventions for neonatal drug addiction include:
- initiating preventive measures
- identifying babies at risk
- assessing the baby
- providing supportive care.

Stop addiction before it starts

Preventing maternal drug use is the ideal approach to eradicating the problem of neonatal drug addiction. Parental teaching and support are essential. To identify a mother and baby at risk for drug addiction:
- obtain a detailed maternal prescription and nonprescription drug history
- assess the social habits of the parents.

Screen those on the scene

To screen for drug exposure, perform maternal and infant assessments. Maternal findings that may indicate a need for neonatal drug testing include:
- lack of antenatal care
- previous unexplained fetal demise
- precipitous labour
- altered nutrition
- placental abruption
- hypertensive episodes
- severe mood swings
- stroke
- myocardial infarction (MI)
- recurrent spontaneous abortions.
  Neonatal characteristics that may be associated with maternal drug use include:
- preterm labour
- cardiac defects
- unexplained intrauterine growth retardation
- neurobehavioural abnormalities
- urogenital anomalies
- atypical vascular incidents (cerebral haemorrhage, myocardial infarction or necrotising enterocolitis in an otherwise healthy term neonate).
  Ongoing neonatal assessment should include monitoring for changes in:
- respiratory system
- reflexes (including suck, swallow and gag)
- CNS
- feeding and growth
- vital signs.

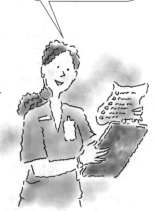

Obtaining a detailed drug history is the first step in identifying those at risk for drug addiction.

Aiding the addicted

Supportive care of the baby with a drug addiction includes:
- maintaining the baby's airway
- assessing breath sounds frequently

- supporting and monitoring ventilation
- providing supplemental oxygen
- managing mechanical ventilation
- making sure that resuscitative equipment is available
- monitoring pulse oximetry (and arterial blood gas [ABG] studies if pulse oximetry is abnormally low)
- decreasing CNS excitability by keeping the baby tightly wrapped (swaddling) – monitor temperature carefully!
- offering a pacifier for nonnutritive sucking
- using a vest/babygro with hand mittens to decrease facial scratching
- aspirating nasal mucus as needed
- organising care to decrease stress due to handling
- decreasing stimuli by reducing light in the room
- monitoring the baby with seizures
- preventing trauma
- administering medications as ordered and noting the responses
- promoting rest
- promoting nutritional intake
- feeding in small, frequent amounts with the head elevated and the nipple positioned correctly so that sucking is effective
- maintaining fluid and electrolyte balance
- monitoring intake and output
- giving supplemental fluids as ordered
- evaluating serum electrolytes as ordered
- maintaining skin integrity and providing skin care
- changing the baby's position
- reporting signs of distress.

Fetal alcohol syndrome

A cluster of birth defects that are caused by in utero exposure to alcohol is referred to as fetal alcohol syndrome. It can result in abnormalities in the CNS, growth retardation and facial malformations.

What causes it

FAS is caused by the exposure of a fetus to alcohol in utero. Although antenatal alcohol exposure doesn't always result in FAS, the safe level of alcohol consumption during pregnancy isn't known.

Midwives advise women not to drink any alcohol while pregnant. Based on the best evidence to date, the Royal College of Obstetricians and Gynaecologists recommends that the only way to be absolutely certain that the unborn baby is not harmed by alcohol is not to drink at all during pregnancy or while couples are trying for a baby. Further information on alcohol and pregnancy are available at http://www.rcog.org.uk/index.asp?PageID=1816

Alcohol crosses through the placenta and enters the fetal blood supply, and it can interfere with the healthy development of the fetus. In fact, birth defects associated with antenatal alcohol exposure can occur in the first 3–8 weeks of pregnancy, before a woman even knows she's pregnant. Variables that affect the extent of damage caused to the fetus by alcohol include the amount of alcohol consumed, the timing of consumption and the pattern of alcohol use.

What to look for

Affected neonates may display these signs within the first 24 hours of life:
- difficulty establishing respirations
- irritability
- lethargy
- seizure activity
- tremulousness
- opisthotonos
- poor sucking reflex
- abdominal distention.

Overalls

Overall signs of FAS include CNS dysfunction, abnormal development of the midline structures of the brain, growth deficiency and a characteristic set of minor facial abnormalities that tend to normalise as the child grows. (See *Common facial characteristics of FAS*.)

Common facial characteristics of FAS

This illustration shows the distinct craniofacial features associated with fetal alcohol syndrome (FAS).

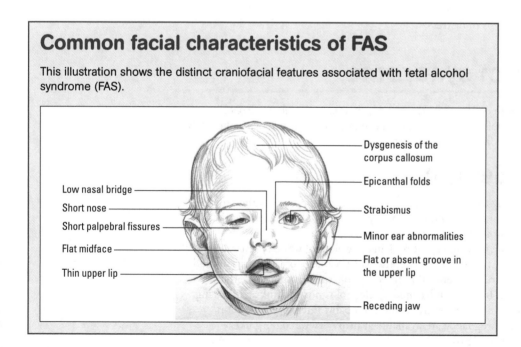

Low nasal bridge

Short nose

Short palpebral fissures

Flat midface

Thin upper lip

Dysgenesis of the corpus callosum

Epicanthal folds

Strabismus

Minor ear abnormalities

Flat or absent groove in the upper lip

Receding jaw

Typical CNS problems for neonates with FAS may include:

- mental retardation
- microcephaly
- poor coordination
- decreased muscle tone
- small brain
- behavioural abnormalities
- irritability
- tremors
- poor feeding.

Growth deficiencies may manifest in a failure to thrive or a disproportionate decrease in adipose tissue. Length and weight in babies with FAS typically measures 3% less than the average newborn baby.

Hits to the other systems

Abnormalities may also be seen in the cardiac system, skeletal system, urogenital system and skin. Potential complications include:

- cardiac murmurs
- limited joint movement
- finger and toe deformities
- aberrant palmar creases
- kidney defects
- labial hypoplasia
- haemangiomas.

As children and adults, individuals with FAS also commonly display:

- defects in intellectual functioning
- difficulties with memory, attention and problem solving
- learning disabilities
- problems with mental health
- difficulties with social interaction.

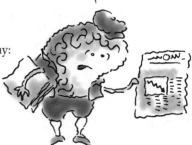

Not so great news. FAS can cause mental retardation and behavioural abnormalities.

What tests tell you

Identifying clinical problems and assessment findings characteristic of FAS leads to diagnosis. Respiratory distress and neurological dysfunction may be present. Feeding difficulties may also be noted. Radiographic studies may be used to reveal renal or cardiac defects.

How it's treated

Treatment of FAS is supportive and depends on the individual neonate. The initial difficulties may be managed by preventing stimulation that may precipitate seizures, administering sedative or anticonvulsant medications and providing supportive measures. Because the effects of alcohol in utero vary, care must be individualised to focus on the neonate's specific abnormalities and deficits.

What to do

A fundamental nursing intervention for FAS is helping to prevent it. This can be achieved by:
- increasing public awareness
- increasing women's access to preconceptual and antenatal care
- providing educational programmes
- screening women of reproductive age for alcohol problems
- using appropriate resources and strategies for decreasing alcohol use.

FASe out respiratory problems

Caring for neonates with FAS involves preventing or treating respiratory distress:
- Place the baby on a cardiac monitor and set the alarms.
- Assess breath sounds frequently and be alert for signs of distress.
- Suction as needed.
- Place the baby in a position in which he displays the least distress.

EmFASize nutrition

Special emphasis should be placed on following weight gain, assessing feeding behaviours and devising strategies to increase nutritional intake:
- Encourage feeding to promote bonding with the parents.
- Elevate the baby's head during and after feeding.
- Evaluate different teats to find one that makes feeding easy.
- Burp the baby well during and after feedings.
- Monitor the baby's weight.
- Measure intake and output.

FAScillitate bonding

To promote mother–infant attachment:
- encourage visits
- encourage physical contact
- educate parents about the infant's complications
- provide emotional support.

Gestational size variations

Whether they're preterm, term or postterm, babies are classified by weight in three ways:

Large for gestational age (LGA) babies are above the 90th percentile for weight.

Appropriate for gestational age (AGA) babies are between the 10th and 90th percentile for weight.

Small for gestational age (SGA) babies are below the 10th percentile for weight.

What causes it

Variations in gestational size are caused by different factors.

SGA babies

Factors that can contribute to a baby being SGA include:
- congenital malformations
- chromosomal anomalies
- maternal infections
- gestational hypertension
- advanced maternal diabetes due to decreased blood flow to the placenta
- intrauterine malnutrition due to poor placental function or maternal malnutrition
- maternal smoking
- maternal drug or alcohol use
- multiple gestation.

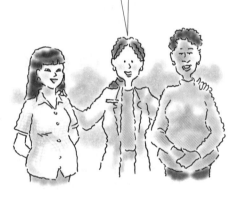

Congenital abnormalities or maternal infections can result in LGA babies.

LGA babies

Babies may become LGA because of genetic factors. For example, babies tend to be larger if they're male, if their parents are larger or if the mother is a multipara. Babies of mothers with diabetes also tend to be LGA because high maternal glucose levels stimulate continued insulin production by the fetus. This constant state of hyperglycaemia leads to excessive growth and fat deposition.

What to look for

Assessment findings depend on whether the baby is SGA or LGA.

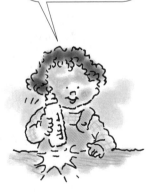

Time to eat yet? SGA babies have higher caloric needs and benefit from frequent feedings.

SGA babies

SGA babies are more likely to experience respiratory distress and hypoxia. They may also appear wide-eyed and alert at birth because of prolonged antenatal hypoxia. In addition, SGA babies are prone to meconium aspiration because fetal hypoxia allows meconium to pass through a relaxed anal sphincter, thus causing the fetus/baby to experience reflexive gasping. Hypoglycaemia can occur in SGA babies and can be noted from birth to day 4 of life. Decreased subcutaneous fat and a large ratio of body surface area to weight put the SGA baby at risk for problems with thermoregulation.

LGA babies

LGA babies generally weigh more than 4,000 g (8 lb, 13 oz) and appear plump and full faced. The LGA baby may experience hypoxia during labour and be exposed to excessive trauma, such as fractures and intracranial haemorrhage, during vaginal delivery. Hypoglycaemia may be noted at birth and during the transition period.

What tests tell you

Babies of mothers with diabetes should have laboratory work to determine their haematocrit and glucose, calcium and bilirubin levels. They should also be monitored for hypoglycaemia, hyperbilirubinaemia and respiratory distress syndrome (RDS).

How it's treated

Treatment of gestational age size abnormalities varies depending on whether the baby is SGA or LGA.

SGA babies

Treatment of the SGA baby should be supportive and individualised with nutrition being the primary focus. SGA babies have higher caloric needs and benefit from frequent feedings. Care of the SGA baby also includes glucose monitoring and careful respiratory assessments.

LGA babies

During delivery of an LGA baby, the mother may need additional help, such as an episiotomy, change in position or the use of forceps or a vacuum. After birth, glucose monitoring and evaluation of jaundice is essential in LGA babies. Any birth traumas also need to be managed.

What to do

Nursing interventions for SGA and LGA babies include:
- supporting respiratory efforts
- providing a neutral thermal environment
- protecting the baby from infection
- providing appropriate nutrition
- maintaining adequate hydration
- conserving the baby's energy
- assessing glucose levels
- preventing skin breakdown
- facilitating growth and development
- keeping parents informed
- providing support to the entire family.

Preterm neonates

A baby is considered preterm if he's born before 37 weeks' gestation. The preterm baby is at risk of complications because his organ systems are immature. The degree of complications depends on gestational age. The closer the baby is to 40 weeks' gestation, the easier will be the transition to extrauterine life.

What causes it

Some mothers go into labour early and the cause may never be discovered. It may be necessary to deliver a baby before term if evidence of a maternal complication exists. For example, pre-eclampsia is a condition that can develop in the second or third trimester of pregnancy. Signs of pre-eclampsia include elevated blood pressure, fluid retention and protein in the urine. The only treatment for pre-eclampsia is to deliver the baby to prevent life-threatening conditions for the mother. Kidney disease, heart disease, diabetes or infection in the mother may also require premature delivery of the baby.

Additional risk factors for a preterm baby include:
- multiple pregnancy
- adolescent pregnancy
- lack of antenatal care
- substance abuse
- smoking
- previous preterm delivery
- high, unexplained alpha-fetoprotein level in second trimester
- abnormalities of the uterus
- cervical incompetence
- premature rupture of membranes
- placenta praevia
- gestational hypertension.

What to look for

Preterm babies have characteristics that are distinctive at various stages of development. These characteristics can give clues to the baby's gestational age and physiological capabilities.

First findings

Initial assessment findings typical of preterm neonates include:
- low birthweight
- minimal subcutaneous fat deposits
- proportionally large head in relation to body
- prominent sucking pads in the cheeks
- wrinkled features
- thin, smooth, shiny skin that's almost translucent

- veins that are clearly visible under the thin, transparent epidermis
- lanugo (soft, downy hair) over the body
- sparse, fine, fuzzy hair on the head
- soft, pliable ear cartilage
- minimal creases in the soles and palms
- skull and rib bones that feel soft
- closed eyes
- few scrotal rugae (males)
- undescended testes (males)
- prominent labia and clitoris (females).

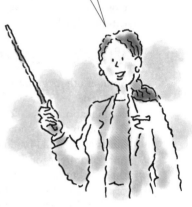

Low birthweight and wrinkled features are typical findings in a preterm baby.

Physical findings

Physical examination findings include:
- inability to maintain body temperature
- limited ability to excrete solutes in the urine
- increased susceptibility to infection
- periodic breathing, hypoventilation and periods of apnoea
- increased susceptibility to hyperbilirubinaemia
- increased susceptibility to hypoglycaemia
- ability to bring the baby's elbow across the chest when eliciting the scarf sign
- ability to easily bring the baby's heel to his ear.

System signs

The baby's neurological status is assessed by observing:
- active movements
- response to stimulation
- response to passive movements.
  CNS evaluation may reveal:
- inactivity (although he may be unusually active immediately after birth)
- extension of extremities
- absence of suck reflex
- weak swallow, gag and cough reflexes
- weak grasp reflex.

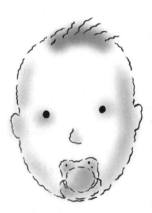

What tests tell you

These tests may indicate the extent of physiological maturity and may assist caregivers in the management of the premature baby:
- chest x-ray
- ABG analysis
- head ultrasounds (particularly the ventricles)
- echocardiography (looking for patent ductus arteriosus [PDA] and other problems)
- eye examination by a retinal specialist (oxygen can damage eyes)
- serum glucose

- serum calcium
- serum bilirubin
- full blood count – especially haemoglobin, haematocrit, platelets and white cell count (WCC).

How it's treated

Preterm babies are cared by a specially trained staff in the neonatal intensive care unit (NICU). The top priority in treating a preterm baby is supporting the cardiac and respiratory systems as needed. If he isn't breathing or respiratory efforts are poor, an endotracheal (ET) tube may be inserted and mechanical ventilation started. Supplemental oxygen may also be given. Medications to increase the heart rate or maintain blood pressure may be administered as part of the resuscitative effort. Other essential interventions include providing thermoregulation and starting I.V. or gavage nutrition.

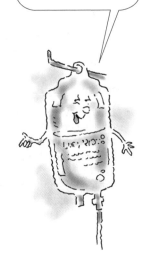

Help is on the way! I.V. nutrition is an essential intervention for preterm babies.

Three goals

Meticulous care and observation in the NICU is necessary until the baby:
- receives oral feedings
- maintains body temperature
- weighs about 2.26 kg (5 pounds).

Preemie problems

Certain complications may occur:
- *Respiratory distress syndrome* (RDS) is a leading cause of morbidity and mortality among preterm neonates. The lungs lack surfactant, which prevents alveolar collapse at the end of respiration. Treatment involves administration of surfactant, oxygen administration and mechanical ventilation.
- *Intraventricular haemorrhage* (IVH) is bleeding in or around the ventricles of the brain. It's most common in babies born before 32 weeks' gestation. Damage to brain function and long-term effects vary.
- *Retinopathy of prematurity* (ROP) is a disease caused by abnormal growth of retinal blood vessels. Prematurity may cause abnormal vessels to grow. Supplemental oxygen is also thought to contribute to this growth. ROP can cause mild-to-severe eye and vision problems. Treatment may involve laser surgery or cryotherapy.
- *Patent ductus arteriosus* (PDA) occurs when the ductus arteriosus reopens after birth due to lowered oxygen tension associated with respiratory impairment. Treatment involves fluid regulation, respiratory support, administration of indomethacin which is a drug that helps close a PDA in premature infants. It works by stimulating the PDA to constrict or tighten, closing the connection. Ibuprofen is a medicine in the same family as indomethacin. It is also used frequently to close a PDA in premature infants and has less side effects. Surgical ligation may be necessary if the baby doesn't respond to other therapies.

A close look at necrotising enterocolitis

Necrotising enterocolitis is an inflammatory disease of the GI mucosa. Here are its causes, pathophysiolgy and signs as well as tests used to diagnose it and ways in which it's treated.

Causes

- Uncertain, appears to occur in babies whose GI tract has suffered vascular compromise.

Pathophysiology

- Blood flow to gastric mucosa is decreased due to shunting of blood to vital organs.
- Mucosal cells lining the bowel wall die.
- Protective, lubricating mucus isn't secreted.
- Bowel wall is attacked by proteolytic enzymes.
- Bowel wall swells and breaks down.

Signs

- Distended abdomen
- Gastric retention
- Blood in stools or gastric contents
- Lethargy
- Poor feeding
- Hypotension
- Apnoea
- Vomiting

Diagnostic tests

- Radiographic studies show intestinal dilation and free air in the abdomen (indicating perforation).
- Laboratory studies show anaemia, leucopenia, leucocytosis and electrolyte imbalance.

Treatment

- Prevention
- Discontinuation of enteral feedings
- Nasogastric drainage
- Administration of I.V. antibiotics
- Administration of parenteral fluids total parenteral nutrition (TPN)
- Surgery

- *Necrotising enterocolitis* (NEC) is an inflammatory disease of the GI mucosa and is common in preterm babies who have an altered blood flow to their GI system, primarily due to other conditions such as RDS or hypoxia. (See *A close look at necrotising enterocolitis.*)
- *Bronchopulmonary dysplasia* (BPD) is also called chronic lung disease. The lungs may be less compliant because of the damage caused by being a preterm baby, due to low-grade infection in the lungs, mechanical ventilation or long-term oxygen therapy. Treatment involves supplying oxygen, maintaining good nutrition and preventing respiratory illness or infection.
- *Apnoea of prematurity* is a common phenomenon in the preterm infant. It occurs because neurological and chemical respiratory control mechanisms are immature in the brain. The number of apnoeic spells tends to increase the more premature the baby is. The condition can be treated with such medications as theophylline and caffeine.

    Additional complications that may occur include:
- infection
- jaundice
- anaemia
- hypoglycaemia
- delayed growth and development.

What to do

Nursing interventions for the preterm baby should focus on maintaining an environment that's similar to the intrauterine environment. Care should be based on knowledge of the preterm baby's physiological problems and the need to conserve energy for growth and repair.

Specific nursing responsibilities include:
- rapid initial evaluation
- resuscitative measures if needed
- thermoregulation
- administration of respiratory support measures
- electronic monitoring
- I.V. parenteral fluids as ordered
- medications as ordered
- blood sample analysis as ordered.

The right touch

Stimulation needs to be individualised to the development and tolerance of each infant. Touch should be smooth and sure. Stroking and rubbing are discouraged. Infant massage is not suitable for every baby in the NICU and parents need to be made aware of their baby's condition so that they watch for his cues and learn to recognise when he is not enjoying stimuli. The baby's head should be supported and the extremities held close to the body during position changes. This type of touch decreases motor disorganisation and stress.

Developmental care

It is vital that developmental care is provided so that the premature baby's brain and other systems are allowed to grow and develop normally with the minimum of stress. Positioning is important in providing comfort, encouraging sleep and reducing pain and stress – it is also vital in reducing developmental problems later on in life such as abnormal gait, walking problems and an inability to sit up, unaided. All premature babies should be positioned in a 'fetal' pose – with arms flexed and hands close to their face; their legs should be flexed and the hips should be abducted, raised and supported when lying prone. The nurse/midwife should provide 'boundaries' around the baby to give him something soft, but firm, to push against – like the uterine walls. Lights should be dimmed, noise kept to a minimum and handling only initiated when absolutely necessary.

Newborn Individualised Developmental Care and Assessment Program (NIDCAP) is used in some hospitals and encourages the use of NIDCAP internationally for supporting the growth and development of premature babies. More information is available from the NIDCAP website: http://www.nidcap.org/

Hard to swallow

Preterm babies born before 34 weeks' gestation aren't coordinated enough to maintain the suck, swallow and breathe regimen necessary for oral

Education edge

Teaching parents of preterm babies

To help the parents of a preterm baby cope with this difficult situation, follow these guidelines.

- Orient them to the neonatal intensive care unit environment and introduce them to all caregivers.
- Orient them to the machinery and monitors that may be attached to their baby. Reassure them that the staff is alert to alarms as well as the cues of their infant.

- Tell them what to expect.
- Teach them the characteristics of a preterm baby.
- Teach them how to handle their baby.
- Instruct them on feeding, whether it's through tube, breast or bottle.
- Inform them of potential complications.
- Offer discharge preparation.
- Make appropriate referrals.

feeding. These babies need to be fed I.V. or by gavage. Be alert for potential complications, such as NEC. Nonnutritive sucking, such as using a pacifier while being fed by tube, may help to ease the transition to oral feeding that occurs later. These babies should also be nursed on a slight tilt during and after a feed to reduce the risk of regurgitation and aspiration.

Keep up the communication

Nursing care also involves keeping the parents informed and educated about what's involved in the care of their preterm neonate. (See *Teaching parents of preterm babies*.)

BLISS is a special care baby charity, providing vital support and care to premature and sick babies across the UK. They also provide education for professionals in neonatal units and parents of premature babies. Their website address is http://www.bliss.org.uk/

Neonatal infection

Infection still remains as one of the main causes of death in the first month of life in premature or high-risk neonates. Term infants are quite susceptible to infection in the first few weeks of life, but the premature baby is even more at risk due to his immature immune system and his sluggish response to infection.

Transmission of bacterial organisms occurs in two ways.

Vertical:
- Ascending – SROM – Group B haemolytic streptococcus (maternal fever)
- Transplacental – TORCH viruses
- Intrapartum – during delivery – Group B streptococcus, herpes, chlamydia.

Horizontal:
- Within 3 days the baby is colonised with microorganisms, e.g. *Staphylococcus aureus*, *S. epidermis*, group A haemolytic streptococcus

- Within 1 week the gastrointestinal tract is colonised with *Escherichia coli*, e.g. artificial *E. coli* and *Lactobacillus bifidus* – B/F
- Infants in NICU are colonised with multiple drug-resistant gram-positive and gram-negative organisms, e.g. *S. epidermis*, *Pseudomonas*, *Klebsiella*, *E. coli*
- Babies in NICU are more at risk of infection due to the environment.

Are you immune?

Development of the immunological responses is initiated early in fetal life; however, many of these functions are inadequate during the neonatal period.

Fetal and neonatal defence systems are capable of an immune response, albeit slow and less effective than that of an older child.

An immune response requires recognition of a pathogen of foreign material and activation of a mechanism to react against it and eliminate it.

There are two types of immune response:

1. Specific (acquired)
   - Humoral immunity (B lymphocytes)
   - Cellular immunity (T lymphocytes)
2. Nonspecific (innate)
   - Skin
   - Mucous membranes
   - Chemical barriers – gastric acid and digestive enzymes
   - Mucus – protective barrier at microvillus surface
   - Resident nonpathogenic organisms
   - Peristalsis
   - Inflammatory response
   - Phagocytes, natural killer cells, interferon, etc.

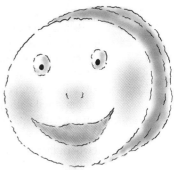

For an individual to become fully immunocompetent, both specific and nonspecific systems are required. The systems are correlated and interdependent.

Let's look at specific (acquired) immunity a little more!

Antigens are specific chemical compounds in each toxin and organism that act as markers on the cell surfaces. They allow identification by the immune system and initiation of specific antigenic immunity by the T and B cells.

Specific immunity can be divided into two groups:

1. Humoral immunity (B-cell immunity)
2. Cellular immunity (T-cell immunity)

Humoral/B-cell immunity

B-cell lymphocytes originate in the bone marrow and make up 5–15% of circulating lymphocytes. They are activated by the presence of antigens and interact with T cells and phagocytes and complement to produce mature plasma cells. B cells produce antibodies carried in the immunoglobulins and stimulate memory B cells; these recognise antigens on subsequent exposure and initiate and escalate the antibody response. B lymphocytes are stored in the bone marrow and lymph tissue.

Types of immunoglobulins:
- Immunoglobulin G (IgG) – These make up around 80% of immunoglobulins and are the only immunoglobulin which can cross the placenta. They provide immunity against bacterial and viral pathogens to which the mother has been exposed and also enhance phagocytosis.

Placental transfer takes place >12–20 weeks, but a majority of transfer takes place >32–34 weeks and increases gradually till term. After 3 months, the baby makes his own IgG, but adult levels are not reached until around the age of 5.
- Immunoglobulin M (IgM) – These are the immunoglobulins that are found in the baby's blood when he has been exposed to a pathogen or foreign matter. They do not cross the placenta but there are detectable levels after 30 weeks' gestation in fetal blood. If detected in cord blood or in high levels in the newborn infant, this indicates intrauterine infection. Levels are 10% of adult level at birth – reaches adult level by 1–2 years of age. They are responsible for protection against gram-negative organisms, e.g. *E. coli* – low levels result in *E. coli* infections in early childhood.

Babies born before 30 weeks' gestation are at increased risk of infection due to poor placental transfer of IgG or low levels of production of IgM.
- Immunoglobulin A (IgA) – The newborn baby does not produce his own IgA till about 4 weeks; therefore, he lacks this initial protection after birth. IgAs are present at the mucosal surfaces (saliva) and guards against respiratory and intestinal pathogens. It does not cross the placenta, but secretory IgA is produced in endocrine glands and secretions very soon after birth. IgAs are not found in tears till after 18–20 days of age and so this may make the newborn infant more liable to eye infections.

There are high levels found in colostrum!
- Immunoglobulin E (IgE) – These are produced in neonatal period. They are present in serum and some secretions and play a major role in allergic reactions by releasing histamines which induce an inflammatory response.

Cellular immunity (T lymphocytes)

T lymphocytes develop and mature in the thymus. Mature T cells leave the thymus and travel to the peripheral tissues and circulate through the lymphatics and vasculature.

T cells can live as long as 10 years and are effective from birth.

Specific cellular immunity is mediated by T lymphocytes which modify the behaviour of phagocytic cells and increase antimicrobial activity.

Types of T cells:
- Helper T cells – They encourage T- and B-cell response to antigens and activate macrophages by recognising antigens that are present on the surface of antigen-presenting cells.

They release lymphokines and cytocynes which stimulate the immune response by recruiting phagocytes, stimulating lymphocytes and macrophages into action. They inhibit viral replication.
- Memory T cells – They remain in the body as an early warning system to the same antigen avoiding any delay in the immune response.

- Suppressor T cells – They repress responses of specific T and B lymphocytes to antigens and 'puts the brakes on after the initial response'.
- Cytotoxic T cells – They kill foreign or virus-infected cells.
- Depressed T-cell function may occur as a result of neonatal viral infection, hyperbilirubinaemia, corticosteroid therapy and maternal medication.

Factors which predispose the neonate infection

Maternal factors
- socioeconomic background
- substance abuse
- maternal illness
- repeated genitourinary infections
- maternal bacteraemia
- maternal fever
- ascending infection (SROM) – group B streptococcus
- prolonged second stage of labour
- transplacental transmission
- poor placental function

Neonatal factors
- prematurity
- IUGR
- male gender
- poor skin integrity
- congenital abnormalities
- immaturity of the immune system
- invasive procedures
- side effects of drugs

Other factors
- environment
- geography
- socioeconomic status

All babies are vulnerable to infection. What starts as a localised infection can quickly spread to become a systemic infection (septicaemia). Sepsis is still one of the biggest killer of babies!

Septicaemia

Septicaemia is an infection of the blood by bacteria or viruses.

The signs may vary depending on whether the sepsis was acquired by vertical transmission (early), where there is usually a rapid onset, or colonisation (late) when there can be a more insidious onset of signs.

What to look for

General presentation:
- baby does not 'look well' or is not his usual self
- may look pale/mottled
- lethargy/hypotonia
- unwilling to feed – intolerance of feeds

Fever

Approximately 50% of babies with proven sepsis are pyrexic, 20% may have hypothermia or temperature instability and 30% may be normothermic. Failure to mount a febrile response may contribute to the poor outlook in neonatal infections. The temperature-regulating centre may be affected by sepsis in the newborn, particularly in the preterm baby.

Other signs

- Tachycardia – inflammatory response leading to vasodilation so blood pressure can fall.
- Respiratory distress – early onset may be identical to RDS.
- Apnoeas with associated bradycardias as condition worsens.
- O_2 saturations may fall – O_2 requirements increase as cardiac and respiratory function become laboured.
- Lethargy, irritability – CNS is affected and so seizures may occur in some cases.
- Vomiting/abdominal distension – decrease in blood pressure means that ischaemia may result making gut motility poor and also rendering the gut wall more susceptible to breakdown and necrosis, which can all predispose to NEC.
- Jaundice – in about 30% of cases, there is increased destruction of RBC leading to high levels of unconjugated bilirubin in the bloodstream.
- Haepatomegaly and splenomegaly due to the excessive breakdown of cells – platelets and RBC.
- Skin lesions – petechiae, raised papular rash, fine macular rash.
- Skin colour becomes progressively worse as condition deteriorates.
- Meningitis – CNS signs – bulging fontanelles, convulsions, irritability, high-pitched cry, cycling, back arching and possible seizures.
- Blood sugar levels may initially be low but as sepsis worsens, hypoglycaemia occurs due to corticosteroid secretion which is antagonistic to insulin, resulting in high blood sugar levels.

What tests will tell you

History and physical examination identifies the high-risk infant and informs you of changes in baby's clinical condition:
- Observations such as temperature, heart rate, respiratory rate, blood pressure, oxygen saturations, blood sugar levels, urinary output and urinalysis. Clinical observations will indicate if the sepsis is worsening or if the baby is responding to treatment.

- Gastric aspirate and swabs to detect the causative organism.
- Blood gases and complete blood count (CBC) (haemoglobin, Urea & Electrolytes [U&E], Serum Bilirubin [SBR]) to detect any other complications such as anaemia, low platelet count or jaundice. If the baby is being ventilated or requires oxygen, it is important to monitor how well he is coping and to find out if he requires greater ventilatory assistance.
- Blood cultures to detect the causative organism.
- White cell count – the total WCC lets us know if infection is present – it may be raised or lowered depending on the infection and how well the baby's immune system is responding. A differential WCC tells us which groups of white cells are raised and which are lowered (neutropenia is good indicator of sepsis), and this can give the doctors vital information in detecting an infection in a clinically unstable baby.
- Platelet count is more likely to be low in sepsis and so it is important to keep an eye on this – the baby could develop clotting disorders – some infected babies develop disseminated intravascular coagulopathy when the blood does not clot effectively, leading to a risk of death.
- C-reactive protein (CRP) is a protein produced by the liver and rises in infection.
- Cerebrospinal fluid (CSF). If a sample of CSF is taken by performing a lumbar puncture, the CSF should look clear. If it looks cloudy, this could be a sign of infection. Blood in the CSF might indicate a bleed within the brain or ventricles. When tested, if there is a raised protein level and a low sugar level, these are usually indicative of infection. The CSF should also render the causative organism.
- Urine can be tested in the neonatal unit for protein and white cells, but ideally it is best to send a sample to the laboratory for testing. Organisms may be found and the number will indicate whether treatment is necessary – also the sensitivities of that organism to various antibiotics. To get a sterile sample, it may be necessary to take a suprapubic sample using a syringe and needle.

Possible complications leading on from sepsis

Necrotising enterocolitis occurs when the gut wall breaks down and bacteria enter through the gut wall into the bloodstream and as the baby becomes more septic, he also suffers from shock due to the leakage of bowel fluid into the peritoneal cavity and his worsening septic state.

Septic shock occurs when the baby's whole system becomes so affected by this overwhelming infection that every cell in his body starts to behave abnormally. His peripheral perfusion worsens and he tries to compensate by pumping blood to his vital organs, but eventually that won't work either and every system begins to fail. As his blood pressure drops even further, he will eventually go into cardiac failure, despite attempts to raise his blood pressure.

Disseminated intravascular coagulation (DIC) disorder – as cell metabolism becomes abnormal, blood pressure falls and every organ begins to suffer, the liver produces less of the essential blood clotting agents. When the baby develops DIC, he does attempt to clot his blood, but the sepsis cause him to consume his clotting products quicker than he can produce them and so his blood does not clot effectively – instead, he produces 'microthrombi' which cannot block bleeding areas and he may eventually bleed from every orifice. The lungs and the brain are particularly susceptible to this disease process.

Death – the baby may never recover from 'overwhelming sepsis' – this is a state where the baby is so premature or sick that his body cannot recover, despite antibiotic therapy, and he succumbs to the infection.

How it's treated

Prevention is better than cure!!
* Try to identify high-risk mothers and screen antenatally for as much as possible, particularly in relation to sexually transmitted diseases, human immunodeficiency virus (HIV) and group B streptococcus.
* Try to treat as many infections antenatally where possible – some mothers may not realise they have had a spontaneous rupture of their membranes and could be infected with group B streptococcus. This can have devastating effects on the newborn infant.

Once the baby is here . . . . .
* Minimal handling – don't touch babies who are sick unless you absolutely have to – every hand carries potential bacterial infection. Parents need to be informed of the risks to their baby.
* Good hand washing – plenty of sinks, good technique, hand rubs for emergencies, education of all staff and visitors coming into the neonatal unit.
* Proper procedures – using approved procedures for carrying out all care, particularly invasive procedures such as passing oral tubes, venupuncture and I.V. cannulation.
* Reduced time in the neonatal unit if possible means the baby is at less risk of catching an infection. If the baby can possibly be nursed in a transitional care unit or a postnatal ward, that is preferable rather than separating mum and baby and nursing him in a more high-risk environment.
* Reduced use of antibiotics will be helpful for the baby in later life. If he is treated with multiple courses of antibiotics as a baby, not only do you kill off his natural 'friendly' bacteria, but you also make him more resistant to antibiotics in the future. The cost of drugs is also spiralling in hospitals so if it's not necessary to treat, don't! When babies are newly admitted to the neonatal unit, they are quite often commenced on antibiotics until a positive diagnosis has been made, but once the test results are back and no organism has been found, antibiotics should be discontinued.

What to do

The infected baby should always be nursed in an incubator; this provides easy access for the nurses, easy observation, good thermal control and a means to isolate the baby in his own environment.

Care

• Carry out clinical observations on an hourly basis – continuous monitoring should be in place.
• Record all fluid intake and output and test urine.
• Regular blood results for oxygen levels, U&E, CBC, blood glucose levels, bilirubin levels, if necessary, CRP, differential WCC, blood cultures.
• Minimal handling and developmental care – comfortable, restful environment to aid recovery.
• Analgesia if required and monitor effects on baby.
• Plan nursing care to reduce handling but not to over stimulate the baby if cluster care is being employed as a method of carrying out the necessary nursing procedures. The baby will be lethargic and may not tolerate a lot of handling.
• Ensure that temperature is monitored – both by the incubator and the nurse – at least 4 hourly.
• Eye care and mouth care as well as nappy area cleansing.
• Encourage parents to stay beside the baby and to spend time with him, keep them up to date with his progress and answer questions honestly.

Human immunodeficiency virus infection

Today, pregnant women have the opportunity to be tested for human immunodeficiency virus (HIV). Such testing has led to an increase in the number of babies known to be exposed to HIV, which in turn has allowed for early diagnosis and treatment.

What causes it

HIV can be transmitted to the newborn infant in one of three ways:

1. Transplacentally during pregnancy
2. During labour and delivery
3. Through breast milk.

Risk factors for perinatal transmission can be either maternal or neonatal. (See *Risk factors for perinatal transmission of HIV*.)

Risk factors for perinatal transmission of HIV

Neonatal and maternal factors can contribute to perinatal transmission of the human immunodeficiency virus (HIV).

Neonatal factors

• Bacterial infection
• Being the first-born twin
• Breastfeeding
• Prematurity

Maternal factors

• Chorioamnionitis
• Low CD4+ count
• High CD8+ count
• High viral load
• New onset of disease
• Ongoing drug abuse
• Prolonged or complicated labour

What to look for

Most infants exposed to HIV are born at term and are of AGA size. Normal physical findings are usually present. Physical findings, such as adenopathy or haepatosplenomegaly, are absent at birth because HIV infection is believed to occur at delivery. These findings may develop later and suggest HIV infection.

What tests tell you

It is recommended that testing for HIV is done within 48 hours of birth, at age 1–2 months and again at age 3–6 months. Two positive tests at different ages are required to make a positive diagnosis. Diagnostic tests used to detect HIV include HIV deoxyribonucleic acid (DNA) polymerase chain reactions (PCR), HIV p24 antigen assay, HIV antibody, HIV culture and immunological testing.

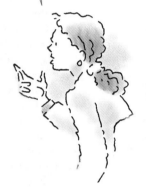

Physical findings of HIV infection aren't usually present at birth, but they may develop later.

PCR preferred

The HIV DNA PCR test is the preferred method for diagnosing HIV in neonates. It's highly sensitive and specific. Positive results can be detected in 93% of infected infants by day 14 of life. This test should be performed at birth and between ages 1 and 2 months. The test should be repeated at age 4 months if the infant remains asymptomatic and the previous test results were negative.

Assay you, assay me

HIV p24 antigen assay may be used to assess HIV infection in infants older than 1 month, but the sensitivity is less than PCR testing. The absence of the p24 antigen, however, doesn't rule out HIV infection.

Antibody home?

The HIV antibody test uses enzyme-linked immunosorbent assay and Western blot analysis to determine whether HIV antibodies are present as a result of exposure to the virus. However, this test doesn't differentiate between maternal and neonatal infection. In addition, diagnosis can be complicated by the presence of the maternal, anti-HIV IgG antibody in the baby. Because of this complication, cord blood should never be used for HIV testing.

A positive HIV antibody test obtained at age 18 months (after the maternal IgG in the baby has broken down) indicates infection. For infants exposed to HIV whose previous testing was negative, a final HIV antibody test at age 24 months is recommended.

An uncommon culture

An HIV culture is a test that isn't readily available. It's also expensive to perform, requires a large blood sample and the results may not be available for 2–4 weeks. If performed, an HIV culture should be taken at birth and again between ages 1 and 2 months. If the initial result is positive, the test should be repeated immediately to confirm. If an infant remains asymptomatic after testing negative, repeat the HIV culture at age 4 months.

More monitoring

Immunological testing, including lymphocyte subsets (CD4$^+$, CD8$^+$, CD4$^+$–CD8$^+$ ratio) and quantitative immunoglobulins (IgG, IgM, IgA) should be performed on all neonates born to HIV-positive mothers. Children born to HIV-infected mothers should also undergo haematological monitoring. This includes assessing CBC, differential leucocyte count and platelet count during the first 6 months of life. Monitoring should continue in infected children and in those whose infection status is undetermined at age 6 months.

To be free from HIV

A baby is considered uninfected with HIV when:
- no physical findings consistent with HIV are present
- immunological test results are negative
- virologic tests are negative
- after 12 months, two or more HIV antibody tests are negative.

How it's treated

To help prevent perinatal transmission of HIV, zidovudine (Retrovir) is given to HIV-positive women during the second and third trimesters of pregnancy as well as during labour and delivery. The drug is also given to infants born to HIV-positive mothers during the first 6 weeks of life. Such treatment has been shown to dramatically decrease perinatal transmission of HIV. Zidovudine therapy is discontinued at age 6 weeks. (See *Complications of zidovudine therapy in the neonates*.)

But wait, there's more

After zidovudine therapy is completed, prophylaxis for *Pneumocystis carinii* pneumonia (PCP) should start. PCP prophylaxis is recommended for all neonates born to HIV-infected women – regardless of the infant's initial test results – because PCP infection commonly occurs between ages 3 and 6 months, when many HIV-exposed infants haven't yet been identified as being infected. PCP prophylaxis should be initiated at age 6 months (after completion of zidovudine regimen). It should then continue until at least age 12 months – even if the infant's infection status hasn't been determined.

Cotrimoxazole (Bactrim) is the recommended chemoprophylaxis regimen for PCP in infants. When initiating therapy, first obtain a baseline CBC, differential leucocyte count and platelet count. These measurements should be checked monthly while the infant receives prophylaxis treatment. If this regimen isn't tolerated, dapsone may be used.

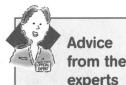

Advice from the experts

Complications of zidovudine therapy in the neonates

Zidovudine may cause transient anaemia. To monitor for this adverse effect, a complete blood count and differential leucocyte count should be performed at birth as a baseline and again at ages 4 and 6 weeks.

Education edge

Caring for a neonate exposed to HIV

When teaching a woman and her family about caring for a neonate exposed to human immunodeficiency virus (HIV), emphasise the need for:

- frequent follow-up
- testing to determine infection status
- zidovudine (Retrovir) administration to decrease the risk of infection
- prophylaxis for PCP
- taking precautions to prevent the spread of HIV infection.

Parent teaching should also include signs of possible HIV infection in the neonate, including:

- recurrent infections
- unusual infections
- failure to thrive
- haematologic manifestations
- renal disease
- neurological manifestations.

What to do

Whether the HIV-infected woman is delivering vaginally or by caesarean birth, follow standard precautions. Be sure to wear gloves, a gown and protective eyewear. Prompt and careful removal of blood and amniotic fluid from the infant's skin is important. Isolation, however, isn't required. Inform the mother that breastfeeding isn't recommended, and instruct her and her family on caring for the infant exposed to HIV. (See *Caring for a neonate exposed to HIV.*)

Hydrocephalus

Hydrocephalus is an excessive accumulation of CSF within the ventricular spaces of the brain. This accumulation of fluid forces the ventricles to dilate, which can put harmful pressure on brain tissue. Such pressure on brain tissue and cerebral blood vessels may lead to ischaemia and, eventually, cell death.

Are we communicating?

Hydrocephalus may be communicating or noncommunicating. Communicating hydrocephalus occurs because CSF isn't absorbed properly. Noncommunicating hydrocephalus occurs because normal CSF flow is obstructed. Congenital hydrocephalus is present at birth. Acquired hydrocephalus develops at the time of birth or later in life (premature babies may develop the condition as a result of intraventricular haemorrhage and the subsequent blockage of the ventricles).

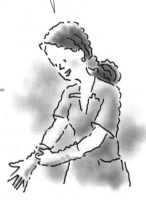

If a pregnant woman is infected with HIV, follow standard precautions during delivery.

What causes it

The cause of hydrocephalus isn't exactly known. Possible causes include:
- genetic inheritance
- neural tube defects, such as spina bifida and encephalocele
- complications of premature birth such as intraventricular haemorrhage
- meningitis
- tumours
- traumatic head injury
- subarachnoid haemorrhage
- antenatal maternal infections.

What to look for

Assessment findings vary. Be aware that a baby's ability to tolerate the accumulation of CSF differs from an adult's – the newborn baby's skull can expand because the sutures haven't yet closed.

On the lookout

Findings in babies that may suggest hydrocephalus include:
- rapid increase in head circumference or an unusually large head size disproportionate to infant's growth
- distended scalp veins
- bulging fontanelles
- thin, shiny, fragile-looking scalp skin
- downward deviation of the eyes ('sunsetting' eyes)
- sluggish pupils with unequal response to light
- seizures
- high-pitched, shrill cry
- irritability
- projectile vomiting
- feeding problems (because the head is 3 cm larger than the chest).
  In addition, the baby may cry when picked up or rocked and be quiet when still.

What tests tell you

Hydrocephalus is diagnosed by clinical assessment and imaging techniques, such as:
- ultrasound
- computed tomography
- magnetic resonance imaging
- pressure monitoring techniques.
  The appropriate diagnostic tool should be chosen based on age, clinical presentation and the presence of known or suspected abnormalities of the brain or spinal cord.

How it's treated

Hydrocephalus is commonly treated with the surgical insertion of a shunt. The shunt, consisting of a catheter and a valve, leads from a ventricle in the brain to the peritoneum or an atrial chamber of the heart, thus allowing CSF to drain to an area where it can be absorbed into the circulation. The valve maintains one-way flow and regulates the rate at which CSF is drained.

Potential complications of shunt systems include:
- mechanical failure
- infection
- obstruction
- need to lengthen or replace catheter.

Infants with surgically implanted shunt systems require regular medical follow-up.

What to do

The infant with diagnosed or suspected hydrocephalus must be observed carefully for signs of increasing intracranial pressure (ICP). The midwife/nurse must be alerted for:
- irritability
- lethargy
- seizure activity
- altered vital signs
- altered feeding behaviour.

> If hydrocephalus is suspected, watch closely for signs of increasing ICP.

Caution

Flexible and frequent feedings

Another aspect of nursing care for the infant with hydrocephalus is maintaining adequate nutrition. Keep feeding schedules flexible to help accommodate for various procedures. Offer small, frequent feedings, and allow extra time for feeding in case the infant has difficulty.

Support after surgery

Postoperative care involves:
- positioning the infant on the side opposite the shunt
- observing for signs of increased ICP
- monitoring intake and output carefully
- preventing infection
- providing skin care.

On the home front

Hydrocephalus poses risks to the baby's cognitive and physical development. The prospect of dealing with chronic disabilities or delayed development can be overwhelming to parents. Providing support to the family is crucial to helping them cope. Encourage them to express their concerns, and refer them to appropriate resources and rehabilitation services, as needed.

Hyperbilirubinaemia (jaundice)

Hyperbilirubinaemia is an excess of bilirubin in the blood that results in serum bilirubin levels above 85.5 μmol/L (5 mg/dl). The elevated levels are due to unconjugated bilirubin depositing in the mucous membranes and on the skin, resulting in jaundice – which can be physiological or pathological. Physiological jaundice is hyperbilirubinaemia that results from delayed bilirubin metabolism. It usually resolves in 7–10 days.

In pathological jaundice, total bilirubin levels and total serum bilirubin levels increase.

If left untreated, hyperbilirubinaemia may result in bilirubin encephalopathy, a neurological syndrome caused by unconjugated bilirubin depositing in the brain cells. Survivors may develop cerebral palsy, epilepsy or mental retardation, or they may have only minor after-effects, such as perceptual motor disabilities and learning disorders.

What causes it

As erythrocytes break down at the end of their neonatal life cycle, haemoglobin separates into globin (protein) and haeme (iron) fragments. Haeme fragments form unconjugated bilirubin. Unconjugated bilirubin then binds with albumin and is transported to liver cells to conjugate with glucuronide and form direct bilirubin. During this process, unconjugated bilirubin (fat soluble or indirect) may escape to extravascular tissue, causing hyperbilirubinaemia. Normally, once the bilirubin has been conjugated it becomes water soluble (direct) and is excreted by the gut and the kidneys.

Developing news

Several factors may affect whether a baby develops hyperbilirubinaemia:
• Certain drugs (such as aspirin, tranquillisers, oxytocin [syntocinon] and sulphonamides) or conditions (such as hypothermia, anoxia, hypoglycaemia and hypoalbuminaemia) can disrupt conjugation and usurp albumin-binding sites.
• Decreased haepatic function can result in reduced bilirubin conjugation.
• Increased erythrocyte production or breakdown or Rh or ABO incompatibility can accompany haemolytic disorders.
• Maternal enzymes present in breast milk can inhibit the baby's glucuronosyltransferase conjugating activity.
• If the baby has glucose-6-phosphate dehydrogenase deficiency, he has an increased risk of developing jaundice.

What to look for

The predominant sign of hyperbilirubinaemia is jaundice, which doesn't become clinically apparent until serum bilirubin levels reach about 120 μmol/L (7 mg/dl).

Physiological jaundice

Physiological jaundice typically develops within 3–4 days after birth in 60% of term babies and in 80% of preterm babies. It generally disappears by day 7 in term babies and by day 9 or 10 in preterm babies. Throughout physiological jaundice, the serum unconjugated bilirubin levels decline rapidly over the first week after birth. Most babies have been discharged by the time the jaundice peaks (72 hours).

Pathological jaundice

Pathological jaundice appears within the first 24 hours of life when the total serum bilirubin level increases by more than 85 µmol/L (5 mg/dl) per day and the total bilirubin level is higher than 290 µmol/L (17 mg/dl) in a full-term neonate. This is likely to be caused by Rh isoimmunisation or ABO incompatibility or some factor that is causing haemolysis.

Pathological jaundice can also be caused by obstruction of the bile duct. This means that conjugated bilirubin is produced but cannot get to the gut for excretion. The result is that:
- the baby's direct bilirubin level rises
- the baby has prolonged jaundice that lasts for over 2 weeks of age
- the baby's stools will look pale and clay coloured but urine looks normal
- the baby will become lethargic and unable to feed effectively
- a high direct bilirubin (conjugated bilirubin) makes up more than 20% of the total SBR.

Any baby who remains jaundiced for >2 weeks should always be investigated for obstructive jaundice – liver function tests should also be done. This must be done to avoid liver damage, brain damage and organ failure or eventual death.

What tests tell you

Jaundice and elevated levels of serum bilirubin confirm hyperbilirubinaemia. Inspection of the baby in a well-lit room (without yellow or gold lighting) reveals yellowish skin colouration, particularly in the sclerae. To verify jaundice, press the skin on the cheek or abdomen lightly with one finger, then release pressure and observe skin colour immediately. Check the mucous membranes also – this can be useful in babies with coloured skin. Signs of jaundice necessitate measuring and charting serum bilirubin levels every 4–6 hours. Testing may include direct and indirect bilirubin levels, particularly for pathological jaundice. Bilirubin levels that are excessively elevated or vary daily suggest a pathological process.

Connecting the cause

Identifying the underlying cause of hyperbilirubinaemia requires:
- A detailed maternal history (including antenatal history).
- A detailed family history (paternal Rh factor can be done, inherited red blood cell defects).

- Present status of the baby (immaturity, infection).
- Blood testing of the baby and mother (blood group incompatibilities, haemoglobin level, serum bilirubin or transcutaneous bilirubin level, haematocrit). It is important to have a fractionated bilirubin result – direct (conjugated bilirubin) and indirect (unconjugated).
- Remember that as part of the national UK regime, all Rh-negative mothers have anti-D given to them at intervals in the pregnancy to avoid Rh isoimmunisation.

How it's treated

Depending on the underlying cause, treatment may include:
- exchange transfusions
- high-intensity phototherapy
- albumin infusion
- I.V. globulin (in isoimmune haemolytic disease).

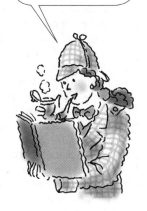

Suspect pathological jaundice if bilirubin levels are excessively high or vary daily.

Uneven exchange

An exchange transfusion replaces the baby's blood with fresh blood (blood that's less than 48 hours old), thus removing some of the unconjugated bilirubin in serum.

Photo albumin

Phototherapy uses fluorescent light to decompose bilirubin in the skin by oxidation. Implemented after the initial exchange transfusion, phototherapy is usually discontinued after bilirubin levels fall below 170 µmol/L and continue to decrease for 24 hours. (See *Administering phototherapy treatment*, page 506.)

Other therapy for excessive bilirubin levels may include albumin administration (1 g/kg of 25% salt-poor albumin), which provides additional albumin for binding unconjugated bilirubin. This may be done 1–2 hours before an exchange transfusion or as a substitute for a portion of the plasma in the transfused blood.

What to do

Nursing interventions for the infant with hyperbilirubinaemia include:
- Assess and record the infant's jaundice and note the time it began. Report the jaundice and serum bilirubin levels immediately to the paediatrician.
- Maintain oral intake. Don't skip feedings because fasting stimulates the conversion of haeme to bilirubin. The baby should be fed 3 hourly if he is clinically able, or breastfed frequently.
- Reassure parents that most babies experience some degree of jaundice.
- Explain hyperbilirubinaemia, its causes, diagnostic tests and treatment.
- Explain to the parents that the baby's stools contain some bile and may be greenish.
- Advise the parents that the community midwife will visit their baby for a few days after discharge but that they should contact the neonatal unit or

Administering phototherapy treatment

To administer phototherapy treatment, follow these steps:

- Set up the phototherapy unit above the baby's cot according to manufacturer's recommendations and verify placement of the light bulb shield. If the baby is in an incubator, place the phototherapy unit above the incubator according to the manufacturer's recommendations and turn on the lights. Place a photometer probe in the middle of the cot/incubator to measure the energy emitted by the lights.
- If the bilirubin level is extremely high and needs to be reduced rapidly, it may be necessary to line the sides of the cot/incubator with aluminium foil or white pads and to place a phototherapy unit below the baby.
- Explain the procedure to the parents.
- Record the baby's initial bilirubin level and his axillary temperature.
- Place the opaque eye mask over the baby's closed eyes and fasten securely.
- Undress the baby and place a nappy under him. Cover male genitalia with a surgical mask or small nappy to catch urine and prevent possible testicular damage from the heat and light waves.
- Take the baby's axillary temperature every 4 hours and provide additional warmth by adjusting the warming unit's thermostat.
- Monitor elimination and weigh the baby daily. Watch for signs of dehydration (dry skin, poor turgor, depressed fontanelles) and check urine specific gravity
- Take the baby out of the cot/incubator, turn off the phototherapy lights, and unmask his eyes at least every 3–4 hours with feedings.
- Assess his eyes for inflammation or injury. Clean his eyes and reapply fresh eye mask over closed eyes to avoid corneal damage.
- Reposition the baby every 2–4 hours to expose all body surfaces to the light and to prevent head moulding and skin breakdown from pressure.
- Check the bilirubin level at least once every 24 hours – more often if levels rise significantly. Turn off the phototherapy unit before taking venous blood for testing because the lights may degrade bilirubin in the blood. Notify the doctor if the bilirubin level nears 340 mmol/L in full-term babies or 250 mmol/L in premature babies.

their own general practitioner if they have any concerns. Discharge may need to be delayed if the baby is at risk for severe bilirubinaemia.
- Ensure that all blood results are recorded in the baby's notes and that serum bilirubin levels are plotted on a graph to show the rise/fall of levels over a given period. This graph also indicates when appropriate treatment such as phototherapy or exchange transfusion may be needed.

Meconium aspiration syndrome

Meconium is a thick, sticky, greenish black substance that constitutes the neonate's first stools. It's present in the bowel of the fetus as early as 10 weeks' gestation. Meconium aspiration syndrome results when the baby inhales meconium that's mixed with amniotic fluid. It typically occurs while the fetus is in utero or with the baby's first breath. The meconium partially or completely blocks the baby's airways so that air becomes trapped during exhalation. Also, the meconium irritates his airways, making breathing difficult.

In the thick of it

The severity of meconium aspiration syndrome depends on the amount of meconium aspirated and the consistency of the meconium. Thicker meconium generally causes more damage.

Increased effort

Infants with meconium aspiration syndrome increase their respiratory efforts to create greater negative intrathoracic pressures and improve airflow to the lungs. Hyperinflation, hypoxaemia and acidaemia cause increased peripheral vascular resistance. Right-to-left shunting commonly follows. In some severe cases, these babies may develop persistent pulmonary hypertension of the newborn (PPHN) and require nitric oxide ventilation or even extracorporeal membranous oxygenation (ECMO) in a specialised unit.

What causes it

Meconium aspiration syndrome is commonly related to fetal distress during labour. Meconium is released in utero because the anal sphincter relaxes secondary to a hypoxic episode. Occasionally, healthy babies pass meconium just before/or during the birth. In either case, if the baby gasps or inhales the meconium, meconium aspiration syndrome can develop. The resulting lack of oxygen may lead to brain damage.

Risk factors for meconium aspiration syndrome include:

- maternal diabetes
- maternal hypertension
- difficult delivery
- fetal distress
- intrauterine hypoxia
- advanced gestational age (greater than 40 weeks)
- poor intrauterine growth.

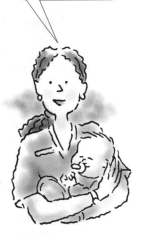

Maternal diabetes and maternal hypertension are some of the risk factors for meconium aspiration syndrome.

What to look for

Signs and symptoms of meconium aspiration syndrome include:

- dark greenish staining or streaking of the amniotic fluid
- obvious presence of meconium in the amniotic fluid
- skin with a greenish stain (if the meconium was passed long before delivery)
- limp appearance at birth
- pallor/cyanosis
- rapid breathing
- laboured breathing
- apnoea
- signs of postmaturity such as peeling skin and long nails
- the skin, cord and nails may be stained with meconium
- low heart rate before birth
- low Apgar score

- hypothermia
- hypoglycaemia
- hypocalcaemia
- nasal flaring
- grunting
- tachypnoea
- irregular gasping respirations.

What tests tell you

The most accurate way to diagnose meconium aspiration syndrome is to observe the vocal cords for meconium staining. Assess breath sounds for coarse, crackly sounds, which are common in infants with meconium aspiration syndrome. ABG analysis helps assess for acidosis (low blood pH and hypoxaemia). A chest radiograph can show patches or streaks of meconium in the lungs and reveal if hyperexpansion and air trapping have occurred.

How it's treated

Paediatricians should be present at a delivery where there has been meconium-stained liquor to resuscitate the infant should aspiration occur. If the infant comes out, cries, begins to breathe normally and pinks up, his nose and mouth should be wiped with sterile gauze and he should be given to his mother. If the baby comes out, white and limp, showing no signs of breathing, he should be removed to the resuscitaire without any stimulation. He should be wrapped in a warm towel and his airways visualised with a laryngoscope. If the meconium is below the level of his vocal cords, he should have them suctioned under direct vision – it may be necessary to intubate the baby so that meconium can be suctioned from deeper within his proximal airways. Tracheal suctioning may be necessary to remove all of the meconium before the first breath is taken. Close monitoring of the infant is necessary after delivery – if the meconium was below his vocal cords, he should be transferred to the NICU immediately, so that he can be observed and treatment intiated.

Additional treatments may include:
- antibiotics
- use of a radiant warmer
- supplemental oxygen
- mechanical ventilation.

If complications arise, further treatments may be necessary. (See *Complications of meconium aspiration syndrome.*)

What to do

Assess risk factors before delivery if possible. Midwifery responsibilities include:
- amniotic fluid assessment
- fetal monitoring
- immediate intervention in delivery room

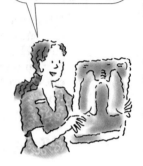

Every picture tells a story. A chest x-ray may reveal patches or streaks of meconium in the lungs.

Advice from the experts

Complications of meconium aspiration syndrome

Meconium aspiration syndrome may cause:

- aspiration pneumonia
- cerebral palsy
- mental retardation
- pneumothorax
- seizures.

- maintaining thermoregulation
- respiratory assessment/clearing airway/suctioning under direct vision
- administering respiratory support, such as oxygen and mechanical ventilation
- being alert for potential complications
- supporting family members by providing education and reassurance and promoting parent–infant attachment.

Transient tachypnoea of the newborn

Transient tachypnoea of the newborn (TTN) is a mild respiratory problem in neonates. It begins after birth and generally lasts about 3 days. TTN is also known as 'wet lungs'.

What causes it

TTN results from the delayed absorption of fetal lung fluid after birth. Before birth, the fetus doesn't use his lungs to breathe. Instead, the fetal lungs are filled with fluid. All of the fetus' nutrients and oxygen come from the mother through the placenta. During the birth process, some of the neonate's lung fluid is squeezed out as he passes through the birth canal. After birth, the remaining fluid is pushed out of the lungs as the lungs fill with air. Fluid that remains is later coughed out or absorbed into the bloodstream. TTN results when fluid remains in the lungs, forcing the baby to breathe harder and faster to get adequate oxygen.

> TTN results when fluid remains in the lungs, forcing the baby to breathe harder and faster to get adequate oxygen.

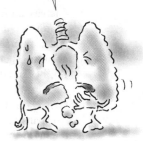

Risk factory

TTN is commonly observed in babies delivered by caesarean birth. These babies don't benefit from the thoracic compression that helps to expel fluid during vaginal delivery. Other risk factors for TTN include:

- preterm delivery
- maternal smoking during pregnancy
- maternal diabetes
- size that's SGA
- macrosomia
- maternal asthma
- maternal drug abuse
- birth asphyxia
- maternal fluid overload (especially with oxytocin administration)
- prolonged labour
- excessive maternal sedation.

Babies who are small or preterm, or who were born rapidly by vaginal delivery, may not have received effective squeezing of the thorax to remove fetal lung fluid.

What to look for

Common signs of TTN include:
- tachypnoea (rate greater than 60 breaths/minute)
- laboured breathing
- expiratory grunting
- nasal flaring
- intercostal and sternal retractions
- cyanosis
- tachycardia.

These signs and symptoms typically occur immediately after birth. However, these could also be indicative of a more serious condition; observe the baby closely.

What tests tell you

Laboratory tests and imaging studies are used to diagnose TTN. For example:
- ABG results may indicate hypoxaemia and decreased carbon dioxide levels.
- Increased carbon dioxide levels may be a sign of fatigue and impending respiratory failure.
- Pulse oximetry is used to noninvasively monitor tissue oxygenation and allow titration of supplemental oxygen.
- A CBC and differential WCC may be done to evaluate for signs of infection.
- Chest x-ray, the diagnostic standard for TTN, will reveal streaking that correlates with lymphatic engorgement of retained fetal lung fluid, hyperexpansion of the lungs, a mild to moderately enlarged heart and flattening of the diaphragm.

Abnormal findings

Abnormalities in diagnostic test results resolve with resolution of the condition, usually within 72 hours.

How it's treated

Specific treatment for TTN depends on:
- the baby's gestational age, overall health and medical history
- the extent of respiratory distress
- tolerance of medical therapies
- expectations for the course of the disease.

Be supportive

Care is mainly supportive as the retained lung fluid is reabsorbed. Treatment may involve:
- monitoring heart rate, respiratory rate and oxygen levels
- providing supplemental humidified oxygen
- maintaining continuous positive airway pressure (CPAP)

- monitoring intake and output
- using mechanical ventilation
- providing proper nutrition.
  Generally, a baby with TTN is supported with I.V. fluids or gavage feedings. The increased respiratory rate and increased work of breathing make oral feeding difficult because he must coordinate the mechanisms of sucking, swallowing and breathing. The rapid respiratory rate puts the baby at high risk for aspiration.

Minimal meds

Medication use in TTN is minimal. Antibiotic therapy may be administered until sepsis is ruled out. The regimen usually consists of penicillin and an aminoglycoside (usually gentamicin) or a cephalosporin (usually cefotaxime).

What to do

A baby with TTN may be cared for in an NICU. Nursing interventions include:
- monitoring heart and respiratory rates and oxygenation
- providing respiratory support
- maintaining a neutral thermal environment
- minimising stimulation by decreasing lights and noise levels
- administering medication as ordered
- providing proper nutrition
- providing parental education and emotional support.
  Symptoms typically resolve within 72 hours. The baby usually recovers completely and has no increased risk of further respiratory problems.

Respiratory distress syndrome

RDS occurs when the lungs are immature. It's seen almost exclusively in preterm babies and carries a high risk of long-term respiratory and neurological complications.

What causes it

RDS is characterised by poor gas exchange and ventilatory failure. It's caused by a lack of pulmonary surfactant, a phospholipid secreted by the alveolar epithelium that normally appears in mature lungs. Surfactant coats the alveoli, keeping them open so that gas exchange can occur. In preterm babies, the lungs may not be fully developed and, therefore, may not have a sufficient amount of surfactant. This leads to:
- atelectasis
- increased work of breathing
- respiratory acidosis
- hypoxaemia.

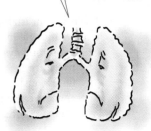

Low surfactant. Poor gas exchange. Looks like we're in trouble!

Changing the flow of the things

As atelectasis worsens, pulmonary vascular resistance increases, which decreases blood flow to the lungs. Blood then shunts from right to left, perpetuating fetal circulation by keeping the foramen ovale and ductus arteriosus patent.

One membrane too many

The alveoli may become necrotic, and the capillaries may become damaged. Ischaemia allows fluid to leak into the interstitial and alveolar spaces, causing a hyaline membrane to form. This membrane hinders respiratory function by decreasing the compliance of the lungs.

Risk factors for RDS include:
- preterm birth
- maternal diabetes
- stress during delivery that produces acidosis in the neonate.

What to look for

RDS can produce respiratory distress acutely after birth or over a period of a few hours. Initial assessment may reveal:
- increased respiratory rate
- retractions (sternal and intercostal)
- satisfactory colour
- good air movement on auscultation.

Obvious observations

As respiratory distress becomes more obvious, the nurse/midwife may note:
- further increase in respiratory rate
- laboured breathing
- more pronounced substernal retractions
- fine rales on auscultation
- expiratory grunting
- nasal flaring
- cyanosis.

It gets worse

If treatment isn't started or if the baby isn't responding to treatment, the nurse/midwife may observe:
- worsening cyanosis
- flaccidity
- unresponsiveness
- apnoeic episodes
- decreased breath sounds.

What tests tell you

Results of laboratory data, such as hypoxaemia, hypercapnia and acidosis, are nonspecific to RDS. Specific tests must be carried out to evaluate the infant for complicating factors. These include:
- blood, urine and CSF cultures
- blood glucose analysis
- serum calcium
- ABG measurements.
    Radiographic evaluation reveals:
- alveolar atelectasis (a diffuse, granular pattern that resembles ground glass) over lung fields
- dilated bronchioles (appear as dark streaks within the granular pattern)
- an air bronchogram is apparent
- the cardiac border is difficult to define
- the 'whiter' the lungs look, the more serious the condition is – this indicates poor air entry.

Phospholipid lingo

Antenatal tests can evaluate lung maturity while the fetus is in utero. This is done by evaluating the lecithin and sphingomyelin ratio of the amniotic fluid. Lecithin and sphingomyelin are two surfactant phospholipids. Evaluation of fetal lung maturity gives insight into how the fetus will fare after birth and may precipitate treatment of the mother to delay labour or to mature the baby's lungs before delivery.

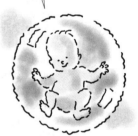

Since prevention of preterm delivery decreases my chance of suffering from RDS, I think I'll hang out here a while longer.

How it's treated

Because RDS is a disease related to gestational age and lung maturity, one management technique is to prevent preterm delivery. If that isn't possible, surfactant production can be stimulated before the baby is born by administering corticosteroids to the mother before birth.

Supportive steps

RDS treatment after birth is mainly supportive and includes general measures used to treat preterm babies, including:
- thermoregulation
- oxygen administration
- mechanical ventilation if needed
- prevention of hypotension
- prevention of hypovolaemia
- correcting respiratory acidosis by ventilatory support
- correcting metabolic acidosis with the administration of sodium bicarbonate
- parenteral feedings.

Oral feeds aren't recommended during the acute stage of RDS because such situations that increase respiratory rate or oxygen consumption should be avoided.

Respiratory remedies

Respiratory support can be given by:
- oxygen administration via nasal cannula
- CPAP
- mechanical ventilation

Sometimes the use of a high-frequency oscillator is needed; these ventilators cause less barotrauma to the airways and lungs. Positive end-expiratory pressure (PEEP) may be used via mechanical ventilation. PEEP prevents alveolar collapse during expiration, thereby allowing more time for gas exchange to occur.

The goals of oxygen therapy are to:
- maintain adequate oxygenation to the tissues
- prevent lactic acidosis
- avoid toxic effects of oxygen.

Complications of oxygen therapy and mechanical ventilation may occur despite efforts to prevent them. They include:
- pneumothorax
- pneumomediastinum
- ROP
- BPD
- infection
- IVH.

Myriad of meds

Management of RDS also includes the administration of surfactant directly into the lungs. Surfactant can prevent atelectasis and contribute to fluid clearance from the alveoli. Other medications that are commonly used to treat neonates with RDS include antibiotics, sedatives, paralytics and diuretics.

What to do

Continuous monitoring of the baby with RDS is essential because of the constant threat of hypoxaemia. Nursing responsibilities include:
- collecting blood samples
- monitoring pulse oximetry
- suctioning (only when absolutely necessary)
- implementing thermoregulation
- monitoring nutrition and blood glucose levels
- administering medication
- providing eye, mouth and skin care
- providing developmental care
- minimising stimuli and/or pain and distress.

Do not disturb

To help decrease oxygen consumption, make efforts to limit how often the baby with RDS is disturbed. Feeding is generally given parenterally during the acute phase of the disease. Keep him in a dark, quiet, thermal neutral environment as much as possible.

In addition to the general teaching for parents of preterm babies, parents of babies with RDS need to be educated about the syndrome, especially during the acute stage. Refer the parents to social services, a chaplain and other sources of support as needed.

There are some excellent websites for parents to access – these are provided by parents who have gone through the experience of having a premature baby in the NICU. http://www.kerri.thomas.btinternet.co.uk/home.html

http://www.babycentre.co.uk/
http://www.tommys.org/

Oxygen administration

Oxygen relieves neonatal respiratory distress, which can be caused by cyanosis, pallor, tachypnoea, nasal flaring, bradycardia, hypothermia, retractions (intercostal, subcostal marginal, suprasternal), hypotonia, hyporeflexia or expiratory grunting.

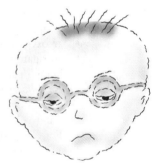

Too much of a good thing?

No matter how it's administered, oxygen therapy can be hazardous to the neonate. When given in high concentrations and for prolonged periods, it can cause ROP, which may result in blindness in preterm babies, and can contribute to BPD. Because of the baby's size and special respiratory requirements, oxygen administration commonly requires special techniques and equipment.

Hands-on in an emergency

In emergency situations, give oxygen through a manual resuscitation bag or via the 'Neopuff', using a mask of appropriate size until more permanent measures can be initiated.

A method for every occasion

When the infant merely requires additional oxygen above the ambient concentration, it can be delivered using a headbox or directly into the incubator. (Headboxes are rarely used nowadays.) When the infant requires CPAP to prevent alveolar collapse at the end of an expiration, as in RDS (hyaline membrane disease), administer oxygen through nasal prongs or an ET tube connected to a manometer. If the infant can't breathe on his own, deliver oxygen through a ventilator. Oxygen must be mixed with air, warmed and humidified to prevent hypothermia and dehydration, to which the neonate is especially susceptible.

The right tools for the job

To begin oxygen therapy, you'll need:
- an oxygen source (wall, cylinder or liquid unit)
- a compressed air source
- flowmeters
- large and small bore sterile oxygen tubing
- a blood gas analyser
- a stethoscope
- a orogastric tube (OGT).

For handheld resuscitation bag and mask delivery, you'll also need:
- a specially sized mask with handheld resuscitation bag and pressure release valve
- a manometer with connectors

'Neopuffs' are especially good because the pressures are preset on the equipment and there is no danger of overfilling a bag or overinflating a newborn baby's lungs. It is easier to use, as the practitioner only has to cover a small hole in the tubing to deliver the desired gases to the baby.

For delivery via a headbox, you'll need:
- an appropriate-sized headbox
- an oxygen analyser
- corrigated tubing
- humidifier

For delivery through nasal prongs, other equipment includes:
- nasal prongs
- water-soluble lubricant.

For CPAP delivery, you'll also need:
- a manometer with connectors
- a nasopharyngeal or ET tube, or nasal CPAP prongs
- water-soluble lubricant
- hypoallergenic tape

For delivery with a ventilator, you'll need:
- a ventilator unit with temperature probe in the tubing
- specimen tubes for ABG analysis
- an ET tube
- a pulse oximeter or transcutaneous oxygen monitor.

Be prepared

To prepare for oxygen administration, wash your hands and gather and assemble the necessary equipment. To calibrate the oxygen analyser, turn the analyser on and read the results. Room air should be about 21% oxygen. Expose the analyser probe to 100% oxygen, adjust the sensitivity, and recheck the amount of oxygen in room air.

By hand

To use a handheld resuscitation bag and mask:
- Place the assembled resuscitation bag and mask in the cot/incubator.
- Turn on the oxygen and compressed air flowmeters – the total flow should be 5 L/min and place the mask over the baby's nose and mouth.
- Check pressure settings and mask size.
- Have another staff member available to assist.
- Provide 40–60 breaths/minute, using enough pressure to cause a visible rise and fall of the chest. Provide enough oxygen to maintain pink nail beds and mucous membranes.
- Continuously watch the infant's chest movements and listen to breath sounds, avoiding over ventilation. If the infant's heart rate falls below 100 beats/minute, continue to use the handheld resuscitation bag until the heart rate rises to 100 beats/minute or greater.
- Insert an orogastric tube to drain air from the infant's stomach.

Headbox

To use a headbox:
- Attach the headbox to the corrigated tubing.
- Activate oxygen and compressed air source, if needed, at ordered flow rates.
- The mixed gases should pass through a heater/humidifier so that gases are heated and moistened before entering the baby's airways.
- Place the headbox over the baby's head.
- Measure the amount of oxygen he is receiving with the oxygen analyser. Be sure to place the analyser probe close to the baby's nose.
- Adjust the oxygen to the prescribed amount.

By prongs

When using nasal prongs:
- Match the prong size to the baby's nose.
- Apply a small amount of water-soluble lubricant to the outside of the prongs.
- Turn on the oxygen and compressed air, if necessary.
- Connect the prongs to the oxygen source.
- Insert the prongs into the nose and secure them.
- Be sure to keep the prongs clean to ensure patency.

By CPAP

If the baby needs CPAP to prevent alveolar collapse at the end of each breath (as in RDS), he may receive this through an ET or nasopharyngeal tube or nasal CPAP prongs. To use CPAP:
- Position the baby on his back with a rolled towel under his neck to keep the airway open, avoid hyperextending the neck.
- Assist with intubation if necessary.
- Turn on the oxygen and compressed air source and attach the delivery system to the ET tube or nasal CPAP prongs.

- If the ET tube is in the correct place – secure it with tape.
- Insert an orogastric tube to keep the stomach decompressed and leave the tube open to air unless the neonate is receiving milk feeds.

   To use a ventilator:

- Turn on the ventilator and set the controls as ordered.
- Help with ET tube insertion and attach it to the ventilator.
- Confirm placement of the ET tube and tape it securely.
- Watch the ventilator monitor to maintain pressure at the prescribed level and monitor for correct temperature.

Knowing the know-how

Know how to perform neonatal chest auscultation correctly to pick up subtle respiratory changes. Also, be able to identify signs of respiratory distress and perform emergency procedures. If required, perform chest physiotherapy and percussion as ordered and follow with suctioning to remove secretions (this is rarely done in the NICU).

Monitor ABG levels at reasonable intervals, or after any changes in oxygen concentration or pressures. If ordered, monitor oxygen levels via a transcutaneous PO_2 monitor, perfusion by pulse oximetry and umbilical vein for blood gases. Keep the doctor aware of ABG levels so he can order appropriate changes in oxygen concentration and ventilation.

When the baby eventually begins to cope on his own, or his lungs recover or mature, he will require his O_2 concentrations to be reduced and eventually discontinued. Repeat ABG measurements 20–30 minutes after discontinuing oxygen and thereafter as ordered by the doctor or unit policy.

On the watch

Assess the baby for complications of oxygen administration, including:
- signs and symptoms of infection
- hypothermia
- metabolic and respiratory acidosis
- pressure ulcers on the his head, face and nose (apparatus/tape)
- signs of a pulmonary air leak, including pneumothorax, pneumomediastinum, pneumopericardium and interstitial emphysema.

Safety first

When administering oxygen, always take safety precautions to avoid fire or explosion. Take measures to keep the infant warm because hypothermia impedes respiration.

For the record

When documenting oxygen administration, be sure to include:
- type of respiratory distress requiring oxygen administration
- oxygen concentration given
- oxygen delivery method used

- each change in oxygen concentration
- routine checks of oxygen concentration
- baby's FiO$_2$ (as measured by the oxygen analyser)
- ABG values, noting the time each sample was obtained
- each time suctioning is performed
- amount and consistency of mucus
- type of continuous oxygen monitoring, if any
- temperature of gases
- complications
- baby's condition during oxygen therapy, including respiratory rate, breath sounds and signs of additional respiratory distress

Quick quiz

1. Testing a neonate for drug exposure while in utero involves collecting and analysing:
  A. urine and meconium.
  B. blood and urine.
  C. CSF and meconium.
  D. CSF and blood.

Answer: A. Urine and meconium specimens are collected when testing a neonate for drug exposure.

2. Neonates classified as SGA have a birthweight that's:
  A. below the 5th percentile.
  B. below the 10th percentile.
  C. below the 15th percentile.
  D. below the 20th percentile.

Answer: B. Neonates classified as SGA have a birthweight below the 10th percentile.

3. Which option is a neonatal risk factor for HIV transmission?
  A. Being born preterm
  B. Being a second-born twin
  C. Being bottle-fed
  D. Being born postterm

Answer: A. Preterm birth is neonatal risk factor for HIV infection.

4. Downward deviation of the eyes (sunsetting eyes) is a classic assessment finding of:
  A. FAS.
  B. hydrocephalus.
  C. preterm birth.
  D. HIV infection.

Answer: B. Downward deviation of the eyes is a characteristic finding in neonates with hydrocephalus.

5. Which is the most accurate diagnostic tool for meconium aspiration syndrome?

    A.   Chest x-ray
    B.   ABG analysis
    C.   Evaluation of the vocal cords using a laryngoscope
    D.   Amniotic fluid testing for meconium

Answer: C. The most accurate way to diagnose meconium aspiration syndrome is to evaluate the vocal cords for meconium staining using a laryngoscope.

6. What's the role of surfactant in the lungs?

    A.   It coats the alveoli to help keep them open so that gas exchange can occur.
    B.   It increases pulmonary capillary blood flow.
    C.   It increases respiratory rate to correct acidaemia.
    D.   It prevents bronchospasm.

Answer: A. Surfactant is a phospholipid secreted by the alveolar epithelium that coats the alveoli, keeping them open so that gas exchange can occur.

7. Which maternal disorder increases the chances that the mother will have a neonate who develops TTN?

    A.   Sickle cell anaemia
    B.   Hyperemesis gravidarum
    C.   Macrosomia
    D.   Asthma

Answer: D. Maternal disorders that increase the risk of having a neonate who develops TTN include a history of asthma, drug abuse, diabetes, excessive sedation, prolonged labour and fluid overload.

Scoring

☆☆☆ If you answered all seven questions correctly, ooh la la! You have a definite flair for neonatal care!

☆☆ If you answered five or six questions correctly, magnifique! You've outfitted yourself with a fine knowledge of high-risk neonates!

☆☆ If you answered fewer than five questions correctly, très bien! You can go back and look this over in your own fashion to get a better view of this chapter!

Appendices and index

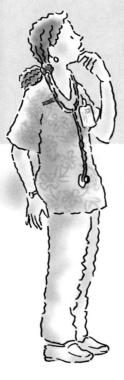

Laboratory values for pregnant and nonpregnant women

	Pregnant	Nonpregnant
Haemoglobin	11.5–14 g/dl	12–16 g/dl
Haematocrit	32–42%	37–47%
White blood cells	5,000–15,000 μl	4,500–10,000 μl
Neutrophils	60% + 10%	60% of WBC
Lymphocytes	15–40%	38–46% of WBC
Platelets	150,000–350,000 μl	150,000–350,000 μl
Serum calcium	7.8–9.3 mg/dl	8.4–10.2 mg/dl
Serum sodium	Increased retention	136–146 mmol/L
Serum chloride	Slight elevation	98–106 mmol/L
Serum iron	65–120 μg/dl	75–150 μg/dl
Fibrinogen	1.8–2 g/dl	4.2 g/dl
Fasting blood glucose	65 mg/dl	70–80 mg/dl
2-hour postprandial blood glucose	<140 mg/dl (after a 100 g carbohydrate meal)	60–110 mg/dl
Blood urea nitrogen	Decreased	1–3 mmol/L
Serum creatinine	Decreased	0.5–1.1 mg/dl
Renal plasma flow	Increased by 25%	490–700 ml/minute
Glomerular filtration rate	Increased by 50% to 160–198 ml/minute	105–132 ml/minute
Serum uric acid	Decreased	2–6.6 mg/dl
Erythrocyte sedimentation rate	30–90 mm/hour	20 mm/hour
Prothrombin time	Decreased slightly	20–40 seconds
Partial thromboplastin time	Decreased slightly during pregnancy and again during second and third stages of labour (indicating clotting at placental site)	18–30 seconds

Normal neonatal laboratory values

This chart shows laboratory tests that may be ordered for neonates, including the normal ranges for full-term infants. Note that ranges may vary among institutions. Because test results for preterm neonates usually reflect weight and gestational age, ranges for preterm neonates vary.

Test	Normal range
Blood	
Albumin	3.6–5.4 g/dl
Alkaline phosphatase	(1 week) SI, 150–400 units/L
Alpha-fetoprotein	Up to 10 mg/L, with none detected after 21 days
Ammonia	9–34 µmol/L
Amylase	5–65 units/L
Bicarbonate	20–25 mmol/L
Bilirubin, conjugated	0–3.4 µmol/L
Bilirubin, total	Less than 34 µmol/L (cord blood)
• 0–1 day	Less than 103 µmol/L (peripheral blood)
• 1–2 days	Less than 137 µmol/L (peripheral blood)
• 3–5 days	Less than 205 µmol/L (peripheral blood)
Bleeding time	2 minutes
Arterial blood gases	
• pH	7.35–7.45
• $PaCO_2$	35–45 mmHg
• PaO_2	50–90 mmHg
Venous blood gases	
• pH	7.35–7.45
• PCO_2	41–51 mmHg
• PO_2	20–49 mmHg
Calcium, ionised	1.12–1.23 mmol/L
Calcium, total	1.75–3 mmol/L

Test	Normal range
Blood (continued)	
Chloride	1.75–3 mmol/L
Clotting time (2 tube)	5–8 minutes
Creatine kinase	76–600 units/L
Creatinine	27–88 µmol/L
Digoxin level	Greater than 2 ng/ml possible; greater than 30 ng/ml probable
Fibrinogen	2–4 g/L
Glucose	1.1–6.1 mmol/L
Gamma glutamyltransferase	0–130 units/L
Haematocrit	56% 51% (cord blood)
Haemoglobin	18.5 g/dl 16.5 g/dl (cord blood)
Immunoglobulins	
• IgG	6.4 to 16 g/L
• IgM	0.06–0.24 g/L
• IgA	0–0.5 g/L
Iron	20–48 µmol/L
Iron-binding capacity	10.6–31.3 µmol/L
Lactate dehydrogenase	160–1,500 international units/L
Magnesium	0.75–1 mmol/L
Osmolality	285–295 mmol/kg
Partial thromboplastin time	40–80 seconds
Phenobarbital level	15–40 mcg/dl
Phosphorus	1.36–2.91 mmol/L
Platelets	100,000–300,000 µl
Potassium	3.5–6 mmol/L
Protein, total	50–71 g/L
Prothrombin time	12–21 seconds
Red blood cell count	5.1–5.8 (1,000,000 µl)
Reticulocytes	3–7% (cord blood)
Sodium	135–145 mmol/L
Theophylline level	5–10 mcg/ml
Thyroid-stimulating hormone	0–17.4 microunits/L (cord blood)
Thyroxine, (T_4) (total)	95–168 mmol/L (cord blood)

Test	Normal range
Blood (continued)	
Urea nitrogen	2–7 µmol/L
White blood cell (WBC) count	18,000 µl
• eosinophils-basophils	3%
• immature WBCs	10%
• lymphocytes	30%
• monocytes	5%
• neutrophils	45%
Urine	
Casts, WBC	Present first 2–4 days
Osmolality	50–1,200 mOsm/kg
pH	5–7
Protein	Present first 2–4 days
Specific gravity	1.006–1.008

Glossary

aberration: a deviation from what's typical or normal

acme: the peak of a contraction

adnexal area: accessory parts of the uterus, ovaries and fallopian tubes

agenesis: failure of an organ to develop

amnion: the inner of the two fetal membranes that forms the amniotic sac and houses the fetus and the fluid that surrounds it in utero

amniotic: relating to or pertaining to the amnion

amniotic fluid: fluid surrounding the fetus, derived primarily from maternal serum and fetal urine

amniotic sac: membrane that contains the fetus and fluid during gestation

analgesic: pharmacological agent that relieves pain without causing unconsciousness

anaesthesia: use of pharmacological agents to produce partial or total loss of sensation, with or without loss of consciousness

anomaly: an organ or a structure that's malformed or in some way abnormal due to structure, form or position

artificial insemination: mechanical deposition of a partner's or donor's spermatozoa at the cervical os

autosomes: any of the paired chromosomes other than the X and Y (sex) chromosomes

basal body temperature: temperature when body metabolism is at its lowest, usually below 36.7°C before ovulation and above 36.7°C after ovulation

Bishop score: method of assessing cervical dilation, effacement, station, consistency and position to determine readiness for induction of labour

c-peptide: an enzyme predictor of early hyperinsulinaemia

cephalocaudal development: principle of maturation that development proceeds from the head to the tail (rump)

chorion: the fetal membrane closest to the uterine wall; gives rise to the placenta and is the outer membrane surrounding the amnion

conduction: loss of body heat to a solid, cooler object through direct contact

congenital disorder: disorder present at birth that may be caused by genetic or environmental factors

convection: loss of body heat to cooler ambient air

corpus luteum: yellow structure formed from a ruptured graafian follicle that secretes progesterone during the second half of the menstrual cycle; if pregnancy occurs, the corpus luteum continues to produce progesterone until the placenta assumes that function

cotyledon: one of the rounded segments on the maternal side of the placenta, consisting of villi, fetal vessels and an intervillous space

cryptorchidism: undescended testes

cul-de-sac: pouch formed by a fold of the peritoneum between the anterior wall of the rectum and the posterior wall of the uterus; also known as Douglas' cul-de-sac

decidua: mucous membrane lining of the uterus during pregnancy that's shed after birth

dilation: widening of the external cervical os

dizygotic: pertaining to or derived from two fertilised ova, or zygotes (as in dizygotic twins)

doll's eye sign: movement of a neonate's eyes in a direction opposite to which the head is turned; this reflex typically disappears after 10 days of extrauterine life

Down's syndrome: abnormality involving the occurrence of a third chromosome, instead of the normal pair (trisomy 21), that characteristically results in mental retardation and altered physical appearance

dystocia: difficult labour

effleurage: gentle massage to the abdomen during labour for the purpose of relaxation and distraction

effacement: thinning and shortening of the cervix

embryo: conceptus from the time of implantation to 8 weeks

endometrium: inner mucosal lining of the uterus

engagement: descent of the fetal presenting part to at least the level of the ischial spines

Epstein's pearls: small, white, firm epithelial cysts on the neonate's hard palate

evaporation: loss of body heat that occurs as fluid on the body surface changes to a vapour

fetus: conceptus from 8 weeks until term

follicle-stimulating hormone: hormone produced by the anterior pituitary gland that stimulates the development of the graafian follicle

fontanelle: space at the junction of the sutures connecting fetal skull bones

gamete intrafallopian tube transfer: placement of an ovum and spermatozoa into the end of the fallopian tube via laparoscope; also called in vivo fertilisation

gene: factor on a chromosome responsible for the hereditary characteristics of the offspring

general anaesthesia: use of pharmacological agents to produce loss of consciousness, progressive central nervous system depression and complete loss of sensation

haematoma: collection of blood in the soft tissue

hereditary disorder: disorder passed from one generation to another

heterozygous: presence of two dissimilar genes at the same site on paired chromosomes

Homans sign: calf pain on leg extension and foot dorsiflexion that's an early sign of thrombophlebitis

homozygous: presence of two similar genes at the same site on paired chromosomes

human chorionic gonadotropin: hormone produced by the chorionic villi that serves as the biologic marker in pregnancy tests

hyperinsulinaemia: prediabetic state marked by insulin resistance

hypoxia: reduced oxygen availability to tissues or fetus

increment: period of increasing strength of a uterine contraction

induction of labour: artificial initiation of labour

informed consent: written consent obtained by the doctor after the client has been fully informed of the planned treatment, potential adverse effects and alternative management choices

intensity: the strength of a uterine contraction

interval: period between the end of one uterine contraction and the beginning of the next uterine contraction

intervillous space: irregularly shaped areas in the maternal portion of the placenta that are filled with blood and serve as the site for maternal–fetal gas, nutrient and waste exchange

in vitro fertilisation: fertilisation of an ovum outside the body, followed by reimplantation of the blastocyte into the woman

involution: reduction of uterine size after delivery, may take up to 6 weeks

karyotype: schematic display of the chromosomes within a cell arranged to demonstrate their numbers and morphology

lanugo: downy, fine hair that covers the fetus between 20 weeks' gestation and birth

lecithin: a phospholipid surfactant that reduces surface tension and increases pulmonary tissue elasticity; presence in amniotic fluid is used to determine fetal lung maturity

lecithin–sphingomyelin ratio: measurement of the relation of lecithin (which rises sharply around 35 weeks' gestation) and sphingomyelin (which remains stable) that's used as an indicator of fetal lung maturity, also known as L/S ratio

leucorrhoea: white or yellow vaginal discharge

lie: relationship of the long axis of the fetus to the long axis of the maternal spine

linear terminalis: imaginary line that separates the true pelvis from the false pelvis

local anaesthesia: blockage of sensory nerve pathways at the organ level, producing loss of sensation only in that organ

lochia: discharge after delivery from sloughing of the uterine decidua

luteinising hormone: hormone produced by the anterior pituitary gland that stimulates ovulation and the development of the corpus luteum

meiosis: process by which germ cells divide and decrease their chromosomal number by one-half

mifepristone: a progesterone antagonist that prevents implantation of fertilised egg; also called RU-486

mitosis: process of somatic cell division in which a single cell divides but both of the new cells have the same number of chromosomes as the first

moulding: shaping of the fetal head caused by shifting of sutures in response to pressure exerted by the maternal pelvis and birth canal during labour and delivery

myometrium: middle muscular layer of the uterus that's made up of three layers of smooth, involuntary muscles

neonate: an infant between birth and the 28th day

nidation: implantation of the fertilised ovum in the uterine endometrium

Nitrazine paper: a treated paper used to detect pH used in determining if amniotic fluid is present

NuvaRing: vaginal contraceptive ring that contains oestrogen and progesterone

oligohydramnios: severely reduced and highly concentrated amniotic fluid

oocyte: incompletely developed ovum

oogenesis: formation and development of the ovum

ovum: conceptus from time of conception until primary villi appear (approximately 4 weeks after the last menstrual period)

perimetrium: outer serosal layer of the uterus

polyhydramnios: abnormally large amount (more than 2,000 ml) of amniotic fluid in the uterus

premonitory: serving as a warning

primordial: existing in the most primitive form

puerperium: interval between delivery and 6 weeks after delivery

radiation: loss of body heat to a solid cold object without direct contact

regional anaesthesia: blockage of large sensory nerve pathways in an organ and its surrounding tissue, producing loss of sensation in that organ and in the surrounding region

ripening: softening and thinning of the cervix in preparation for active labour

Ritgen manoeuvre: manual pressure applied through the perineum to the occiput of the head as the fetus is extending and emerging during birth

rugae: folds in the vaginal mucosa and scrotum

semen: white, viscous secretion of the male reproductive organs that consists of spermatozoa and nutrient fluids ejaculated through the penile urethra

smegma: whitish secretions around the labia minora and under the foreskin of the penis

sperm: male sex cell

spermatogenesis: formation and development of spermatozoa

sphingomyelin: a general membrane phospholipid that isn't directly related to lung maturity but is compared with lecithin to determine fetal lung maturity; levels remain constant during pregnancy

station: relationship of the presenting part to the ischial spines

strabismus: condition characterised by imprecise muscular control of ocular movement

subinvolution: failure of the uterus to return to normal size after delivery

surrogate mothering: conceiving and carrying a pregnancy to term with the expectation of turning the infant over to contracting, adoptive parents

sutures: narrow areas of flexible tissue on the fetal scalp that allow for slight adjustment during descent through the birth canal

teratogen: any drug, virus, irradiation or other nongenetic factor that can cause fetal malformation

tocolytic agent: medication that stops premature contractions

tocotransducer: an external mechanical device that translates one physical quantity to another, most often seen in capturing fetal heart rates and transmitting and recording the value onto a fetal monitor

trisomy: condition where a chromosome exists in triplicate instead of in the normal duplicate pattern

Wharton's jelly: whitish, gelatinous material that surrounds the umbilical vessels within the cord

X chromosome: sex chromosome in humans which exist in duplicate in the normal female and singly in the normal male

Y chromosome: sex chromosome in the human male that's necessary for development of the male sex glands, or gonads

zygote intrafallopian tube transfer: fertilisation of the ovum outside the mother's body, followed by reimplantation of the zygote into the fallopian tube via laparoscope

Selected references

Côté-Arsenault, D., *et al.* (2006). Watching & worrying: early pregnancy after loss experiences. *Maternal Child Nursing* 31(6):356–363.

Heaman, M. (2006). Breastfeeding support and early cessation. *MCN American Journal of Maternal Child Nursing* 31(5):336.

Kyle, T. (2007). *Essentials of Pediatric Nursing*. Philadelphia: Lippincott Williams & Wilkins.

Leifer, G. (2006). *Introduction to Maternity and Pediatric Nursing*. Philadelphia: W.B. Saunders Co.

Logsdon, M.C. and Hutti, M.H. (2006). Readability: an important issue impacting healthcare for women with postpartum depression. *Maternal Child Nursing* 31(6):350–355.

Lowdermilk, D. and Perry, S. (2006). *Maternity & Women's Healthcare*, 9th edn. St. Louis: Mosby.

Maternal–Neonatal Nursing Made Incredibly Quick, 2nd edn. Philadelphia: Lippincott Williams & Wilkins, 2008.

Pillitteri, A. (2006). *Maternal and Child Health Nursing Care of the Childbearing and Childrearing Family*, 5th edn. Philadelphia: Lippincott Williams & Wilkins.

Scott-Ricci, S. (2006). *Essentials of Maternity, Newborn, and Women's Health Nursing*. Philadelphia: Lippincott Williams & Wilkins.

Shorten, A., *et al.* (2005). Making choices for childbirth: a randomized controlled trial of a decision-aid for informed birth after cesarean. *Birth* 32(4):252–261.

Symon, A. (2007). *Risk and Choice in Maternity Care*. London: Churchill Livingstone.

Zwelling, E., *et al.* (2006). How to implement complementary therapies for laboring women. *Maternal Child Nursing* 31(6):364–370.

Index

i refers to an illustration; t refers to a table; **bold type** refers to colour pages

i refers to an illustration; t refers to a table; **bold type** refers to colour pages

i refers to an illustration; t refers to a table; **bold type** refers to colour pages

i refers to an illustration; t refers to a table; **bold type** refers to colour pages

i refers to an illustration; t refers to a table; **bold type** refers to colour pages